The Nutritional Trace Metals

The Nutritional Trace Metals

Conor Reilly
BSc, BPhil, PhD, FAIFST
Emeritus Professor of Public Health
Queensland University of Technology, Brisbane, Australia

Visiting Professor of Nutrition
Oxford Brookes University, Oxford, UK

Blackwell
Publishing

Editorial Offices:
Blackwell Publishing Ltd, 9600 Garsington Road, Oxford OX4 2DQ, UK
Tel: +44 (0)1865 776868
Blackwell Publishing Professional, 2121 State Avenue, Ames, Iowa 50014-8300, USA
Tel: +1 515 292 0140
Blackwell Publishing Asia Pty Ltd, 550 Swanston Street, Carlton, Victoria 3053, Australia
Tel: +61 (0)3 8359 1011

First published 2004 by Blackwell Publishing Ltd

Library of Congress
Cataloging-in-Publication Data
Reilly, Conor.
The nutritional trace metals/Conor Reilly.
p. cm.
Includes bibliographical references and index.
ISBN 1-4051-1040-6 (hardback : alk. paper)
1. Trace elements in nutrition. 2. Trace elements in the body.
I. Title.

QP534.R456 2006
613.2′8–dc22

2004004232

ISBN 1-4051-1040-6

A catalogue record for this title is available from the British Library

Set in 10/12 pt Times
by Kolam Information Services Pvt. Ltd, Pondicherry, India
Printed and bound in India
by Gopson Papers Ltd, Noida

The publisher's policy is to use permanent paper from mills that operate a sustainable forestry policy, and which has been manufactured from pulp processed using acid-free and elementary chlorine-free practices. Furthermore, the publisher ensures that the text paper and cover board used have met acceptable environmental accreditation standards.

For further information on Blackwell Publishing, visit our website:
www.blackwellpublishing.com

Contents

Preface

This book is intended to cover a somewhat neglected area of human metabolism and nutrition. Historically, the interest of writers of nutrition textbooks has mainly been in the role of organic substances in human metabolism. The inorganic nutrients, lumped together as 'minerals', have usually been given scant attention. Though the situation has changed in recent years, the nutritionally significant inorganic components of food, especially those that occur in very small amounts in the diet, still receive only a limited share of the space in textbooks. They are no better treated in many university nutrition courses. Yet, there are few, if any, functions of tissues and cells of the human body that are not dependent on the presence of these elements. Without an adequate supply of nutritional trace metals, human life would cease.

This book is intended to draw attention to the roles played by trace metals in human metabolism. Its structure and content are largely based on the approach I have adopted, during more than three decades of teaching nutrition to a wide range of undergraduate and postgraduate students, in dietetics, food science, medicine, pharmacology and related fields of study. In addition to providing basic information on the nature and functions of the trace metals, it draws on reports from specialist literature to highlight current thinking about their significance to human health. It is not, strictly speaking, a textbook, though it could well serve in that capacity for a dedicated course on trace elements. It is hoped that *Nutritional Trace Metals* will be of value as a reference work, as well as recommended background reading for undergraduate and postgraduate students of human nutrition. I have adopted a style of writing that I hope will make it easy to read, and not demand more than a reasonable undergraduate level of scientific knowledge to follow its reasoning. Where necessary, explanations of chemical and physiological matters that might not be familiar to some readers, but can be omitted by others who have a stronger scientific foundation, are provided to compensate for inadequacies in background knowledge. My hope is that those who use this book will gain a level of knowledge of the nutritional trace metals that will enrich their understanding of a fascinating area of human nutrition, at a level that will meet their professional needs, satisfy their curiosity and at the same time encourage them to expand their knowledge by following up at least some of the many references provided.

Nutritional Trace Metals is aimed at a wide audience. It should be particularly useful for undergraduates in dietetics and nutrition courses but also, it is hoped, be of value to medical, pharmaceutical and other health professionals, including alternative health practitioners. It could also serve as a reference book for food scientists and technologists, as well as for administrators and others in the food industry, who need to know more about the nutritional trace metals that occur in processed and other foods either naturally or added in fortification. Even non-professionals, whose background in science is minimal, but who wish to expand their knowledge of an area of nutrition in which there is, today, considerable media and general interest, will, I hope, find it a reliable and readable resource book.

My gratitude is owed to many people for the help they have given me in writing this book: to my wife, Ann, as ever encouraging and tolerant; to the librarians at Oxford Brookes University and the Bodleian Library, Oxford University; to many academic and professional colleagues, especially to Professor Jeya Henry, Dr Ujang Tinggi and Professor John Arthur, and several others who remain anonymous; not least to the helpful and encouraging production team at Blackwell Publishing.

Conor Reilly
Enstone, Oxfordshire
January 2004

Chapter 1
Introduction

1.1 The role of metals in life processes – a belated recognition

It is only in relatively recent years that the metallic elements, other than those usually classified under the term *bulk minerals*, began to receive more than passing attention in textbooks on human nutrition. Though iron had been recognised as a constituent of the human body in the early eighteenth century, another 100 years were to pass before inorganic elements began to be accepted as more than minor players in human biology[1]. Even today, to judge by the number of pages assigned to them in some widely used textbooks, their roles in human nutrition and metabolism are often less than adequately appreciated. The truth is that metal ions regulate a vast array of essential physiological mechanisms with unprecedented specificity and selectivity[2]. Indeed, in the absence of the nutritional trace metals, life would cease.

Da Silva and Williams[3] have noted that our understanding of the chemistry of life has been seriously hampered by the ways in which chemists have, traditionally, looked upon living organisms. This is because of a tendency to concentrate on the organic molecules that make up biological substrates and genetic material. As a result, they largely neglect the mineral elements of life, particularly those metals that are found in biological catalysts.

To some extent, this failure to appreciate the fact that metals have an important role to play in living organisms can be traced back to the beginnings of modern chemistry in the late eighteenth and early nineteenth centuries. This was a period of extraordinary progress in understanding of the composition of the world. New elements were being discovered at an impressive rate. The French pioneering scientist, Lavoisier, listed 23 elements in his 1789 publication, *Traité élémentaire de chimie*. Half a century later, Gmelin was able to include a total of 61 elements, of which 49 were metals, in his *Handbook of Chemistry*. Several of these new metals, including selenium, thorium, cerium, vanadium and lithium, were discovered in the laboratory of the Swedish chemist, Berzelius. Yet, in spite of his great interest in metals, Berzelius must bear at least some of the responsibility for the neglect of the role of metals in life processes, as a result of the distinction he made in his writings between organic and inorganic chemistry. According to him, the former was concerned only with substances produced by living matter, whereas the inorganic concentrated on the non-living[4]. The barrier he thus helped establish between the two fields of study was not easily breached by his successors[5].

A partial breakthrough was made, however, when the German chemist, von Liebig grasped the significance of Lavoisier's concept of life as a chemical function. In 1842, von

Leibig published his *Chemistry of Animals*, in which he proposed the theory that humans were nourished by three classes of food: carbonaceous, or energy-building (we call them carbohydrates and fats), nitrogenous (proteins) and mineral salts essential for the construction of bones and teeth[6]. Unfortunately, in spite of the significance of his recognition of the importance of minerals in nutrition, von Liebig's subsequent research concentrated on the so-called organic components of food, particularly protein. Minerals, which were to be found in the residue left after food was incinerated, were largely ignored by him and by those who followed in his footsteps. As one commentator has put it, there was another division of foodstuffs 'to which some, on rare occasions, slurringly referred. They called this fourth division "ash". The division "ash" was always exasperatedly ignored'[7].

It would, however, be unfair, and inaccurate, to blame chemists alone for the neglect of the mineral components of food. Biologists and nutritionists could also be accused of failing to pay sufficient attention to the role of inorganic elements in the human body. But to do so would be anachronistic. Until well into the twentieth century, scientists did not have very much information about the distribution and functions of trace elements in foods and body tissues. It was a laborious task, using the equipment then available, to determine with accuracy the concentrations of even a limited range of the metals present in biological samples. It was far easier, using techniques learned from 'wet' chemistry, to investigate the organic compounds of nutritional importance. As a result, and, in contrast to the limited progress being made in the area of the minerals, there was an impressive expansion of understanding of the functions of the vitamins as well as of the larger organic nutrients. This imbalance in nutrition knowledge was reflected in the textbooks published during that period, with only a small fraction of the texts devoted to minerals.

That situation no longer exists. The days when 'ash' was exasperatedly ignored are gone forever. The central role of trace metal nutrients and other inorganic elements in human metabolism and nutrition is now fully accepted by the majority, if not by all who work in the field of human biology. This change in attitude has been encouraged by the growing recognition that trace element deficiencies are major causes of illness throughout the world. Indeed, as has been noted by one expert in the area of micronutrient studies, 'taken together, mineral and vitamin deficiencies affect a greater number of people in the world than does protein-energy malnutrition'[8].

1.1.1 Bioinorganic chemistry

Though detailed knowledge of the intricacies of bioinorganic chemistry is by no means necessary, some appreciation of this relatively new and burgeoning field of investigation may help more biologically inclined readers of this book to appreciate the reason why there is a high level of interest among scientists in the nutritional trace metals. Bioinorganic chemistry has attracted the attention of a wide range of scientists from a variety of disciplines, from inorganic chemistry and biochemistry to spectroscopy, molecular biology and medicine. It deals with problems that are at the interface of chemistry, biology, agriculture, nutrition, food science and medicine[9]. Among major developments to which studies in the field have contributed is our rapidly growing knowledge of the role of metals in life processes. Using skills and techniques that were primarily developed in the field of inorganic chemistry, bioinorganic chemists have been able to shed light on the mechanisms of many activities that metals perform in living organisms. These include such chemical transformations as nitrogen fixation, conversion of water into dioxygen in photosynthesis, and utilisation of oxygen, hydrogen, methane and nitric oxide in metabolism[10]. They have shown moreover that ribosomes, though made entirely of ribonucleic acid and not proteins, can function as metalloenzymes, for example by catalysing reactions in the phosphodiester backbone of RNA[11]. No less important is the discovery that in addition to regulation of gene expression by 'zinc finger' proteins, a group of proteins that exert metal-responsive control of genes is intimately involved in respiration, metabolism, and metal-specific homeostasis, such as iron uptake and storage, copper efflux and mercury detoxification[12].

Kaplin, in an interesting paper on the contribution made by inorganic chemists to our understanding of metalloenzymes[13], has made the observation that it was the distinctive ligation and coordination geometries, many with unusual colours and spectral characteristics, of the metal cores of these functional proteins that first drew the attention of physical chemists and other non-biologists to the subject of bioinorganic chemistry. Chemists with an interest in industrially important small molecules were attracted to the investigation of metalloenzymes known to use these same molecules in catalytic reactions under conditions considerably milder and more specific than equivalent industrial processes. According to Kaplin, it was by applying their inorganic model approach that the chemists were able to highlight the diverse array of protein and metal coordination sites found in biological systems. It also revealed how nature uses basic recurring structures for different functions, by, for example, coordination of different amino acid side chains to the metal or by modulating the hydrophobicity, hydrogen bonding, or the local dielectric constant in the vicinity of the active site.

1.1.2 A brief review of the metals

It will be an advantage, before proceeding further, to review briefly what we know about the metals. This review will not enter into great detail, since it is not necessary to have a specialist understanding of metal chemistry to appreciate the significance of the different reactions and chemical forms in which these elements occur in the natural surroundings of living matter. The information provided here should be enough to help readers with even a limited background in chemistry to understand why it is that metals have a special role to play in the functions of life. For those who require further information, a variety of dedicated bioinorganic textbooks are available. The study jointly published by da Silva and Williams[14] and the somewhat more chemically inclined text by the husband-and-wife team of Wilkins and Wilkins[15] are recommended. For those with a strong chemical interest, the text by Shriver and Atkins may be consulted[16].

1.1.2.1 What are the metals?

About 80 of the 103 elements listed in the Periodic Table of the Elements are metals. The uncertainty as to the exact number arises because the borderline between what are considered to be metals and non-metals is ill-defined. While all the elements in the *s*, *d* and *f* blocks of the Table are known to be metals, there is some doubt about the elements of the *p*-block. Usually, seven of these (aluminium, gallium, indium, thallium, tin, lead, and bismuth) are included among the metals, but the dividing line between them and the other 23 *p*-block elements is uncertain. These divisions are illustrated in Fig. 1.1. It is easy in most cases to distinguish between metallic and non-metallic elements by their physical characteristics. Metals are typically solids that are lustrous, malleable, ductile and electrically conducting, while non-metals may be gaseous, liquid or non-conducting solids. However, there is also an intermediate group of elements, known as *metalloids* or, to use the term preferred by the International Union of Pure and Applied Chemistry (IUPAC), *half-metals*, which are neither clearly metals nor non-metals, but share characteristics of both. The metallic characteristics of the elements decrease and non-metallic characteristics increase with increasing numbers of valence electrons. In contrast, metallic characteristics increase with the number of electron shells. Thus, the properties of succeeding elements change gradually from metallic to non-metallic from left to right across the periodic table as the number of valence electrons increases, and from non-metallic to metallic down the groups with increasing numbers of electron shells. There is, as a consequence, no clear dividing line between elements with full metal characteristics and those that are fully non-metallic. It is in this indistinct border area that the metalloids occur.

1.1.2.2 Chemical properties of the metals

It is not the metals as such, in their bulk, elemental form, but rather their chemical compounds that are of significance in the context of metabolism and nutrition. In their metallic state, they are insoluble in water and therefore cannot be used by biological systems. Neither can living matter use the electrical conductivity of metals to carry messages. While elemental metals are used industrially as catalysts in a wide variety of chemical reactions, this is normally done at high temperatures and requires considerable energy inputs. Living cells, which could not survive such conditions, are, however, able to use compounds of metals as enzymes in extremely sophisticated catalytic processes developed over millions of years of evolution[17].

There are considerable differences between the chemical properties of metals and non-metals. Atoms of non-metals, for instance, are generally electronegative and can readily fill their valence shells by sharing electrons with, or transferring electrons from, other atoms. Thus, a typical non-metal, such as chlorine, can combine with another atom by adding one electron to its outer shell of seven, either by taking the electron from another atom or by sharing an electron pair. In contrast, a typical metal, such as sodium, is electropositive, with positive oxidation states, and enters into chemical combination only by the loss of its single valence electron. There are other important differences between metals and non-metals, relating to reduction/oxidation potential, acid/base chemistry and structural or ligand coordination properties, which have considerable consequences for their roles in biological processes.

1.1.2.3 Representative and transition metals

The metals are classified by chemists, in terms of their electronic structure, into two subgroups that are important in relation to their biological functions. Metals such as sodium and lead that have all their valence electrons in one shell are known as *representative* metals, while those such as chromium and copper that have valence electrons in more than

Key: Atomic number / Symbol / Atomic weight

Period	1	2	3	4	5	6	7	8	9	10	11	12	13	14	15	16	17	18
1	1 H 1																	2 He 4
2	3 Li 6.9	4 Be 9											5 B 10.8	6 C 12	7 N 14	8 O 16	9 F 19	10 Ne 20.2
3	11 Na 23	12 Mg 24.3											13 Al 27	14 Si 28.1	15 P 31	16 S 32.1	17 Cl 35.5	18 Ar 39.9
4	19 K 39.1	20 Ca 40.1	21 Sc 45	22 Ti 47.9	23 V 50.9	24 Cr 52	25 Mn 54.9	26 Fe 55.8	27 Co 58.9	28 Ni 58.7	29 Cu 63.5	30 Zn 65.4	31 Ga 69.7	32 Ge 72.6	33 As 74.9	34 Se 79	35 Br 79.9	36 Kr 83.8
5	37 Rb 85.5	38 Sr 87.6	39 Y 88.9	40 Zr 91.2	41 Nb 92.9	42 Mo 95.9	43 Tc [98]	44 Ru 101.1	45 Rh 102.9	46 Pd 106.4	47 Ag 107.9	48 Cd 112.4	49 In 114.8	50 Sn 118.7	51 Sb 121.8	52 Te 127.6	53 I 126.9	54 Xe 131.3
6	55 Cs 132.9	56 Ba 137.3	57 La 138.9	72 Hf 178.5	73 Ta 180.9	74 W 183.8	75 Re 186.2	76 Os 190.2	77 Ir 192.2	78 Pt 195.1	79 Au 197	80 Hg 200.6	81 Tl 204.4	82 Pb 207.2	83 Bi 209	84 Po [209]	85 At [210]	86 Rn [222]
7	87 Fr [223]	88 Ra [226]	89 Ac [227]															

Period														
6	58 Ce 140.1	59 Pr 140.9	60 Nd 144.2	61 Pm [145]	62 Sm 150.4	63 Eu 152	64 Gd 157.2	65 Tb 158.9	66 Dy 162.5	67 Ho 164.9	68 Er 167.3	69 Tm 168.9	70 Yb 173	71 Lu 175
7	90 Th 232	91 Pa [231]	92 U 238	93	94	95	96	97	98	99	100	101	102	103

Metals (plain box) · Non-metals (bold box: H, He, C, N, O, P, F, S, Cl, Se, Br, I, Ne, Ar, Kr, Xe, Rn) · Metalloids (diagonal line: B, Si, Ge, As, Sb, Te, Po, At)

Figure 1.1 Periodic table of the elements.

one shell are *transition* metals. Representative metals that have one or two valence electrons have one oxidation state (e.g. sodium, +1; calcium, +2) while those with three or more valence electrons have two oxidation states (e.g. lead, +2 and +4; bismuth, +3 and +5). In contrast, transition metals exhibit a variety of oxidation states. Manganese, for instance, which has two electrons in its outermost shell and five electrons in the next underlying *3d* shell, exhibits oxidation states of +1, +2, +3, +4, +6 and +7.

There is another difference between representative and transition metals which is of significance in relation to their biological functions. Because succeeding elements in the transition series differ in electronic structure by one electron in the first underlying valence shell, the properties of succeeding elements do not differ greatly from left to right across the periodic table. It is this property that accounts for the ability of some transition elements to replace other elements in certain metalloenzymes. In contrast, since their electronic structures differ by one electron in the outer shell, the properties of succeeding representative metals in a period differ considerably from one another and do not possess the same biological flexibility as the transition elements.

The metal zinc is, strictly speaking, in terms of the definition of transition and representative metals, a representative metal. However, it has many characteristics analogous to those of the transition metals and often functions like them in biological systems. Consequently, it is often classified along with the transition elements. It has one difference from them that can be of some importance to the analyst. Most of the transition metal ions with incomplete underlying electron shells are coloured, both in solid salts and in solution. The colour depends on the oxidation state of the metal. However, when as is the case with zinc, and generally with all representative metals, the underlying electron shell is filled, the substance containing the ion is colourless.

1.1.2.4 The biological functions of trace metals

In living organisms, metal ions regulate an array of physiological mechanisms with considerable specificity and selectivity, as components of enzymes and other molecular complexes. The reactivities of the complexes depend both on the specific properties of the particular biological protein, or other organic molecule to which the metals are joined, and on the variety and flexibility of the metals' own specific chemical properties[18].

It is in the metalloenzymes that what has been described as 'the subtle interplay between macromolecular ligands and metal ions' can be best appreciated[19]. About 30% of all enzymes have a metal atom at their active site. Metalloenzymes occur in each of the six categories of enzymes listed by IUPAC. The biological reactions in which they take part include acid-catalysed hydrolysis (hydrolases), redox reactions (oxidases) and rearrangements of carbon–carbon bonds (isomerases and synthetases). The specificity of a metalloenzyme is determined both by the nature of the non-metal partner and by a metal ion which has an appropriate size, stereochemical preference and other individual chemical characteristics.

The activity of certain metalloenzymes depends on the ability of metal ions to function as what are known as Lewis acids. These are substances that can form a covalent bond with a base by accepting a pair of electrons from it. This property is exploited by enzymes that utilise acid catalysis. An example is the zinc-containing metalloenzyme alkaline phosphatase responsible for the hydrolysis of phosphate esters, relying on the Lewis acid properties of the zinc ion.

Oxidation/reduction properties of metals are utilised by many metalloenzymes, especially those that contain transition metals. Redox catalysis can involve electron, atom or group transfers. Examples of the first two types of transfers are provided by the iron-containing metalloproteins. The cytochromes and flavoproteins are haem enzymes responsible for controlled oxidation within tissues by the transfer of electrons down a chain of metalloproteins of decreasing standard potential from substrate to oxygen. Atom transfer is utilised by cytochrome P-450, an iron-porphyrin metalloprotein, to join an oxygen atom to hydrophobic compounds as part of the body's defences against toxic compounds. Group transfer is illustrated by the enzyme system methionine synthetase, which uses the metal cobalt, in the form of methylcobalamin, to transfer a CH_3 group to homocysteine to make methionine[20]. The *d*-block transition metals play a particularly prominent part in enzyme activities of living organisms. Their wide variety of oxidation states, extensive bonding patterns and chemical flexibility allow them to participate extensively in catalysis. The facility with which iron, copper and molybdenum, for instance, can undertake one or two electron changes accounts for their importance in the oxidoreductase enzymes. All of the first-row transition metals, as well as zinc, are represented among the hydrolase, lyase and isomerase classes of enzymes.

1.2 The metal content of living systems

Though only a small proportion of the approximately 2 million species of plants, animals and other forms of life found in the world today have been analysed for their elemental composition, there is little doubt that all living organisms have the ability to concentrate preferentially certain elements from the environment. This process has been described as 'a natural selection of chemical elements by biological systems, which involves a readjustment of the element distribution of the earth's local scale by utilising energy ultimately provided by the sun'[21].

When the ash of tissue taken from an organism is analysed, the presence of most, if not all, of the metallic elements will normally be detected. Most of the elements will be at barely detectable *trace* levels, while others will be in significant amounts, reflecting their concentrations in the original organism. In spite of the many differences between species, the composition of ash is remarkably uniform between organisms, not necessarily in quantity, but in the variety of elements it contains. Present in the greatest quantities will be calcium, sodium, potassium and magnesium. In addition to these *macro elements*, there will also be a wide range of *trace elements.*

The ash of all living organisms, apart from a few types of *Lactobacilli* bacteria, will contain iron in significant quantities. Present also, though at lower concentrations, will be zinc, copper, manganese, nickel, molybdenum, cobalt and a few others. In only a few cases will there be more than minute amounts of other metals. Exceptions will occur if the organism has been exposed to environmental contamination or possesses the rare ability of being able to accumulate in its tissues certain elements normally excluded by living organisms.

1.2.1 Metals in human tissue

Analysis of human tissue shows that, like other organisms, the body contains a wide range of metals, as seen in Table 1.1. Most of these metals, apart from calcium and the other so-called *bulk metals*, are present in μg/kg or lesser concentrations, and of these, only a handful play significant metabolic roles in the body. At the present time, nine metals (iron, zinc, chromium, cobalt, nickel, copper, manganese, molybdenum and selenium) are generally included in this group of essential trace metals. It is highly probable that some others, such as vanadium, may also be nutritionally important, though as yet, their essentiality has not been fully established.

Table 1.1 Metals in the human body.

Metal	Concentration (mg/kg)
Calcium	14000
Potassium	2000
Sodium	1400
Magnesium	270
Iron	60
Zinc	33
Copper	1.7
Aluminium	0.9
Manganese	0.2
Selenium	0.2
Titanium	0.2
Tin	0.2
Nickel	0.1
Molybdenum	0.1
Gold	0.1
Chromium	0.09
Lithium	0.04
Antimony	0.04
Tellurium	0.04
Bismuth	0.03
Silver	0.03
Vanadium	0.03
Cobalt	0.02
Caesium	0.02
Tungsten	0.01
Uranium	0.01
Radium	4×10^{-10}

Based on Schroeder, H.A. (1973) *The Trace Elements and Nutrition*, Faber & Faber, London; Reilly, C. (2002) *Metal Contamination of Food*, 3rd ed. Blackwells, Oxford.

1.2.2 Essential and non-essential elements

There are a number of reasons why there is uncertainty about the true number of essential trace metals in humans. Not least are the analytical difficulties encountered in trying to determine concentrations, particularly at the very low levels at which many of them are normally found in tissues. Possibly equally important is the problem of classification. Deciding whether an element is essential or non-essential implies, as has been pointed out, a prescriptive definition of 'essentiality', which may not be acceptable to all and may have to be modified as a result of new findings[22].

A number of definitions of the concept of essentiality have been proposed by different investigators. One of the simplest is that an essential element is a 'metabolic or functional nutrient'[23]. A somewhat more sophisticated definition is that an essential element is one that is required for the maintenance of life, and its deficiency causes an impairment of a function from optimal to suboptimal[24]. The impairment can lead to disease, metabolic anomalies or perturbations in development[25].

Many nutritionists adopt a more precise and detailed definition that can be summarised as follows: to be considered as essential, a trace element must:

(1) be present in healthy tissue
(2) its concentration must be relatively constant between different organisms
(3) deficiency induces specific biochemical changes
(4) the changes are accompanied by equivalent abnormalities in different species
(5) supplementation with the element corrects the abnormalities[26].

The location in the periodic table of those elements, non-metals as well as metals, is shown in Fig. 1.1. Two observations can be made from a study of the figure. The first is that nearly all the essential elements are found among the lighter elements. Only iodine, a non-metal, and molybdenum, which, though a metal, in many instances behaves chemically like a non-metal, have atomic numbers greater than 34. The second is that the essential elements occur in all the chemical groups, except for groups 3, 4 and 18 (the inert gas group). The significance of this is that all kinds of chemical processes are associated with the processes of life. Life is, as was pointed out by Lavoisier long ago, a chemical function, and the essentiality of an element can be explained in terms of its chemical and physical properties[27].

1.2.3 The essentiality of trace metals

It is important when considering the properties and biological roles of the essential trace elements to realise that, between them, they make less than 0.1% of the total composition of the human body. Four non-metallic elements, hydrogen, oxygen, carbon and nitrogen, account for 99% of all the elements, not just in the human, but in all biological systems. Another seven elements, the so-called *major elements*, sodium, potassium, calcium, magnesium, phosphorus, sulphur and chlorine, provide approximately another 0.9% of the total. The essential trace metals share the remaining 0.1% with all the other elements, metals and non-metals[28].

Why, it can be asked, out of all the elements of the periodic table which were available to living organisms during the course of evolution, were only about one-third selected as essential and the others rejected as inessential or even as positively detrimental to life? Henry Schroeder, who was one of the pioneer investigators who did much to bring the trace elements to the attention of nutritionists, summarised a number of key points which should be taken into account when considering this question. In his now classic paper, *The Trace Elements and Nutrition*[29], he noted that an essential element must have been (1) abundant when life began, in sea water; (2) reactive, that is, able to join up or bond with other elements; (3) able to form an integral part of a structure; and (4) in the case of the metals, soluble in water, reactive of itself with oxygen, and able to bond to organic material. These qualities are found in 23 elements of the first 42 elements of the periodic table.

As has already been noted, the essential elements are the lighter elements. They are also abundant on earth, on both land and sea[30]. Life almost certainly began in an aquatic environment, possibly three thousand million years ago. Today, most life chemistry takes place in aqueous media. All cells are composed of 80–90% water[31]. As a consequence, only processes that are compatible with the presence of water are possible, which puts strict limits on the range of redox potentials, pH and temperature that may be used in metabolism. Metallic elements therefore cannot be used in their metallic state, but only as their soluble compounds. Moreover, since temperatures and pH ranges are strictly limited, life processes involving the essential elements can only be carried out using highly sophisticated catalytic systems.

The primitive ocean contained the same elements as does seawater today, though in much lower concentrations. This difference, however, does not affect the fact that, generally, biological elements are still those that are the most universally abundant[32]. What actually determined the suitability of an element for an essential role was not simply abundance in the primitive ocean, but its availability in aqueous solution. Availability depends largely on the ability of an element to form compounds that are soluble in water at pH 7.0. The elements, sodium, potassium, calcium and magnesium, of groups 1 and 2, can do this and, as a consequence, are available for uptake by living organisms. In contrast, scandium, titanium and other elements of groups 3 and 4 form compounds of low solubility and do not have a biological role[33]. The essential non-metals oxygen and sulphur, as well as the metalloid selenium, in group 16, also form soluble compounds in neutral aqueous solution, as do in general the transition metals of groups 6–12.

The term 'economical utilisation of resources', has been used by da Silva and Williams to describe the manner in which Nature responds to abundance and availability in its selection of chemical elements. These authors believe that Nature follows a principle of choosing elements that are less costly in terms of energy required for uptake, 'given the function for which they are required'[34]. They stress, however, that the principle should not be considered as other than dynamic because, since life first appeared on earth, environmental conditions have undergone many modifications which have had an effect on the uptake and distribution of elements. Apart from changes in surface waters, such as an increase in sodium in the oceans and a fall in pH, dramatic changes have occurred in the composition of the atmosphere.

The atmosphere under which life first began was rich in carbon dioxide and methane. However, once plants had evolved and developed the ability to use solar energy to take in carbon dioxide, release oxygen and combine carbon atoms with water to make carbohydrates, the situation altered. The atmosphere gradually changed from a carbon dioxide-rich, reducing atmosphere to the one we know today that allows oxygen-dependent animals and plants to survive[35].

The change in the atmosphere from reducing to oxidising must have had a dramatic effect on the anaerobic forms of life in the primitive oceans. Those that could not adapt to the aerobic conditions would have been eliminated, unless they were able to find a niche which provided the environment they needed to survive. This is what, in fact, a very small number did. Some primitive protozoa and algae accumulated high concentrations of the sulphates of barium and strontium, both high density metals, which allow them to exist in deep anaerobic waters of relatively high density[36].

Of more immediate interest in the context of this book was the effect of the change from a reducing to an oxidising atmosphere on the availability of iron. In the primitive ocean, the element was present in the Fe^{2+}, ferrous form as the soluble cation or a soluble anion, such as FeO_4^{2-}. Under today's oxidising conditions, iron is only present in very low concentrations in water in the Fe^{3+}, ferric state, which precipitates as insoluble $Fe(OH)_3$. The resulting lack of availability of the metal has serious consequences for human nutrition, as we will see in detail later.

1.3 Metals in food and diets

It should be no surprise to find that the human body contains a great variety of metals, since its inorganic composition reflects the make up of the food we consume. This, in turn, depends on the environment in which we live. Using modern multielement equipment, it is possible for an analyst to detect the presence of most, if not all, of the metallic elements in samples of a normal diet. The UK Government's food surveillance programme regularly monitors levels of 30 metals and metalloids in foods and estimates population exposure to them (Table 1.2). Similar monitoring programmes are conducted by government and other agencies in many other countries. From the data they produce, as well as from the considerable number of research findings published in the scientific literature, it is possible to obtain an overall idea of the levels of metal elements in foods consumed commonly throughout the world. This is seen in Table 1.3, which lists the average concentrations of 33 different metals and metalloids in four of the major food groups. Though the table is mainly based on UK findings, a comparison between it and data from other countries shows a surprising level of uniformity of intake of the elements across the world. Thus, in the case of the three metals iron, copper and zinc, for instance, there is little difference between concentrations in three types of vegetable that are commonly consumed in the US and the UK, as can be seen in Table 1.4. This uniformity in elemental composition of foodstuffs between countries means that people whose food consumption habits are broadly comparable, though they live in different countries, will generally have similar levels of dietary intake of trace metal nutrients. Thus, for example, Australian adults can be expected to have an intake of zinc of approximately 11 mg/d[37], while that of a UK adult is between 9 and 12 mg[38]. Similarly, daily intakes of nickel are on average 0.12 mg in the UK[39], 0.13 mg in Finland[40] and 0.17 mg in the US[41].

Table 1.2 Dietary intake of metals in the UK.

Metal	Intake (mg/d)
Aluminium	11
Antimony	0.003
Arsenic	0.063
Barium	0.58
Bismuth	0.0004
Boron	1.5
Cadmium	0.014
Calcium	775
Chromium	0.34
Cobalt	0.012
Copper	1.2
Germanium	0.004
Gold	0.001
Iridium	0.002
Iron	14
Lead	0.024
Lithium	0.016
Manganese	4.9
Mercury	0.004
Molybdenum	0.11
Nickel	0.13
Palladium	0.001
Platinum	0.0002
Rhodium	0.0003
Ruthenium	0.004
Selenium	0.043
Strontium	1.3
Thallium	0.002
Tin	2.4
Zinc	8.4

Adapted from Ysart, G., Miller, P., Crews, H. *et al.* (1999) Dietary exposure estimates of 30 elements from the UK Total Diet Study. *Food Additives and Contaminants,* **16**, 391–403.

1.3.1 Variations in metal concentrations in foods

Though, in general, levels of trace metal nutrients in most of the main foodstuffs can be expected to be broadly similar in most countries, there can also be significant differences in certain situations. An example is seen in the case of selenium, as shown in Table 1.5, which summarises data on levels of the element in wheat from several countries. The differences in concentrations in the grain are due to differences between soil selenium concentrations in the areas in which the wheat was grown[42]. As we shall see in a later section, differences in selenium levels in cereals resulting from differences in soil levels

Table 1.3 Metal concentrations in foods (mg/kg, fresh weights).

Metal	Cereals	Meat	Dairy products	Vegetables	References
Al	78	3.2	0.64	1.8	1
Sb	0.004	0.004	0.001	<0.001	1
As	0.01	0.004	0.003	0.003	1
Ba	0.79	0.27	0.31	0.38	1
Bi	0.003	0.0003	0.001	0.0007	1
B	0.9	0.4	0.4	2.0	1
Cd	0.02	0.007	0.002	0.006	1
Ca	731	350	2320	379	1
Cr	0.1	0.2	0.9	0.2	1
Co	0.01	0.008	0.004	0.009	1
Cu	1.8	1.5	0.45	0.84	1
Ge	0.004	0.002	0.002	<0.002	1
Au	0.002	0.001	0.0004	<0.0004	1
Ir	0.002	<0.001	<0.001	<0.001	1
Fe	32	23	12	11	1
Pb	0.02	0.11	0.01	0.01	1
Li	0.02	0.01	0.005	0.01	1
Mn	6.8	1.4	0.27	2.0	1
Hg	0.004	0.003	0.002	0.002	1
Mo	0.23	0.12	0.07	0.15	1
Ni	0.17	0.06	0.02	0.11	1
Pd	0.0009	0.0006	0.0004	0.0006	1
Pt	0.0001	<0.0001	0.0001	0.0001	1
Rh	0.0001	<0.0001	0.0001	<0.0001	1
Ru	<0.002	<0.002	0.002	<0.002	1
Se	0.03	0.12	0.05	0.01	1
Sr	1.3	0.64	1.0	1.6	1
Te	<0.005	<0.005–0.01	<0.010	0.100	2
Tl	0.001	0.001	0.001	0.003	1
Sn	0.02	0.31	0.31	0.02	1
Ti	0.002	0.002	0.001	0.002	3
V	0.023	0.10	0.001	0.006	4
Zn	8.6	25	14	3.4	1

1. Ysart, G., Miller, P., Crews, H. *et al.* (1999) Dietary exposure estimates of 30 elements from the UK Total Diet Study. *Food Additives and Contaminants,* **16**, 391–403.
2. Kron, T., Hansen, C.H. & Werner, E. (1991) Tellurium ingestion with foodstuffs. *Journal of Food Composition and Analysis,* **4**, 196–205.
3. Shimbo, S., Hayase, A., Murakami, M. *et al.* (1996) Use of a food composition database to estimate daily dietary intakes of nutrients or trace elements in Japan, with reference to its limitations. *Food Additives and Contaminants,* **13,** 775–86.
4. Pennington, J.A.T. & Jones, J.W. (1987) Molybdenum, nickel, cobalt, vanadium and strontium in total diets. *Journal of the American Dietetics Association,* **87**, 1644–50.

Table 1.4 Iron, copper and zinc levels in US and UK vegetables.

	Metal (mg/kg, fresh (weight)		
Vegetable	Iron	Copper	Zinc
Broccoli			
US	1.1	0.03	0.27
UK	1.5	0.07	0.6
Brussels sprouts			
US	1.5	0.1	0.87
UK	0.7	0.06	0.5
Carrot			
US	0.7	0.08	0.52
UK	0.6	0.08	0.4

Data adapted from American Dietetics Association (1981) *Handbook of Clinical Dietetics,* Yale Univerity Press, New Haven; Paul, A.A. & Southgate, D.A.T. (1978) *McCance and Widdowson's The Composition of Foods.* HMSO, London.

Table 1.5 Selenium levels in wheat from different countries.

Country of origin	Selenium levels (μg/g, wet weight)
Australia	0.15
China – high soil Se area	0.30
China – low soil Se area	0.02
USA	0.33

Data adapted from Reilly, C. (1996) *Selenium in Food and Health.* Blackie/Chapman & Hall, London

can be highly significant with major implications for health, since cereals are the principal source of this essential nutrient for most consumers.

Variations in the trace metal composition of foods can be due to several other causes besides soil composition, such as genetic diversity. For example, a study of nine essential elements in seeds of eight cultivars of the common bean *Phaseolus vulgaris* found considerable variability in levels of several of the elements, as shown in Table 1.6. The findings of this study have significance with regard to proposals for the use of plant breeding as a strategy for combating widespread trace element deficiencies in certain parts of the world[43].

Even within a single sample of a food, metals may not be distributed evenly, so there can be differences in their concentrations in different parts. A whole grain of wheat can contain 7.4 μg/g of copper, but with only 2.0 μg/g of this in the endosperm. It is for this reason that refining or fractionation of cereals during milling affects the amount of metals in the food as consumed, as illustrated in Table 1.7[44].

Table 1.6 Mean concentrations of boron, iron and zinc in different bean cultivars.

	Cultivar							
Trace metal (μg/g)	1	2	3	4	5	6	7	8
Boron	10.1	13.3	12.8	12.3	11.4	11.7	12.7	12.0
Iron	58	69	54	53	56	59	61	62
Zinc	29	29	29	24	25	28	32	29

Adapted from Moraghan, J.T. & Grafton, K. (2001) Genetic diversity and mineral composition of common bean seed. *Journal of the Science of Food and Agriculture*, **81**, 404–8.

Table 1.7 Changes in concentrations of trace metals in wheat following processing.

	Metal content (μg/g, wet weight, mean ± SEM)			
Cereal	Mn	Fe	Zn	Cu
Wheatgerm	194 ± 11	105 ± 4	92 ± 0	14.7 ± 0.8
Whole wheat	67.2 ± 2	35.4 ±0.7	21.0 ± 0.4	3.32 ± 0.03
White flour	12.9 ± 0.2	12.4 ± 0.2	9.18 ± 0.13	1.63 ± 0.01

Data adapted from Booth, C., Reilly, C. & Farmakalidis, E. (1996) Mineral composition of Australian ready-to-eat breakfast cereals. *Journal of Food Composition and Analysis*, **9**, 135–47.

1.3.1.1 Chemical forms of metals in food

It should be noted that the figures given in the previous sections on the metal content of various foods are for total concentrations of these elements. Most of the data published in official tables, such as those for the US and thc UK Total Diet Studies, are presented in the same way. In only a few instances are data given for different chemical forms of the elements, and then usually only for certain types of food. This is the case with mercury and tin, where levels of organic mercury and organotin compounds in fish and a few other foods are published. Most other data published in the scientific literature and by official agencies will refer only to total concentrations of metals in foods.

The reason for such limitations in published data on food composition is twofold. First, it is relatively easy to analyse foodstuffs for their total metal content, whereas the determination of individual chemical species in a complex biological matrix requires expertise and equipment not yet widely available in analytical laboratories. Moreover, such determinations are generally time-consuming and expensive. Second, it is only recently that the significance of the different chemical species of metals in nutrition and health has come to be recognised. If essential trace elements are to exert a physiological effect on the body, they must be biologically available. Though bioavailability is affected by a number of factors, such as the individual's physiological response, as well as the presence of other components in the diet, primarily it depends on the element's chemical form or speciation. This will determine how the element is absorbed and behaves in the gastrointestinal tract, and how it is subsequently metabolised.

Crews has commented, in an informative review, that the study of human nutrition and health requires considerably more information than is available at present on chemical speciation of trace elements in the diet[45]. This information should, she believes, include data on valency states, metal–ligand complexes and chemical compounds, since the nature of the chemical species and its subsequent effect(s) vary from element to element. Cobalt, for instance, is only biologically active in the human body in its organic form as cyanocobalamin (vitamin B_{12}), while chromium(III) has a number of important biological activities, and in its hexavalent form as Cr(VI), it is toxic: in the case of iron, its bioavailability depends to a great extent on whether it is present in food as the Fe(II) or Fe(III) form.

1.3.2 Determination of levels of trace metals in foods

Were it not for the skills of analytical chemists who, over the years, have developed procedures and equipment of ever-increasing precision and refinement, our knowledge of the nutritional trace metals would be meagre. Our tables of food composition would still list 'ash' or 'minerals', rather than the precise concentrations, down in some cases to microgram and even nanogram per kilogram levels, of a wide range of metals they include today. There would be few publications of research findings on the elemental composition or on the roles of trace metals in the diet if investigators still had to rely on time-consuming gravimetric and colorimetric analytical methods rather than on modern equipment and procedures.

It has to be stressed that the use of precise analytical equipment does not, of itself, guarantee the reliability of results. When, in the mid-1950s, the atomic absorption spectrophotometer first became commercially available, following its development by Walsh in Australia and Alkemade and Milaz in the Netherlands[46], it was welcomed as a replacement for the simple flame emission spectrophotometers and other equipment then in use. The new instrument was not difficult to use, even by inexperienced analysts. It was also relatively cheap and allowed rapid determination of a wide range of elements, many at levels of concentration previously unattainable. Different brands of instrument were developed, ranging from simple manual to sophisticated, automated models, many with the addition of background correction and a variety of modes which further expanded the range and sensitivity of the method. Atomic absorption (AA) quickly became the most widely used technique for the determination of metals in food and other materials. It remains so today, in spite of the arrival of a wide range of far more sophisticated equipment.

Unfortunately, though the use of AA has allowed considerable advances to be made in the study of trace elements in biology, its very popularity among investigators and its accessibility have not always contributed to progress in the field. Some investigators failed to recognise that no matter how advanced technically or how modern their equipment and procedures, the quality of the data generated by them must always be checked by a quality assurance programme. It was this failure that prompted two of the leaders in the field of trace element analysis to make the comment that much of the data on mineral composition of foods published as recently as the late 1970s is unreliable[47]. There is much evidence to support this statement. In the case of the non-nutritional element aluminium, for instance, failure to take into account high levels of contamination was probably responsible for reports of high dietary intakes which are not supported by more recent studies[48]. Other analytical problems most probably account for the contradictory reports on levels of intake of selenium in Glasgow, one of 234 μg[49], the other 30 $\mu g/day$[50]. The situation has improved. Journal editors are reluctant to accept for publication reports based on analytical data that have not been subjected to acceptable checks for accuracy and reliability and do not give adequate details of analytical procedures. No reputable analytical laboratory would think of operating today without having a quality assurance programme in place to validate the accuracy of its data[51].

1.3.3 How do metals get into foods?

Whatever the chemical form it has when it finally becomes part of the human diet, the primary source of most metals in food is the soil from which food is produced. There is an intimate connection between soil and the metals we consume and incorporate into our bodies. It is appropriate, then, to give some attention to the nature and composition of soil and especially how it contributes to the metal content of food.

1.3.3.1 Metals in soils

Soils are complex mixtures of solids, liquids and gases[52]. The solid portion includes both primary and secondary minerals, ranging in size from $< 2\,\mu m$ in diameter (gravel) to > 2 mm diameter (rocks). The minerals are inorganic compounds of the different metallic elements. Primary minerals, such as quartz (SiO_2), are those which have not been chemically changed by weathering or other natural activities, in contrast to secondary minerals, such as kaolin, $Al_2Si_2O_6(OH)_4$, which have undergone physical, chemical and structural changes. The inorganic portion can account for up to 90% of the solid matter of soil, with the remaining 10% made up of organic matter.

The metals found in the highest concentrations in soils are aluminium, iron, calcium, potassium, sodium and magnesium. Most of the other metals and metalloids will also be present, though normally at much lower concentrations, as shown in Table 1.8. The actual elemental composition of a particular soil depends primarily on the chemical composition of the parent material from which it was formed. However, the original composition may have been modified by weathering, as well as by mining, industry and farming, and by accumulation from natural biogeochemical processes[53].

1.3.3.2 Soil as a source of trace metals in plants and in human diets

Fertile soils are able to supply plants with all the trace metal nutrients they require for growth. These are boron, cobalt (for legumes), copper, iron, manganese, molybdenum and possibly nickel. Many other elements are also present in soil, as is shown in Table 1.8, and can also be taken up by plants. Some of these, such as selenium and chromium, while not required by the plants themselves, are of nutritional significance to farm animals and humans who consume the crops. Toxic metals, such as cadmium and lead, can also be taken up from some soils.

Table 1.8 Metal concentrations in soil.

Metal	Concentration range (mg/kg)
Aluminium	7–10 000
Barium	<0.1–100
Boron	10–5000
Beryllium	<1–15
Calcium	100–320 000
Cadmium	0.01–2
Cobalt	<3–70
Copper	<1–700
Chromium	1–2000
Lithium	<5–140
Magnesium	50–100 000
Manganese	<2–7000
Molybdenum	<3–15
Selenium	<0.1–4.4
Sodium	<500–100 000
Tin	<0.1–10
Titanium	70–20 000
Uranium	0.29–11
Vanadium	<7–500
Zinc	<5–2900

Adapted from Sparks, D.L. (1995) *Environmental Soil Chemistry*, p. 24. Academic Press, New York; Reilly, C. (2002) *Metal Contamination of Food*, p. 9. Blackwell, Oxford.

1.3.3.3 Effects of agricultural practices on soil metal content

Amendment of soil by the application of top dressings and agrochemicals can result in significant changes in its metal content. Some of these changes can be deliberate, intended to increase levels of desirable nutrients where these are inadequate. Thus, in some countries, such as Finland and New Zealand, in which soil selenium levels are low, the element is applied as a top dressing to increase its levels in fodder and food crops[54]. Unfortunately, toxic rather than nutritional metals can also be added to soil, and thus to foods for human consumption, by agricultural practices. A serious level of cadmium contamination in potatoes and cereals has occurred in some parts of Australia from the use of cadmium-containing phosphate[55].

1.3.3.4 Uptake of trace metals by plants from soil

The actual extent of uptake of metals by plants depends not only on the total elemental composition of the soil in which the plants grow, but also on the availability, or lability, of the elements in the soil. It is their availability for uptake and accumulation by crops that determines whether or not a particular plant can serve as a significant food source of a nutritional trace metal. Availability is determined by a metal's properties, such as chemical species, solubility and ability to complex with organic matter and to become adsorbed on other soil constituents. The plant itself can assist uptake by modifying the chemistry of the surrounding soil solution by exuding hydrogen ions and organic chelating agents.

Once within the plant, some of the absorbed metals will be retained in the roots. Others are translocated upwards to the leaves and into the fruits, seeds and other storage organs. There, the various elements are retained, to provide nutrients for growth and survival into the next generation of the plant itself and, no less important, for animals and humans that feed on them.

1.3.3.5 Accumulator plants

Some plants have the ability to take up certain metals from soil and accumulate them in their tissues to an unusually high concentration. One of these *accumulator plants* of importance in human diets, is the tea plant, *Camellia sinensis*, which can accumulate both manganese[56] and aluminium[57] to levels far higher than are found in other plants. It can also accumulate selenium and for this reason is promoted in China for its nutritional benefits[58].

Nuts, especially tree nuts, are good sources of a number of trace metals, though generally not in the league of the accumulator plants. In the UK's official Table of Food Composition, for instance, levels of iron ranging from 9 to 42 mg/kg, zinc 24 to 42 mg/kg, and copper 1.4 to 11 mg/kg are given for a number of commonly consumed nuts, such as almonds, Brazil, chestnut, peanuts and walnuts[59]. Nuts are also a good dietary source of nickel. However, some other metals, including aluminium and barium[60], which could have adverse health effects, can also be accumulated by them.

1.3.4 Non-plant sources of trace metal nutrients in foods

Though plants are the primary channels for transfer of inorganic nutrients from soil to humans, much of this transfer goes, except in the case of vegetarians, through a secondary step in the bodies of farm animals. This diversion can have important consequences for human health, for example as a result of concentration and metabolism of certain elements in animal tissues. Thus, iron, which in plant tissues is normally at low levels of concentration and in a chemical form which is of limited bioavailability, is concentrated in the animals, especially in organs and muscle tissue. It is also converted to organic forms that are readily absorbed by the human gut. Animal tissues are also far better dietary sources of zinc than are plant foods. Not only does red meat, for instance, have a higher concentration of zinc than do cereals, but it is also free of phytic acid and other components of plants which can inhibit absorption of the metal by the gut.

Fish and other sea foods are not good sources of trace metal nutrients. Though they have the ability to take up inorganic elements in their tissues, the amount and kind accumulated depend on their presence and concentration in the water. The majority of the nutritional trace metals are neither abundant nor soluble to any useful extent in seawater and thus are not accumulated by marine organisms. The only exception is selenium. The element is taken in initially from the water by unicellular and other algae that are grazed by small fish. The algae-eating fish are consumed by larger fish, and these, in turn, are the food of larger fish and so on to the top of the hunting chain. In this way, the selenium originally in the water is passed on and concentrated in the tissues of large carnivorous fish, such as shark and tuna, which may finally become the food of humans. Unfortunately, selenium is not the only metal which can reach the human diet in this way. It is usually accompanied by mercury, not just in high concentrations but in its most toxic organic form. Other toxic elements, especially arsenic, can enter the human food chain by the same route.

1.3.5 Adventitious sources of trace metals in foods

While soil is normally the major source of metals in the human diet, primarily through crops and secondarily through domestic animals fed on them, foods also take up these elements in a variety of other ways. Industrial activity which results in environmental contamination is normally a source of toxic metals, such as cadmium and lead, rather than of nutritionally important metals. However, some technological processes can increase levels of certain nutrient metals in foods. At a very simple level, the use of cast iron cooking pots has been found to increase iron levels in the diet to an appreciable level[61]. There is some evidence that a significant part of our intakes of chromium and nickel comes as leachate from stainless steel used in food processing and storage equipment[62]. Copper, too, can be taken up by food in a similar manner, when brass and copper utensils are used in its preparation. However, though copper, like chromium and nickel, is an essential nutrient, high levels in food prepared in brass vessels may be responsible for liver disease in some children[63].

1.3.6 Food fortification

The addition of certain nutrients, including trace metals, to food and drink is widely practised as a public health measure and a cost-effective way of ensuring the nutritional quality of the food supply[64]. In some countries, it is a legal requirement for certain types of foods. Additions of inorganic and other trace nutrients to processed foods are also made by manufacturers in response to consumer pressure and, not least, to ensure that certain products have a competitive edge in the market place.

During World War II, several countries introduced fortification of wheat flour and bread with iron, and certain other nutrients. This was a legal requirement designed to combat nutritional deficiencies expected to result from wartime food shortages. The requirements were retained after the war and are still in force today in some countries, including the UK and the USA. Several other foods besides flour and bread are required by UK law to be fortified with iron. These include infant formulae and processed foods used as substitutes for meat. In addition, the law allows for voluntary fortification with iron of several different types of food such as breakfast cereals, infant weaning foods and meal replacements[65]. Other minerals may also be added to foods provided that the addition is not injurious to health, and the product is correctly labelled[66]. In the USA, a wide variety of additives may be used to fortify foods under the GRAS (Generally Recognised as Safe) system[67]. Some countries, such as Australia and New Zealand, have adopted a more restrictive policy, which allows fortification of specified foods with a limited number of minerals[68]. The result of these and similar regulations in other countries is that foods fortified with a variety of trace metals are available to consumers in most parts of the world.

Fortification of foods by the addition of trace elements has had a remarkable effect on nutrition in many countries. The earliest example, iodisation of salt, which was first introduced in the 1920s, resulted in the elimination of iodine deficiency in several countries. Iodisation of salt and some other foodstuffs has been adopted as one of the most efficient and cost-effective methods of combating IDD in areas of the world where iodine deficiency is endemic[69]. Iron fortification of flour and flour products has also had considerable success in preventing nutritional deficiencies of the element, but it has not totally overcome the problem. Iron deficiency anaemia (IDA), like IDD, in spite of continuing availability of fortified foods, persists as a major public health problem throughout the world[70].

Fortification of what are known as ready-to-eat, or RTE, breakfast cereals, though not designed initially to combat any specific disease, has also made a major contribution to nutritional health for many. RTE cereals are, in fact, an extraordinary success story of modern food technology. Their growth in popularity in many countries from their introduction at the beginning of the twentieth century, has been remarkable. They have replaced, for great numbers especially in the English-speaking world, the traditional cooked breakfast of bacon and eggs and even of oatmeal porridge[71]. In Australia, which is believed to have the third highest consumption of RTE cereals in the world, after Ireland and the UK[72], 80% of the population consume them at least once a week, with 50% consuming them every day. Americans are also big eaters of these products[73]. It has been shown that RTE breakfast cereals can make a significant contribution to intake of several trace elements, such as iron, zinc and copper, in countries where consumption is high, such as Ireland[74]. Similar findings have been reported in Australia[75], the UK[76] and the US[77].

Most of the cereals used to manufacture such RTE products, such as maize and rice and refined wheat, are naturally poor dietary sources of trace elements. It is the added minerals that account for the high levels of nutrients listed on the package and are a major selling point. How significant nutritionally these increased levels can be may be gathered from the fact that a normal serving of cornflakes produced by one of the major companies is capable of supplying 29% of the iron, 2.5% of the copper, 3% of the manganese, and 1% of the zinc requirement of an (Australian) adult[78].

1.3.7 Dietary supplements

Many people do not rely on food to supply the trace metal nutrients they consume. This is, in some cases, because they believe that much of the food available in the marketplace has been depleted of nutrients as a result of intensive farming and processing. Others do so because they are convinced that the maintenance of good health and the need to ward off cancer and other diseases requires a higher intake of nutrients than can be met by consuming ordinary food. Supplements are consumed to make up this perceived shortfall.

The market for dietary supplements is enormous. Total sales in what is known as the over-the-counter (OTC) healthcare sector in the UK were estimated to be worth £343 million in 1996[79]. In the same year, consumers in the US spent $6.5 billion on supplements. This was twice the expenditure reported in 1990–1991[80]. Similar levels of spending occur in other countries, with a continuous expansion of the OTC supplement market worldwide[81].

The contribution made to total dietary intake of trace metals and other micronutrients by consumption of self-selected supplements is considerable for many individuals. In addition to self-selection, supplements are frequently prescribed by physicians to treat recognised deficiency conditions. Iron, in various chemical forms and types of preparation, is commonly prescribed for the prevention and treatment of iron deficiency anaemia. Selenium supplements are used to prevent selenium deficiency-related cardiomyopathy in certain parts of China. The element is also increasingly used as a preventative and treatment for prostate and other forms of cancer. In poorer countries, zinc supplements are given frequently to children to reduce morbidity and help improve the growth rate. In all these, and other similar cases, the supplements are intended to compensate for dietary inadequacies of particular trace metal nutrients. An examination of the shelves of any pharmacy or health-food store will reveal the wide range of supplements and health preparations, which include many other trace elements which are either recognised as essential nutrients or believed to have some beneficial effect on health that are available, without prescription, to consumers. The elements include, in addition to the most widely used iron and zinc, boron, chromium, cobalt, manganese, nickel, selenium and vanadium. They are usually available either as individual metals or as multielement preparations.

1.3.8 Bioavailability of trace metal nutrients in foods

Trace metals occur in foods in different chemical forms, as inorganic or organic compounds or complexes with various organic compounds such as amino acids and proteins. This, as has been noted a number of times, has important consequences for bioavailability. If, for example, a metal is present in food only as an insoluble chemical form, it is unlikely to be absorbed to any significant extent from the gastrointestinal tract and will be excreted, unabsorbed and unutilised. This can have good and bad consequences for health. As little as 1% of the aluminium occurring naturally in food, mainly as the insoluble hydroxide or phosphate, is absorbed in the human gut, and thus potentially toxic uptake of the element is prevented[82]. Iron, which occurs especially in plant foods in the very insoluble inorganic Fe^{3+}, ferric form, is, like inorganic aluminium, absorbed by the human gut only to a limited extent. In this case, the consequences are undesirable.

While it is clear, however, that the bioavailability and concentration of a nutritional trace element are not always the same thing, a distinction that should be well known to nutritionists, it is not always recognised in practice. As was noted by Greger, nearly two decades ago, official food-composition tables and dietary recommendations for trace metals and other micronutrients list them in quantities down to fractions of milligrams. The result is that 'not surprisingly, consumers and sometimes nutritionists are so awed by all the figures that they forget that evaluating a diet nutritionally is more than simply adding the amounts of nutrients in individual foods and comparing the sum to a recommended intake'[83].

1.3.9 Estimating dietary intakes of trace metals

It can be a difficult task to estimate the dietary intake of any trace element in the diet. There is no single technique for doing so which can be considered a universal method of choice. An idea of the considerable number of different procedures that have been employed to do so by investigators is given by the bibliography produced by Krantzler *et al.*, which covers more than 80 different studies[84].

1.3.9.1 A hierarchial approach to estimating intakes

If, as has been recommended by Rees and Tennant, a combination of procedures, rather than a single method is used, many of the usual difficulties experienced in the estimation of dietary intakes can be overcome[85]. This *hierarchical* approach follows World Health Organisation (WHO) guidelines[86] and is conducted at three different levels (or hierarchies), depending on the needs and resources available, as follows:

(1) *Per capita estimation of intake*: Obtained by multiplying per capita food consumption by the estimated concentration of the particular food component of interest. The raw data needed for the estimation are normally available from a number of sources in most countries. The method is the simplest and most cost-effective, and provides an estimate of average intake of everyone in the whole population. While results allow comparisons to be drawn between intakes in, for example, different countries and can be useful in highlighting potential problems for further investigation, they do not apply to individual and non-average consumers.

(2) *Total Diet Studies (TDS)*: Also known as the Market Basket Survey (MBS) because it is based on a basket of food representing the total diet of consumers. The foods are separated into groups, and each group is analysed for its components. The method provides information on intakes and overall background levels, and can be used to pinpoint food groups which are of particular interest. It does not give information on individual foods, and its findings apply to the average, not the extreme consumer.

(3) *Hypothetical diets:* A 'model diet' approach can be used when there is insufficient information for a TDS. It can be a cost-effective way of estimating intakes, especially when a particular food is of major interest. The model diet approach can be refined by constructing various scenarios to reflect different cases and is particularly useful in predicting trends and pinpointing 'at-risk' groups.

1.3.9.2 Other methods for assessing intakes

Other methods for assessing intakes which provide more precise results than can be obtained by the hierarchical approach are normally more expensive to use, since they require considerable input of professional expertise and other resources. *Surveillance methods,* for example, which are used in major national studies, such as the UK National Dietary Survey[87] and the US Nationwide Food Consumer Survey[88], require reliable food consumption data combined with validated data on food composition. The consumption data are obtained from *food frequency questionnaires (FFQ)* or *weighed food diaries (WFD)*.

A *duplicate diet (DD)* method is particularly useful for obtaining information about the intake of individual consumers who have been identified at being 'at-risk' of deficiency, or excess. In theory, this is the ideal method for assessing the intake of a particular food component, since it allows direct measurements to be made on groups of special interest.

However, its accuracy depends on the reliability of individuals in dividing their meals between themselves and the duplicate plate. It can also be an expensive operation and demand a high degree of motivation from subjects[89].

1.3.10 Recommended allowances, intakes and dietary reference values

Knowing how much of a particular food component is consumed by a population group, or by an individual, does not by itself tell us much about its significance for health, unless we have further information about its nutritional value. It is for this reason that health authorities over the past half century have issued recommendations and guidelines on intakes of nutrients and other food components.

1.3.10.1 The US RDAs of 1941

Though some advice on nutrition had been issued by health authorities during World War I in an effort to counteract possible ill effects of food rationing, it was not until World War II that the first of what we know as Recommended Dietary Allowances (RDAs) were produced in the US. In 1940, the Food and Nutrition Board (FNB) of the US National Research Council (NRC) was given the responsibility for developing dietary standards that could be used to evaluate the dietary intakes of the population and to provide a guide for practical nutrition and the planning of agricultural production. In 1941, *Recommended Dietary Allowances* was published[90]. The document has subsequently gone through many revisions, has become 'the leading authoritative guide to the nutrient needs of the US populace and has been used in an extraordinary variety of applications'[91]. Its influence can be seen in the dietary recommendations published in nearly 50 countries during the latter half of the twentieth century[92].

The experts who developed the RDAs recognised that the inadequate information they had on many of the nutrients made it impossible to propose exact nutritional requirements. Nevertheless, they believed that a need did exist for standards and that even if their recommendations were subsequently found to be inaccurate, it was better to have at least interim standards than none at all[93].

The data on which the RDAs were based were obtained from (1) surveys to determine the presence or absence of disease in relation to nutrient intake by different populations, (2) controlled feeding experiments of humans and (3) metabolic studies with animals. These are still the bases on which modern recommendations largely depend.

The 'allowances' were numerical expressions of quantities which, on the basis of the best scientific evidence available at the time, were believed to be adequate to meet the known nutritional needs of practically all healthy persons. Recommendations were made for both sexes and for different age groups. They were not estimates of average requirements, since these apply only to half the population. They included a 'margin of safety' of two standard deviations above the mean, to allow for individual physiological variations, provide a buffer against increased need due to stress, and take account of growth and other factors.

The use of the term *allowance* was deliberate and was intended to avoid any implication of finality. It also allowed for re-evaluation of the figures as more information on which to base estimates became available. Later, some commentators objected to the term on the grounds that it had paternalistic overtones, and in some other countries, the term *Recommended Dietary Intake* (RDI) was adopted[94].

The first recommendations, in 1941, were for energy, protein, calcium, vitamins A, C and D, thiamin, riboflavin and niacin, as well as for a single trace element, iron. Over the years, additional nutrients have been added, including several more trace metals. The determination of recommendations regarding trace element nutrients has presented particular problems, as was noted by the WHO Expert Committee on Trace Elements in 1973[95]. Though most nutritionists at that time considered the major problems of developing countries to be deficiency of energy and protein, the Committee emphasised the need, also, for an adequate intake of certain trace elements. There was growing evidence, for example, of the nutritional importance of zinc and chromium, in addition to indications that 'new trace elements' also had significant roles to play in the maintenance of human health.

1.3.10.2 Estimated Safe and Adequate Daily Dietary Intakes

The WHO Expert Committee on Trace Elements believed that it did not have enough reliable information to allow it to make precise intake recommendations for the trace elements. Instead, estimated ranges that were believed to cover requirements under different circumstances were proposed. This was the approach adopted in the US in the 1980 (9th) edition of the *Recommended Dietary Allowances,* which introduced ranges of *Estimated Safe and Adequate Daily Dietary Intakes* (ESADDI) for six trace elements, as well as for three vitamins and three electrolytes[96]. Though, as has been noted by Mertz[97], these ESADDI were put forward as 'tentative and evolutionary', they represented, in fact, an important development in that they 'can be considered the first approach to the total dose response that recognises the homeostatic regulations of the organism and sets upper limits of intake'.

Even today, considerably more attention is paid by many nutritionists to requirements than to the important question of the safety of high intakes of nutrients, especially of trace elements. Yet, as far back as 1912, the French scientist Gabriel Bertrand had established and mathematically formulated dose–response curves for trace elements[98]. These bell-shaped curves describe biological function in relation to exposure. Though the shape and width of the curves vary from element to element, and even from individual to individual, all the curves have two extremes, one representing deficient and the other toxic exposure. Both are incompatible with life. Between the two extremes is a plateau that represents a range of exposures in which homeostatic regulation can maintain optimal function. It is into this range that the ESADDI falls.

Though it would seem obvious that the upper ranges of dose–response curves should be as important for nutritionists as the lower end, there is not much evidence that this was a guiding principle in many of the deliberations that took place about recommended intakes of nutrients until well towards the end of the last century[99]. Instead, the upper ranges tended to be the preserve of toxicologists, who concentrated largely on questions of safety. As a result, recommendations for intake developed by experts in the two fields tended to diverge, with the toxicologists setting stringent safety standards based on minimal risk, while nutritionists were satisfied with smaller safety factors. Thus, for example, the US Food and Nutrition Board set an ESADDI for manganese for adults of 2–5 mg/d, while the

Environmental Protection Agency (EPA) estimated an adult lowest-observable-adverse-effect level (LOAEL) for manganese in drinking water to be 4.2 mg/d. Thus, anyone consuming the amount of manganese recommended by the ESADDI could consume apparently excessive amounts if much of the trace metal came from water. There is a similar conflict between the standards set by the NRC Food and Nutrition Board for chromium and the guidance value used by the EPA for what is known as the reference dose (RfD) for the same element. For a 70 kg adult, the RfD is 70 mg/d, while the ESADDI range is 0.05–0.20 mg[100]. In contrast, the RfD for another essential trace metal, zinc, is in the same range as the RDA[101]. As has been remarked by Greger, conflicting standards of this sort lead to alarm and/or cynicism among the public and scientists[102]. They were also responsible for the decision by the American Society for Nutritional Sciences (ASNS) in 1997 to organise a symposium with the very apposite title *Between a Rock and a Hard Place: Dietary and Toxicological Standards for Essential Minerals.*

Though, as we shall see, efforts to set intake standards for the essential trace elements still fall between the rock and the hard place, much progress has been made in recent years as cooperation has improved between nutritionists and toxicologists. The results can be seen in the emergence of new concepts and the introduction of the novel terms and definitions. However, there still remain problem areas, especially with regard to the nutritional trace metals. There are several reasons for this.

Merk, in a keynote paper presented at the 1998 ASNS Symposium[103], made the significant observation that any standard of safe or adequate intakes of a nutrient is valid only for the conditions under which it was determined, because of the many modifying factors that affect the reaction of the organism to a given exposure. These factors include the chemical form of the nutrient, the route and timing of intake, and dietary interactions. Each of these can change an intake that is adequate under one condition to a deficient or excessive intake under another.

In the case of the metallic elements, the valence of the element determines both bioavailability and toxicity. Chromium, for instance, in its trivalent state acts as a nutrient but is toxic in its hexavalent form. Organically bound iron, as well as the inorganic divalent ion, is more easily absorbed from the diet than is its trivalent form. There are differences, also, between the effects of elements consumed in food and as supplements outside meals. Zinc and iron supplements can cause irritation of the gastrointestinal tract, and thus restrict absorption, whereas when consumed as part of food, they do not have this effect. A further consideration that has to be taken into account is the possibility of interactions between trace elements and other components of the diet. Apart from interactions that can occur between individual trace elements, for example between zinc and iron, the presence of other substances such as phytate which can reduce the bioavailability of trace elements, can be significant. For these reasons, an RDA may be valid only for one type of diet, not another[104].

1.3.11 Modernising the RDAs

Though collaboration between nutritionists, toxicologists and other scientists and health administrators in many countries had, over the 50 years since they were first introduced, done much to improve the usefulness and reliability of official dietary recommendations, by the final decades of the twentieth century, the need for a new approach became apparent. One of the major reasons for this was a change of emphasis away from the old concept of essentiality[105]. In the original RDAs, essentiality of a nutrient was considered to involve only prevention of a clinically distinct deficiency state. Now, with increasing interest in the role of nutrients in prevention of development of chronic diseases, a new paradigm began to emerge which took into account both the prevention of overt nutritional deficiencies and the provision of specific health benefits.

1.3.11.1 The US Dietary Reference Intakes for the twenty-first century

In the late 1990s, the Food and Nutrition Board of the Institute of Medicine, US National Academy of Sciences, set up an expert committee, which included a representative of Health Canada, to undertake a comprehensive review of dietary reference values for Americans[106]. The Committee, whose long title, Standing Committee on the Scientific Evaluation of Dietary Reference Intakes, was fortunately shortened to the DRI Committee, noted that since the publication of the 10th edition of the US RDAs in 1989 and the Canadian RNIs in 1990[107], there had been 'a significant expansion of the research base, an increased understanding of nutrient requirements and food constituents, and a better appreciation for the different types of nutrient data needed to address the application of dietary reference values for individuals and population groups'[108]. It was essential, the Committee believed, to reassess the nutrient requirement estimates for various purposes, how estimates of nutrient requirements should be developed and how these values can be used in various clinical and public health settings. The Committee intended to undertake this review and thus help to eliminate some of the limitations, misinterpretations and misuses of the old RDAs. To achieve this purpose, a number of expert panels with responsibility for different groups of nutrients were set up. Each panel was to be responsible for (1) reviewing the scientific literature on its assigned nutrients, (2) considering the roles of these nutrients in decreasing risk of chronic and other diseases and conditions, and (3) interpreting the current data on intakes in North America. The panels were to report back to the Committee, which would determine the DRI values to be included in a final report.

The Committee had from the beginning decided against simply updating and replacing the 1989 edition of the RDAs. Instead, it would be replaced in its entirety by a new series of publications. These would be published as the deliberations of the various nutrition panels were completed and would become the accepted dietary recommendations for North America and, it was hoped, a framework for the development and harmonisation of DRIs internationally.

The North American dietary references for the trace metal nutrients will be considered in detail in later chapters on the individual metals. Here, it will be sufficient to draw attention to the overall implications of the changes resulting from the replacement of the old terms and concepts. Though, superficially, there appear to be many similarities between RDAs and DRIs, there are, in fact, significant differences[109]. The term itself, *Dietary Reference Intake*, refers to at least four nutrient-based reference values, that have been introduced to cover quantitative estimates of nutrient intakes and can be used for planning and assessing diets and for many other purposes. The reference values, collectively called the DRIs, include the following values:

(1) *Recommended Dietary Allowance* (RDA), the average daily intake sufficient to meet the needs of nearly all (97–98%) healthy persons of a particular age and sex. Unlike the original RDA, in the DRI framework this is the sole use of the RDA.
(2) *Estimated Average Requirement* (EAR), an amount estimated to meet the requirements of 50% of healthy persons in a group. The EAR is used to assess adequacy of intakes of population groups and, along with knowledge of the distribution of requirements, to develop RDAs, which are set at 2SD above the EAR.
(3) *Adequate Intake* (AI), an amount based on observed or experimentally determined approximations. It is used when an RDA cannot be determined.
(4) *Tolerable Upper Intake Levels* (UL), the highest level of daily intake that is likely to pose no risk of adverse health effects to almost all individuals in the general population. Above the UL, toxicity is likely to occur.

The first of the reports published by the DRI Committee, based on the work of the expert panel on calcium and related nutrients (vitamin D, phosphorus, magnesium and fluoride) and incorporating the new concepts and terms, was published in 1997. Subsequently, several more have appeared, two of which include several of the trace metal nutrients which will be considered in detail in later chapters. These are selenium, which was considered by the panel responsible also for vitamins C and E, β-carotene and other carotenoids, and a group of trace metals (chromium, copper, iron, manganese, molybdenum, nickel, vanadium and zinc), which was the responsibility of the panel which looked also at vitamins A and K.

1.3.11.2 The UK's Dietary Reference Values

North America was not the only part of the world in which serious attention was being given to the need for revision of current dietary intake recommendations. In the UK, for instance, a report by the Committee on Medical Aspects of Food Policy (COMA) of the Department of Health in 1991 proposed that, in addition to updating data, recommendations needed to be restated and the original single-figure RDA replaced by different values appropriate to different situations and groups[110]. A new term, *Dietary Reference Value* (DRV) was introduced to replace the original term of RDA. This, like its predecessor, was to apply to groups of healthy persons, not the ill or those with metabolic abnormalities. It differed from the old RDA, however, in having four different categories:

(1) *Estimated Average Requirement* (EAR), which is the average estimated requirement for everyone and assumes a normal distribution of variability. In a normal population, some people will need more, and some less, than the EAR.
(2) *Reference Nutrient Intake* (RNI), which is the EAR + 2SD. It is the amount of nutrient that is enough for almost every individual. If the RNI is consumed, it is most unlikely that deficiency will occur.
(3) *Lower Reference Nutrient Intake* (LRNI), 2SD below the EAR. The LRNI will be enough for only a small number of people with low needs. If the LRNI is habitually consumed, deficiency is almost certain to occur.
(4) *Safe Intake* (SI) is used for nutrients for which there is not as yet enough information to allow an EAR to be made. It is given as a range of intakes within which there is no risk of deficiency and above which there is a risk of toxicity.

As well as providing values for energy, proteins, fats, carbohyrdrates and nine different vitamins, the DRVs gave RNIs for 11 minerals. These included the four trace elements, iron, zinc, copper and selenium, for which the COMA Group believed there was sufficient information to permit them to estimate an RNI. In addition, SIs were provided for three other trace metals, manganese, molybdenum and chromium. For these elements, there was inadequate information to allow more precise recommendations to be made. The Expert Group also considered several other trace elements, including aluminium, antimony, arsenic, boron, cobalt, nickel and vanadium, but concluded that convincing evidence for their essentiality was lacking.

1.3.11.3 Australian and New Zealand Nutrient Reference Values

In 1998, arrangements were made for a joint Australian–New Zealand review of recommended nutrient intakes used in the two countries[111]. It has been agreed that the new recommendations will be called *Nutrient Reference Values* (NRVs) for Australia and New Zealand. Within the NRVs, there will be six reference values: *Reference Nutrient Intake* (RNI), *Estimated Average Requirement* (EAR) or *Adequate Intake* (AI) if an EAR cannot be estimated, *Critical Low Intake* (CLI), *Upper Safe Limit* (USL), *Provisional Functional Range* (PFR), and *Toxic Threshold* (TT). In general, the categories correspond to those used in the US/Canadian DRIs, with some word modifications, with the addition of the PFR. This value takes into account possible additional health benefits of higher intakes than are recommended in the EAR. As in the US, the proposed NRVs take into account the increasing number of people who take nutrient supplements, often at levels of intake beyond those typically in the diet.

1.3.11.4 Other nutrient intake recommendations

Reviews of nutrient intake recommendations are currently being undertaken in several other countries and by various health organisations resulting in the development of certain new categories and descriptive terms. For example, WHO's *population requirement safe ranges* include *Basal* (lower limit), *Normative* (sufficient to meet normative requirements) and *Maximum* (upper limit)[112]. The term *Recommended Intake* is used for average requirements augmented by a factor that takes into account inter-individual variability[113].

In the European Union, the following terms are used: *Lower Threshold Intake* (LTI), *Average Requirement Intake* (ARI), *Population Reference Intake* (PRI) and *Acceptable Range* (AR). The PRI is equivalent to the UK's RNI and is the mean requirement + 2SD. The AR, like the SI in the US, is a range of safe values given when there is insufficient information to estimate the PRI.

Reference values for nutrient intakes have been developed by expert groups in many other countries, besides the UK, the US, and the European Union. Though all share the common purpose of providing guidelines for the maintenance of the nutritional health of consumers, there are certain significant differences in the values and in their manner of presentation[114]. This is particularly so in the case of the number of life-stage groups identified by different countries. In addition, while two general types of reference values are used, (1) an estimate of average requirements or (2) the intake that will meet the needs of 97–98% of the population, the actual references values differ between countries. These differences are in many cases due to the use of different criteria for estimating average requirements as well as to judgements made when limited data were available. In certain cases, there are country-specific reasons for differences between national recommendations. In those of several Asian countries, including Indonesia, Malaysia, the Philippines and Vietnam, the recommendations for iron intake, for example, are much higher than in other countries. This reflects the differences in composition of the normal national diet, with its effects on iron supply and bioavailability in these Asian countries compared to the high animal protein diet of many other countries, particularly in the West.

As we shall see, differences between DRIs in different countries can have practical implications for nutritionists and others responsible for giving nutritional advice. We will consider this problem in the following chapters on individual nutrients.

References

1. Epstein, E. (1972) *Mineral Nutrition of Plants: Principles and Perspectives*, pp. 9–11. Wiley, New York.
2. Stillman, M.J. & Presta, A. (2000) Characterising metal ion interactions with biological molecules – the spectroscopy of metallothionein, 1. In: *Molecular Biology and Toxicology of Metals* (eds. R.K. Zalups & J. Korpatnick), Taylor & Francis, London.
3. Fraústo da Silva, J.J.R. & Williams, R.J.P. (2001) *The Biological Chemistry of the Elements*. Oxford University Press, Oxford.
4. Hurd, D.L. & Kipling, J.J. (1964) *The Origins and Growth of Physical Science*, Vol. 2, p. 103. Penguin, London.
5. Iyengar, G.V. (1988) Biological trace element research. A multidisciplinary science. *Science of the Total Environment*, **71**, 1–7.
6. Griggs, B. (1988) *The Food Factor: An Account of the Nutrition Revolution*, pp. 12–16. Penguin, London.
7. McCann, A. (1919) *The Science of Eating*, p. 55. Garden City Publishing, New York.
8. Bouis, H. (1996) Enrichment of food staples through plant breeding: a new strategy for fighting micronutrient malnutrition. *Nutrition Reviews*, **54**, 131–7.
9. Lippard, S.J. (1993) Bioinorganic chemistry: a maturing frontier. *Science*, **261**, 699–700.
10. Karlin, K.D. (1993) Metalloenzymes, structural motifs, and inorganic models. *Science*, **261**, 701–8.
11. Pyle, A.M. (1993) Ribozymes: a distinct class of metalloenzymes. *Science*, **261**, 709–14.
12. O'Halloran, T.V. (1993) Transition metals in control of gene expression. *Science*, **261**, 715–24.
13. Karlin, K.D. (1993) Metalloenzymes, structural motifs, and inorganic models. *Science*, **261**, 701–8.
14. Fraústo da Silva, J.J.R. & Williams, R.J.P. (2001) *The Biological Chemistry of the Elements*. Oxford University Press, Oxford.
15. Wilkins, P.C. & Wilkins, R.G. (1997) *Inorganic Chemistry in Biology*. Oxford University Press, Oxford.
16. Shriver, D.F. & Atkins, P.W. (1999) *Inorganic Chemistry*, 3rd ed., p. 645. Oxford University Press, Oxford.
17. Fraústo da Silva, J.J.R. & Williams, R.J.P. (2001) *The Biological Chemistry of the Elements*. Oxford University Press, Oxford.
18. Lippard, S.J. (1993) Bioinorganic chemistry: a maturing frontier. *Science* **261**, 699–700.

19. Shriver, D.F. & Atkins, P.W. (1999) *Inorganic Chemistry*, 3rd ed., p. 645. Oxford University Press, Oxford.
20. Wilkins, P.C. & Wilkins, R.G. (1997) *Inorganic Chemistry in Biology*, p. 61. Oxford University Press, Oxford.
21. Fraústo da Silva, J.J.R. & Williams, R.J.P. (2001) *The Biological Chemistry of the Elements.* Oxford University Press, Oxford.
22. Fraústo da Silva, J.J.R. & Williams, R.J.P. (2001) *The Biological Chemistry of the Elements.* Oxford University Press, Oxford.
23. Nicholas, D.J.D. (1961) Minor mineral nutrients. *Annual Review of Plant Physiology*, **12**, 63–86.
24. Mertz, W. (1981) The essential trace elements. *Science*, **213**, 1332–8.
25. Fraústo da Silva, J.J.R. & Williams, R.J.P. (2001) *The Biological Chemistry of the Elements.* Oxford University Press, Oxford.
26. Cotzias, G.C. (1967) Importance of trace substances in environmental health, as exemplified by manganese. In: *Trace Substances in Environmental Health* (ed. D.H. Hemphill), pp. 5–19. University of Missouri Press, Columbia, MO.
27. Fraústo da Silva, J.J.R. & Williams, R.J.P. (1976) *The Uptake of Elements by Biological Systems. Structure and Bonding*, pp. 67–121. Springer, Berlin.
28. Bowen, H.J.M. (1979) *Environmental Chemistry of the Elements.* Academic Press, London.
29. Schroeder, H.A. (1973) *The Trace Elements and Nutrition*, pp. 13–14. Faber & Faber, London.
30. Cox, P.A. (1995) *The Elements on Earth.* Oxford University Press, Oxford.
31. Kobayashi, I.K. & Ponnamperuma, C. (1985) Trace elements in chemical evolution. *Origins of Life*, **16**, 41–55.
32. Williams, R.J.P. & Fraústo da Silva, J.J.R. (1996) *The Natural Selection of the Chemical Elements.* Oxford University Press, Oxford.
33. Fraústo da Silva, J.J.R. & Williams, R.J.P. (2001) *The Biological Chemistry of the Elements.* Oxford University Press, Oxford.
34. Fraústo da Silva, J.J.R. & Williams, R.J.P. (2001) *The Biological Chemistry of the Elements.* Oxford University Press, Oxford.
35. Shriver, D.F. & Atkins, P.W. (1999) *Inorganic Chemistry*, 3rd ed., p. 645. Oxford University Press, Oxford.
36. Hewitt, E.J. & Smith, T.A. (1975) *Plant Mineral Nutrition.* English Universities Press, London.
37. Dreosti, I.E. (1990) Zinc. In: *Recommended Nutrient Intakes Australian Papers* (ed. A.S. Truswell), pp. 257–63. Australian Professional Publications, Sydney.
38. Department of Health (1996) *Dietary Reference Values for Food Energy and Nutrients in the United Kingdom*, p. 169. HMSO, London.
39. Ysart, G., Miller, P., Crews, H. *et al.* (1999) Dietary exposure estimates of 30 elements from the UK Total Diet Study. *Food Additives and Contaminants*, **16**, 391–403.
40. Varo, P. & Koivistonen, P. (1980) Mineral composition of Finnish foods XII. General discussion and nutritional evaluation. *Acta Agricultura Scandinavica*, **S22**, 165–70.
41. Nielsen, F.H. (1984) Fluoride, vanadium, nickel, arsenic and silicon in total parenteral nutrition. *Bulletin of the New York Academy of Medicine*, **60**, 177–95.
42. Reilly, C. (1996) *Selenium in Food and Health*, p. 217. Chapman & Hall, London.
43. Moraghan, J.T. & Grafton, K. (2001) Genetic diversity and mineral composition of common bean seed. *Journal of the Science of Food and Agriculture*, **81**, 404–8.
44. Booth, C.K., Reilly, C. & Farmakalidis, E. (1996) Mineral composition of Australian ready-to-eat breakfast cereals. *Journal of Food Composition and Analysis*, **91**, 135–47.
45. Crews, H.M. (1998) Speciation of trace elements in food, with special reference to cadmium and selenium: is it necessary? *Spectrochimica Acta*, **B53**, 213–9.

46. Cantle, J.E. (1982) *Techniques and Instrumentation in Analytical Chemistry, Vol. 5, Atomic Absorption Spectrophotometry*. Elsevier, Amsterdam.
47. Versieck, J. & Cornelis, R. (1989) *Trace Elements in Human Plasma or Serum*. CRC Press, Boca Raton, FL.
48. Allen, J.L. & Cumming, F.J. (1998) *Aluminium in the Food and Water Supply: An Australian Perspective. Research Report No. 202*. Water Services Association of Australia, Melbourne.
49. Cross, J.D., Raie, R.M., Smith, H. & Smith, L.B. (1978) Dietary selenium in the Glasgow area. *Radiochemical and Radioanalytical Letters*, **35**, 281–90.
50. MacPherson, A., Barclay, M.N.I., Dixon, J. *et al.* (1993) Decline in dietary selenium intake in Scotland and effect on plasma concentrations. In: *Trace Elements in Man and Animals – TEMA 8* (eds. M. Anke, D. Meissner & C.F. Mills), pp. 269–70. Verlag Media Touristik, Gersdorf, Germany.
51. Alvarez, R. (1984) NBS Standard Reference Materials for food analysis. In: *Modern Methods of Food Analysis* (eds. K.K. Stewart & J.R. Whitaker). AVI, Westport, CT.
52. Sparks, D.L. (1995) *Environmental Soil Chemistry*, pp. 35–47. Academic Press, San Diego.
53. McBride, M.B. (1994) *Environmental Chemistry of Soils*, p. 308 ff. Oxford University Press, Oxford.
54. Reilly, C. (1996) Selenium supplementation – the Finnish experiment. *British Nutrition Foundation Nutrition Bulletin*, **21**, 167–73.
55. Bennet-Chambers, M., Davies, P. & Knott, B. (1999) Cadmium in aquatic systems in Western Australia. A legacy of nutrient-deficient soils. *Journal of Environmental Management*, **57**, 283–95.
56. Wenlock, R.W., Buss, D.H. & Massey, R.C. (1979) Trace nutrients. 2. Manganese in British foods. *British Journal of Nutrition*, **41**, 253–61.
57. Saroja, A. & Sivapalan, P. (1990) Aluminium in black tea. *Sri Lanka Journal of Tea Science*, **59**, 4–8.
58. Reilly, C. (1998) Selenium: a new entrant into the functional foods arena. *Trends in Food Science and Technology*, **9**, 114–18.
59. Paul, A.A. & Southgate, D.A.T. (1978) *McCance and Widdowson's The Composition of Foods*, p. 235. HMSO, London.
60. Ysart, G., Miller, P., Crews, H. *et al.* (1999) Dietary exposure estimates of 30 elements from the UK Total Dietary Study. *Food Additives and Contaminants*, **16**, 391–403.
61. Borigato, E.V.M. & Martinez, F.E. (1998) Iron nutritional status is improved in Brazilian infants fed food cooked in iron pots. *Journal of Nutrition*, **128**, 855–9.
62. Smart, G.A. & Sherlock, J.C. (1985) Chromium in foods and diet. *Food Additives and Contaminants*, **2**, 139–47.
63. Tanner, M.S., Bhave, S.A., Kantarjian, A.H. & Pandit, A.N. (1983) Early introduction of copper-contaminated animal milk feeds as a possible cause of Indian childhood cirrhosis. *Lancet*, **ii**, 992–5.
64. Brady, M.C. (1996) Addition of nutrients: current practice in the UK. *British Food Journal*, **98**, 12–18.
65. Fairweather-Tait, S.J. (1997) Iron fortification in the UK: how necessary and effective is it? In: *Trace Elements in Man and Animals – TEMA 9: Proceedings of the Ninth International Symposium on Trace Elements in Man and Animals* (eds. P.W.P. Fischer, M.R. L'Abbé, K.A. Cockell & R.S. Gibson), pp. 392–6. National Research Council Research Press, Ottawa.
66. Ministry of Agriculture Fisheries and Food (1996) *Food Labelling Regulations*. HMSO, London.
67. United States Food and Drug Administration (1987) *Code of Federal Regulations. Title 21. Nutritional Quality Guidelines for Foods*, Part 104.5. Food and Drug Administration, Washington, DC.

68. Australia New Zealand Food Authority (2000) *Draft Food Standards Code: Standard 1.3.2 Vitamins and Minerals.* http://www.anzfa.gov.au/Draft Food Standards/Chapter 1/Part1,3/1.3.2 htm
69. Hetzel, B.S. (1987) An overview of the prevention and control of iodine deficiency disorders. In: *The Prevention and Control of Iodine Deficiency Disorders* (eds. B.S. Hetzel, J.T. Dunn & J.B. Stanbury). Elsevier, Amsterdam.
70. Hurrell, R.F. (1977) Preventing iron deficiency through food fortification. *Nutrition Reviews*, **55**, 210–22.
71. Collins, E.J.T. (1976) Changing patterns of bread and cereal-eating in Britain in the twentieth century. In: *The Making of the Modern British Diet* (eds. D.T. Oddy & D.S. Miller), pp. 26–43. Croom Helm, London.
72. Kellogg Market Research (1995) Kellogg (Australia) Sydney.
73. Pennington, J. & Young, B. (1990) Iron, zinc, copper, manganese, selenium and iodine in foods from the United States Total Diet Study. *Journal of Food Composition and Analysis*, **3**, 166–84.
74. Sommerville, J. & O'Regan, M. (1993) The contribution of breakfast to micronutrient adequacy of the Irish diet. *Journal of Human Nutrition and Dietetics*, **6**, 223–8.
75. Wang, C.Y., Reilly, C., Patterson, C., Morrison, E. & Tinggi, U. (1992) Contribution of breakfast cereals to Australian intake of trace elements. *Food Australia*, **44**, 70–2.
76. Crawley, H. (1993) the role of breakfast cereals in the diets of 16–17 year old teenagers in Britain. *Journal of Human Nutrition and Dietetics*, **6**, 205–16.
77. Pennington, J. & Young, B. (1990) Iron, zinc, copper, manganese, selenium and iodine in foods from the United States Total Diet Study. *Journal of Food Composition and Analysis*, **3**, 166–84.
78. Booth, C.K., Reilly, C. & Farmakelidis, E. (1996) Mineral composition of Australian Ready-to-Eat breakfast cereals. *Journal of Food Composition and Analysis*, **9**, 135–47.
79. Mintel (1997) *Vitamins and Dietary Supplements.* Mineral International Group, London.
80. Gkurtzweil, P. (1998) An FDA guide to dietary supplements. *FDA Consumer*, **32**, 28–35.
81. Kirk, S., Woodhouse, A., Conner, M. & The UKWCS Steering Group (1998) Beliefs, attitudes and behaviour in relation to supplement use in the UK Women's Cohort Study. *Proceedings of the Nutrition Society*, **57**, 54A.
82. Exley, C., Burgess, E. , Day, J.P. *et al.* (1996) Aluminium toxicokinetics. *Journal of Toxicology and Environmental Health*, **48**, 569–84.
83. Greger, J.L. (1987) Mineral bioavailability/New concepts. *Nutrition Today*, **22**, 4–9.
84. Krantzler, N.J., Mullen, B.J., Comstock, E.M. *et al.* (1982). Methods of food intake assessment – an annotated bibliography. *Journal of Nutrition Education*, **14**, 108–19.
85. Rees, N. & Tennant, D. (1994) Estimation of chemical intake. In: *Nutritional Toxicology* (eds. F.N. Kotenis, M. Machey & J. Hjelle) pp. 199–221. Raven Press, New York.
86. World Health Organisation (1985) *WHO Guidelines for the Study of Dietary Intakes of Chemical Contaminants, Prepared by the Joint UNEP/FAO/WHO Global Environmental Monitoring Programme. Offset Publication No. 87.* World Health Organisation, Geneva.
87. Gregory, J., Foster, K., Tyler, H. & Wiseman, M. (1990) *The Dietary and Nutritional Survey of British Adults.* HMSO, London.
88. US Department of Agriculture (1994) *Nationwide Food Consumption Survey, Continuing Survey of Food Intakes by Individuals and Diet Health and Knowledge Survey, 1990, Machine-Readable Data Set, Accession No. PB94-500063.* National Technical Information Service, Springfield, VA.
89. Duffield, A.J. & Thomson, C.D. (1999) A comparison of methods of assessment of dietary selenium intakes in Otago. *British Journal of Nutrition*, **82**, 131–8.
90. National Research Council (1941) *Recommended Dietary Allowances.* National Academy Press, Washington, DC.

91. Lachance, P.A. (1998) International perspective: basis, need, and application of Recommended Dietary Allowances. *Nutrition Reviews*, **56**, S2–S4.
92. Truswell, A.S. & Chambers, T. (1983) IUNS report on recommended dietary allowances around the world. *Nutrition Abstracts and Reviews*, **53**, 939–1119.
93. Guthrie, H.A. (1975) *Introductory Nutrition*, pp. 326–31. Mosby, St. Louis, MO.
94. Truswell, A.S. (1990) Recommended nutrient intakes: some general principles and problems. In: *Recommended Nutrient Intakes: Australian Papers* (ed. A.S. Truswell). pp. 18–24. Australian Professional Publications, Mossman, Australia.
95. World Health Organisation Expert Committee (1973) *Trace Elements in Human Nutrition.* WHO Technical Report Series, No. 532. World Health Organisation, Geneva.
96. National Research Council (1980) *Recommended Dietary Allowances*, 9th ed. National Academy Press, Washington, DC.
97. Mertz, W. (1998) A perspective on mineral standards. *Journal of Nutrition*, **128**, 375S–8S.
98. Bertrand, G. (1912) On the role of trace substances in agriculture. In: *8th International Congress of Applied Chemistry*, Vol. **28**, pp. 30–49. New York, as cited in Mertz, W. (1998).
99. Mertz, W. (1976). Defining trace element toxicities in man. In: *Molybdenum in the Environment* (eds. W.R. Chappell & K.K. Petersen), Vol. 1, pp. 267–86. Dekker, New York.
100. National Research Council (1989) *Recommended Dietary Allowances*, 10th ed. National Academy Press, Washington, DC.
101. Olin, S.S. (1998) Between a rock and a hard place: methods for setting dietary allowances and exposure limits for essential minerals. *Journal of Nutrition*, **128**, 364S–7S.
102. Greger J.L. (1998) Dietary standards for manganese: overlap between nutritional and toxicological studies. *Journal of Nutrition*, **128**, 368S–71S.
103. Mertz, W. (1998) A perspective on mineral standards. *Journal of Nutrition*, **128**, 375S–8S.
104. World Health Organisation (1973) *Trace Elements in Human Nutrition. Technical Report Series No. 532.* WHO, Geneva.
105. Hambidge, M.K. (1996) Overview and purpose of the workshop on new approaches, endpoints and paradigms for RDAs of mineral elements. *Journal of Nutrition*, **126**, 2301S–3S.
106. Institute of Medicine, Food and Nutrition Board (1994) *How Should the Recommended Dietary Allowances be Revised?* National Academy Press, Washington, DC.
107. Health Canada (1990) *Nutrition Recommendations. The Report of the Scientific Review Committee 1990.* Canadian Government Publishing Centre, Ottawa.
108. Institute of Medicine (1997) *Dietary Reference Intakes for Calcium, Phosphorus, Magnesium, Vitamin D, and Fluoride*, p. ix. National Academy Press, Washington, DC.
109. Yates, A.A., Schlicker, S.A. & Suitor, C.W. (1998) Dietary Reference Intakes: the new basis for recommendations for calcium and related nutrients, B vitamins, and choline. *Journal of the American Dietetics Association*, **98**, 699–706.
110. Department of Health (1991) *Report on Health and Social Subjects, 41: Dietary Reference Values for Food Energy and Nutrients for the United Kingdom.* Committee on Medical Aspects of Food Policy. HMSO, London.
111. Thomson, C.D. (2003) Proposed Australian and New Zealand nutrient reference values for selenium and iodine. *Journal of Nutrition*, **133**, Abstracts, 278E.
112. World Health Organisation (1992) *Trace Elements in Human Nutrition.* WHO, Geneva.
113. World Health Organisation (1974) *Handbook on Human Nutritional Requirements.* WHO, Geneva.
114. Anon (1997) Dietary reference intakes. *Nutrition Reviews*, **55**, 319–26.

Chapter 2
Iron

2.1 Introduction

Iron presents nutritional scientists with a fascinating challenge. In spite of more than two centuries of scientific investigation, there are still unanswered questions as to how the body manages its iron economy[1]. Iron has been used in medicine since ancient times. The Greeks believed that Mars, the god of war, had endowed the metal with special properties, including the ability to heal wounds and maintain virility – according to legend, the Argonaut Apollodorus of Iphyclus was cured of impotence by drinking iron rust in wine, a preparation known as Saffron of Mars[2]. Hippocrates, the 'Father of Medicine', used iron to cure chlorosis, a condition which we now know as iron deficiency anaemia. Iron continued to be used to treat various illnesses during the following centuries, but without any real understanding of its function. It remained part of the medical pharmacopoeia, under its ancient name of Mars with as its symbol ♂, until well after the Scientific Revolution of the seventeenth century[3].

By the early eighteenth century, as chemical knowledge and laboratory techniques improved, systematic studies of iron were undertaken by several investigators. In 1713, the French scientist Lemery showed that it was a constituent of blood. In the following year, the Swedish chemist Berzelius showed that iron in blood was neither an alkaline salt nor a phosphate as had been claimed by others, but was what he called an 'organic compound' and contained carbon, nitrogen, hydrogen, phosphorus, oxygen and calcium, as well as iron[4]. In 1825, the red colouring matter of blood was reported to have an iron content of 0.35%, a value very close to that calculated by modern methods[5]. About the same time, anaemia was recognised as being due to low levels of iron in the blood and a reduction in the number of red cells.

One of the earliest attempts to study the relationship between iron in food and the composition of blood was made by the French physician Verdeil about the middle of the nineteenth century. He found that a dog fed a diet of meat had considerably more iron in its blood than when it was fed on bread and potatoes[6]. The nutritional essentiality of iron was proposed in 1872 by another French physician, Boussingault[7]. By the early twentieth century, the connection between anaemia and a low dietary intake of iron was widely recognised. The use of iron-enriched tonics to prevent and treat anaemia, especially in women and children, became standard practice, and iron salts and other forms of iron supplements were commonly prescribed for the same purpose. The practice received official endorsement when, in the early years of World War II, governments in the US and some other countries ordered iron to be added to flour to counteract nutritional deficiencies expected to result from wartime rationing.

Further advances in understanding of the metabolic role of iron and its place in human nutrition have been made over the past half century. Considerable expertise and resources have been committed to these efforts, and much progress has been made. Yet, there remain many baffling problems about the functions of this essential metal.

2.2 Iron chemistry

Iron is the second most abundant metal, and the fourth most abundant element in the earth's crust. The earth's core is believed to be made of a mass of iron and nickel, and, to judge from the composition of meteorites, iron is also abundant elsewhere in the solar system. The importance of the element in the physical world is matched by its importance in human life. We use more of it than of any other metal. Without it, civilisation, as we know it, would not exist.

The human body, like nearly all other living organisms, has, during the course of evolution, come to depend on iron as the linchpin of its existence. Indeed, it has been proposed that life first began within iron sulphide 'cells' that provided a micro-environment in which prebiotic organic systems were able to develop on the floor of primitive oceans[8]. The release and utilisation of energy from food depend on iron-containing enzymes. Iron is used in the synthesis of blood pigments and in many other essential activities of cells. Out of all living organisms, only certain bacteria, of the genera *Lactobacillus* and *Bacillus*, appear to possess no iron-containing enzymes. Nevertheless, in spite of its abundance in the environment, and its almost universal distribution in living matter, iron deficiency is probably the most common nutritional deficiency in the world, even in the most affluent countries[9].

The chemical symbol of iron is Fe, after *ferrum*, its Latin name. It is element number 26 in the periodic table, with an atomic weight of 55.8 and a density of 7.86. The pure metal is white and lustrous but rapidly oxidises in moist air to produce a brown skin of rust. It is relatively hard, ductile and malleable, and has a melting point of 1528°C. It is a good conductor of both heat and electricity. Its physical properties are significantly altered by the presence of even very small amounts of other metals, as well as of carbon, an effect that accounts for one of its most important characteristics, its ability to be transformed into various types of steel. These are the properties that made iron so useful to the metal workers of the Iron Age and still account for its key place in industry today.

The chemistry of iron is complex. It is one of the *d*-block transition elements and can exist in oxidation states ranging from -2 to $+6$. However, in biological systems, these are limited to the ferrous ($+2$), ferric ($+3$) and ferryl ($+4$). Three oxides are known, FeO, Fe_2O_3 and Fe_3O_4, representing the Fe(II) and the Fe(III), as well as the mixed Fe(II)–Fe(III) oxide which occurs in nature as the mineral magnetite. Iron dissolves in acids to form salts. With non-oxidising acids, in the absence of air, ferrous salts are formed. Many iron salts, as well as hydroxides, are insoluble in water. As we shall see, it is this insolubility, particularly of its Fe(III) compounds, that is one of the main contributory factors in the aetiology of iron deficiency anaemia.

Like the other transition metals, with their labile *d*-electron systems, iron has a rich redox chemistry, which allows it to play a role in a variety of oxido-reductase enzyme activities as well as in electron transfers. Iron can also, by virtue of its unoccupied *d*-orbitals, bind reversibly to many different ligands. This ability to form coordination complexes is one of its most important chemical properties, from the biological point of view. Its preferred biological ligands are oxygen, nitrogen and sulphur atoms in cellular components, such as water and small organic molecules, and in the side chains of amino acids. Both the electron spin state and the redox potential of the iron atom can change according to the ligand to which it is bound. Because of this ability to exploit the electronic spin and the redox potential, as well as its oxidation state, which allow iron to adjust its chemical activity, it is able to participate in a wide variety of key biochemical activities[10]. This is seen particularly in its complexes with the porphyrin nucleus in haem pigments, cytochromes and a variety of other functional proteins.

2.3 Iron in the body

The human body contains about 50 mg of iron per kilogram of body weight, or about 3–4 g in an adult. About 60% of the total is present as haemoglobin in erythrocytes, with another 10% in myoglobin of muscle. The remaining 30% occurs in a variety of iron-containing proteins, such as the cytochromes, iron–sulphur enzymes, and in iron storage and transporting proteins. Iron does not occur as free ions in body fluids or tissues.

2.3.1 Haemoglobin

All the mammalian haemoglobins are conjugated proteins with a molecular weight of about 65 000 and are composed of colourless basic proteins, the globins, and ferroprotoporphyrin (haem). They are essentially tetramers, consisting of four polypeptide chains, to each of which is bound the haem group. Normally, humans are capable of synthesising four distinct, but related polypeptide chains, designated α, β, γ, and δ, respectively. In the different haemoglobins, the chains are combined in different patterns. For example normal adult haemoglobin, called HbA, contains two α and two β chains, while in fetal haemoglobin, there are two α and two γ chains.

Though they differ in their protein moiety, all haemoglobins, in humans and other vertebrates, as well as in some invertebrates, contain the same ferroprotoporphyrin, known as protoporphyrin IX (Fe-PP-IX). This same ferroprotoporphyrin occurs also in several other functional conjugated proteins, including human myoglobin, cytochromes, catalase and certain other enzymes and transport proteins[11]. Haem consists of a 16-membered structure formed by four pyrrole rings in which an iron atom replaces the dissociable hydrogen atoms of two of the pyrrole rings and is simultaneously bound by coordinate valencies to the tertiary nitrogen atoms of the other two rings, as illustrated Fig. 2.1. In haemoglobin, the imidazole nitrogen from a histidine residue in each polypeptide chain provides a fifth ligand for the iron atom. The sixth position is occupied either by a water molecule or by oxygen, depending on whether oxygen is available or not. It is this ability to bind reversibly to oxygen that accounts for the special role of haemoglobin.

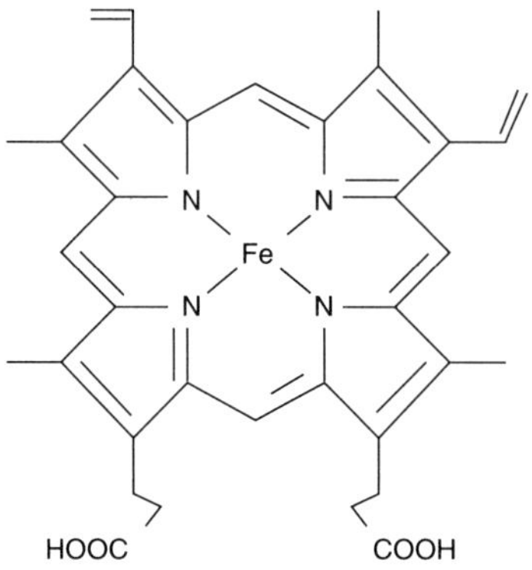

Figure 2.1 Structure of haem.

The unique feature of haemoglobin is not simply its ability to bind oxygen. This can also be done by other, non-haemoglobin ferroprotoporphyrin complexes. In those molecules, however, the iron atom is irreversibly oxidised to the ferric state by molecular oxygen and cannot function as an oxygen carrier. In haemoglobin, this does not occur because the haem moiety is located within a cover of hydrophobic groups of the globin which surrounds and protects it. This allows the formation of a stable oxygen complex in which the iron remains in the ferrous state[12].

The protein moiety plays an important regulatory role in the function of haemoglobin. The coils of the helical protein act like springs that respond to the strain when oxygen binds at one iron porphyrin site and convey the strain to other sites. This helps to increase the oxygen affinity of the second site and enables haemoglobin to bind and release oxygen more effectively[13]. The four subunits of the haemoglobin molecule react cooperatively to convey oxygen from the alveoli/capillary interface in the lung to the red cells and via capillaries to the tissue interface in peripheral tissues where it is released to myoglobin. The efficiency of this transport is modulated specifically by pH, pCO_2, and other environmental factors, including temperature. Uptake of oxygen by haemoglobin is facilitated by the high pH and low pCO_2 of the lung, while downloading is favoured by the lower pH and higher pCO_2 in tissues[14].

2.3.2 Myoglobin

Myoglobin, the red pigment of muscle, is an oxygen-storage protein which provides oxygen to muscle tissue. It is a single-chain haemoprotein homologue of haemoglobin with a molecular weight of 17 000. The porphyrin active site is entwined within the polypeptide chain in a pocket formed from amino acid residues with non-polar side groups and is hydrophobic. These groups protect the iron atom in the haem moiety against irreversible oxidation to the ferric state. This control of the reaction environment by the protein enables the Fe(II) complex to bind and release oxygen.

The transfer of oxygen from haemoglobin to myoglobin at the blood/tissue interface requires that myoglobin has a greater oxygen affinity than haemoglobin at low partial pressures of oxygen. Though the oxygen is bound in both molecules to haem, the two molecules are structurally different, with haemoglobin being essentially a tetramer of myoglobin. As has already been noted, because of cooperativity between the four units, this leads to changes in the shape of the protein in the haemoglobin when oxygen binds to one of the iron atoms, with the result that under conditions of lower pH and higher pCO_2, transfer of oxygen from haemoglobin to myoglobin is promoted[15].

2.3.3 Cytochromes

The oxygen transported to tissues by haemoglobin and stored in muscle cells by myoglobin is utilised in cellular metabolism to produce the energy essential for life. Respiration, in which glucose and other metabolites are oxidised and chemical energy captured in the form of high-energy phosphate bonds of adenosine triphosphate (ATP), is a complex process which depends on the interaction of a series of functional proteins, many of which contain iron. Dioxygen is a powerful and potentially dangerous oxidising agent, and if it is to be utilised in metabolism, a safe distance must be kept between the sites of oxidation by O_2 and the different metabolic reactions. This isolation is brought about by a series of interconnecting proteins of decreasing standard potential, which pass electrons down the chain towards oxygen in the mitochondria in several cautious, discrete steps. The chain of proteins of decreasing potential allows energy released at the different steps to be stored for use elsewhere by coupling the reactions to the formation of ATP from ADP and HPO_4^{2-}. This arrangement of the electron transport chain also allows the process to be organised spatially, from one side of the membrane, where the cytochromes are located, to the other[16]. A schematic representation of the chain is shown in Fig. 2.2.

The most prominent of the participants in this electron transport system in mitochondria are the cytochromes[17]. These are a group of haem proteins, with Fe in a porphyrin-type ligand environment, which act as one-electron transfer agents by shuttling the iron atom between the Fe(II) and the Fe(III) state. There are several different cytochromes that, in collaboration with a number of iron–sulphur as well as copper-containing and other proteins, constitute the respiratory chain.

Classification of the cytochromes is complex, since they differ from organism to organism and even within a particular species. Keilin, who, in 1925, was the first to identify them, recognised three different molecules, which he named *cytochromes a, b,* and *c*[18]. He was able to distinguish between them by spectroscopic examination of tissue suspensions, which showed sharp absorption bands in the presence of oxidisable

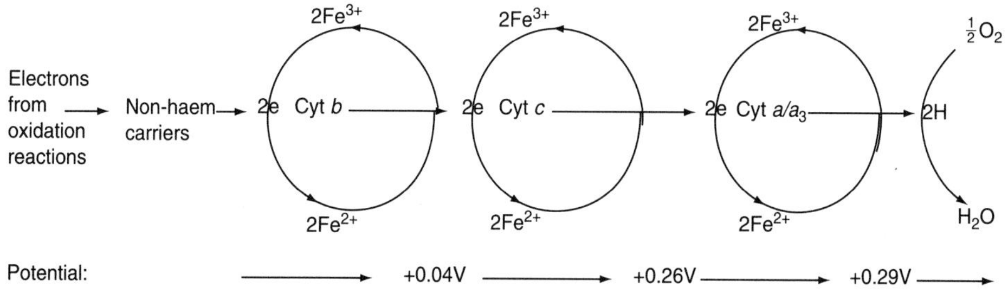

Figure 2.2 Simplified outline of electron transport from substrate oxidation, via FAD and other non-haem carriers down the cytochrome chain of increasing potential to the ultimate electron acceptor, oxygen. The two intermediates, cytochromes *a* and a_3 are known as cytochrome oxidase.

substrates under anaerobic conditions. He observed three different absorption maxima, which he assigned to the three different cytochromes.

Subsequently Keilin's cytochrome *a* came to be known as *cytochrome oxidase*. It also became apparent that there are numerous different kinds of cytochromes, and not just three as originally suggested. As these new cytochromes were identified, they were designated according to which of the original three they were most closely identified with by spectroscopic criteria. These new molecules were named, for example, cytochromes b_1, b_2, b_3, etc. This nomenclature, which is still in use, does not, in fact, necessarily indicate that similarly designated cytochromes are closely related, nor that they have similar oxidation potentials or play equivalent roles.

2.3.3.1 Cytochrome P-450 enzymes

In addition to their role in respiration, there is also what has been called the cytochrome P-450 'super family' of enzymes. These extra-mitochondrial enzymes have iron porphyrin active sites and catalyse the addition of oxygen to a hydrocarbon substrate. The designation 'P-450' refers to the characteristic blue to near-ultraviolet absorption Soret band of the porphyrin that is red-shifted to 450 nm in carbonyl complexes. Some 30 cytochrome P enzymes have been identified in humans, with several hundreds in other species. They are known as 'mixed-function oxidases' and most exhibit broad substrate specifity. The microsomal P-450 enzyme system is involved in the biosynthesis of steroid hormones, as well as of prostacyclin, thromboxane and leucotrienes[19].

Cytochrome P-450 enzymes are part of the body's defence against hydrophobic compounds, such as drugs, steroid precursors and pesticides. This is achieved through use of the insertion reaction, an atom-transfer mechanism which allows the insertion of oxygen into an RH group, converting it to ROH. The hydroxylation makes the molecule more soluble in water and facilitates its excretion from the body.

2.3.4 Iron–sulphur proteins

As illustrated in Fig. 2.2, there are several other electon transfer mediators besides the cytochromes in mitochondria. Among these are the ferrodoxins, an important group of iron–sulphur proteins[20]. These non-haem proteins contain iron in a tetrahedral environment of four S atoms known as iron–sulphur clusters. They are involved in single electron transport by undergoing reversible Fe(II)–Fe(III) transitions. The different iron–sulphur proteins have different side chains, rendering them either lipid- or water-soluble, so that they occur both in cytoplasm and in membranes of the cell. The ferrodoxins include the flavoproteins NADH dehydrogenase and succinic dehydrogenase, found in mitochondria, and aconitase, which occurs in the cell interior.

2.3.5 Other iron enzymes

There is a wide range of peroxidase enzymes in mammals, all of which, with the exception of glutathione peroxidase (a selenoprotein) contain iron. Catalase and peroxidase are both haem proteins. They are widely distributed in the body but are particularly abundant in red blood cells and the liver. They function as part of the body's defences against oxidative damage by degrading hydrogen peroxide. Other oxidases include myeloperoxidase, which forms hypochlorite anion, a cytotoxic molecule produced by neutrophils. Another, thyroperoxidase, is involved in the function of the thyroid gland, with responsibility for conjugation of iodinated tyrosine residues on thyroglobulin.

2.3.6 *Iron-transporting proteins*

Free iron is, as has been noted above, extremely toxic and capable of catalysing many deleterious reactions in cells and tissues. In order to prevent this, the body utilises a number of different proteins to sequester the element, either for storage and possible excretion, or for transporting to locations where it is used for metabolic purposes.

2.3.6.1 *Transferrin*

Transferrin (Tf) belongs to a family of proteins that includes lactotransferrin and ovotransferrin. It is a single-chain, 80-kDa glycoprotein, organised in two homologous polypeptide chains, each of which has a single iron-binding site. Each site is able to bind ferric iron in a complex of protein ligands, bicarbonate and water. Transferrin has a very high affinity for iron at a pH above 7.0. The iron can be released by lowering the pH to less than 5.5[21]. In addition to iron, transferrin can also bind manganese and aluminium[22].

The plasma concentration of transferrin in adults is normally about 2.4 g/l. Each mg of transferrin can bind 1.4 μg of iron. *In vivo* transferrin is normally 25–50% saturated with iron[23]. The transfer of iron from plasma transferrin to immature red cells for haemoglobin synthesis, as well as to other cells, is brought about by specific receptors in the cell membrane[24].

2.3.6.2 *Lactoferrin*

Lactoferrin is a cationic iron carrier glycoprotein very similar to transferrin and is present in human breast milk in high concentrations of about 1 mg/ml. It binds two atoms of ferric iron per molecule and is found on mucosal surfaces as part of their protective coat and in neutrophilic granulocytes.

Lactoferrin plays an important role in the defence of the breast-fed infant against infection by bacteria. It does this, apparently, by depriving the bacteria of iron they need for multiplication and also by contributing iron to generate reactive oxygen radicals used by phagocytes to destroy microorganisms[25].

2.3.6.3 *Ferritin*

Iron is stored in cells as ferritin, which is a soluble spherical protein enclosing a core of iron. The polypeptide apoferritin in humans is made up of 24 polypeptide subunits. At least two distinct isoforms of the subunits exist: what is known as the H isoform is a 22-kDa protein consisting of 182 amino acids; the second, the L isoform, is a 20-kDa protein with 174 amino acids. Combinations of these subunits also occur, allowing for considerable heterogeneity[26]. In humans, the L subunit predominates in liver and spleen ferritin, while in the heart and erythrocytes, the H subunit predominates. The different forms appear to have different properties and functions.

The subunits of ferritin are roughly cylindrical in shape and form a nearly spherical shell that encloses a central core. Theoretically, the core can contain up to 4500 iron atoms, but normally ferritin in most tissues is about 20% saturated (800 out of 4500 iron sites occupied). However, in liver, spleen, heart and kidney, saturation levels are higher with about 1500 iron atoms per molecule. The structure and composition of the core is analogous to a polymer of ferrihydrite ($5Fe_2O_3.9H_2O$) with a variable amount of phosphate[27].

There is some uncertainty about how the ferritin iron core is made. The first step is the entry of ferrous iron into the protein through specific channels. The iron is then oxidised, either within the protein or on the core surface. The H chain is known to have one or more distinct ferro-oxidase sites where oxidation could occur. The L chain does not, apparently, have any such sites, but both it and the H chain are capable of self-loading with iron. It is suggested that the two subunits act cooperatively in the process of iron loading[28]. Some investigators believe that ferritin iron oxidation and loading are brought about by the copper protein caeruloplasmin[29].

2.3.6.4 Haemosiderin

Haemosiderin is an insoluble iron storage protein composed of degraded ferritin. It is produced when tissue iron stores increase to about 4000 iron atoms per ferritin molecule[30]. The ferritin is degraded by lyosomal proteases that cause the protein coat to disintegrate partly and the iron core to aggregate. Haemosiderin consists of about 40% protein, with a core consisting of various forms of iron, including amorphous ferric oxide and ferrihydrite. These forms of iron are less chemically active than those found in ferritin and may be less available for mobilisation. In persons with an adequate iron status, most of the body's storage iron is present as ferritin, but with increasing iron accumulation, the concentration of plasma haemosiderin increases. Its presence in lysosomes, where it is usually found, may be detected under a light microscope after tissue sections are stained with Prussian blue {potassium ferriferrocyanide, $KFe[Fe(CN)_6]$}.

2.4 Iron absorption

Though iron plays a key role in human metabolism, and is abundant in the environment and in foods, the daily intake of a healthy adult is only about 1 mg. This low intake is, in most circumstances, sufficient to meet the body's needs. The reason for this is that the body does not have a regulated mechanism for excreting iron, but is able to retain and reutilize its stores of the metal very efficiently. The relatively small intake from the diet is normally sufficient to replace what has been lost through non-specific mechanisms, such as exfoliation of gut cells, urinary and biliary secretions and menstruation[31]. However, this is not always the case, and iron deficiency remains an intractable primary micronutrient deficiency worldwide. At the same time, paradoxically, it is now becoming increasingly evident that iron overload, in which there is excessive accumulation of iron in the body, is a significant health problem for a large number of people, especially in certain population groups[32]. Thus, the regulation of dietary absorption of iron is the major factor in the maintenance of iron homeostasis in the body.

The absorption of iron from ingested food occurs in the proximal small intestine. None occurs in the oesophagus, or stomach, though preparation for absorption takes place in the latter organ. The subsequent process in which the solubilised iron is transferred from the lumen of the intestine into the mucosal cell and on to the plasma pool can be divided into three sequential stages: (1) uptake from the gut lumen across the apical mucosa; (2) intracellular processing and transport in the enterocytes; (3) storage and extraenterocyte transport across the basolateral (serosal) membrane and into the plasma.

2.4.1 The luminal phase of iron absorption

In general, only a small proportion of the iron in the diet is absorbed from food which has entered the lumen of the gut. This is because of a number of factors, including the chemical form of the element. Iron occurs in food in two chemical forms: as organic, haem iron, and as non-haem, inorganic ferrous and ferric iron, the former mainly in meat and other animal products, the latter in cereals, vegetables and other plant foods[33]. Iron can occur in fortified foods and in dietary supplements in both organic and inorganic forms. It can also be present in food, normally in inorganic form, as adventitious iron picked up from contact with metal containers and cooking utensils.

Though the absorption of iron does not begin to take place until it reaches the small intestine, an important preparation for that process occurs in the stomach. There hydrochloric acid is produced which assists the removal of bound iron during protein degradation. The acid also helps solubilise the iron by reducing it from the ferric to the ferrous state. Reduction is necessary because most of the iron in the diet is in the relatively insoluble ferric form and is poorly absorbed. Just less than 50% of the conjugated iron in food is released, and about 30% of the ferric iron is reduced by the combined action of gastric acid and pepsin in the stomach[34].

Intestinal absorption of dietary iron occurs mainly in the duodenum and upper jejunum[35]. Though there is uncertainty about the full details, and aspects of the process are still controversial, it is clear that many different dietary and other factors are involved in the passage of iron from the intestinal lumen into the mucosal cells of the intestine. Not least of these is the physicochemical form of the iron. Haem and non-haem iron are absorbed by different pathways, with different degrees of efficiency, depending on the presence of other components of the diet and the level of iron stores already present in the body[36]. Absorption of haem iron normally occurs at a fairly constant rate of about 20–30%. Uptake can be reduced to some extent by the simultaneous presence of calcium[37] and increased by protein[38], but it is relatively unaffected by other dietary components[39].

2.4.1.1 Inhibitors of iron absorption

Absorption of non-haem iron, in contrast to haem, can be affected significantly by a variety of factors. Extrinsic intraluminal factors that decrease absorption include components of plant-based foods, such as wheat bran[40], pectin[41], phytates[42], polyphenols[43] and others (see Table 2.1). Absorption is also affected by interactions with other metals. Generally, high levels of divalent cations inhibit absorption[44]. Of particular significance

Table 2.1 Factors influencing iron uptake in the intestine.

pH of intestinal contents
Chemical form of iron
Presence of reducing agents
Presence of food components capable of forming complexes with iron:
(i) Inhibitors:
• Calcium
• Phosphates
• Phytates
• Tannins
(ii) Facilitators:
• Meat
• Ascorbic and other carboxylic acids

Adapted from Roeser, H.P. (1990) Iron. In: *Recommended Nutrient Intakes, Australian Papers* (ed. A.S. Truswell), pp. 244–54. Australian Professional Publications, Sydney.

is calcium, which is the only metal known to inhibit the absorption of both haem and non-haem iron[45]. Iron, in its turn, can also inhibit the absorption of other nutritionally important metals, especially zinc[46].

An unusual cause of interference with iron absorption is geophagia, the deliberate ingestion of soil, which is practised by some people in certain parts of the world, including Turkey, Uganda and Tanzania[47]. In a study of soils used for this purpose, it was found that while they can contribute a significant amount of soluble calcium to the diet, they are also capable of binding iron, as well as zinc[48].

2.4.1.2 Effect of tannin in tea on iron absorption

An example of a food component that can have a significant effect on non-haem iron absorption are the flavonoids in tea. These are polyphenols which occur in tannin, the component which gives tea its brown colour and contributes to its taste. There are several different types of tea flavonoids, all containing two aromatic rings with two or more hydroxyl groups which have strong iron-binding capacities. A cup of black tea, brewed with 2.5 g of tea leaves contains about 200 mg of flavonoids[49]. Non-haem iron absorption from test meals has been shown to be reduced by between 63 and 91% when a cup of tea is consumed along with the food[50].

2.4.1.3 Dietary factors that enhance iron absorption

A large number of dietary variables are known to enhance absorption of non-haem iron. These include ligands, such as citric, ascorbic, malic and other carboxylic acids, amino acids and fructose. Ascorbic acid has been shown to increase absorption from an inhibitory meal as much as 10-fold[51]. These ligands form soluble complexes with the iron and prevent precipitation and polymerisation. Ascorbic acid also functions as a reducing agent and converts inorganic iron from the ferric to the ferrous form, thus increasing absorption. Non-haem iron absorption is also promoted by the presence of meat, fish and poultry[52].

This appears to be due to the formation of readily absorbed iron complexes with amino acids such as cysteine, as well as with polypeptides. Meat also promotes gastric acid production by the stomach, which lowers the pH and increases iron solubility, an effect also brought about by alcohol.

2.4.1.4 Non-dietary factors that affect iron absorption

In addition to these dietary influences, several different factors which are not food-related play significant roles in the absorption of iron from the gut. There is an inverse relationship between levels of iron stored as ferritin in the body and uptake, with a marked increase when stores are low[53]. Efficiency of absorption is also affected by the level of iron to which the intestinal mucosal cells have been previously exposed[54]. The physiological state of the body is also known to affect absorption, especially under conditions in which tissue iron is reduced, such as during growth and pregnancy. Depending on the stage of pregnancy, absorption can increase by more than 30%[55]. Absorption is also affected by the production of gastric acid which is necessary for the solubilisation of non-haem iron. Achlorhydria is known to reduce absorption and utilisation of non-haem, but not haem, iron[56]. Several other physiological conditions that can affect iron absorption are the rate of erythropoiesis (incorporation of iron into red blood cells)[57], tissue hypoxia, including that caused by high altitude[58], and the level of pancreatic, bilary and other intestinal secretions[59].

2.4.2 Uptake of iron by the mucosal cell

The principal way in which the body regulates levels of iron in its tissues and individual cells is by controlling levels of absorption from the diet. There are still many uncertainties about how this is done, since the complete pathway of absorption is still not fully understood, though recent biochemical and genetic studies have begun to clarify several of the steps involved. It is known that transport of iron at the intestinal brush border and into the epithelial cells at the tips of the villi depends on iron-binding moieties, ferrireductase activity and specific transport molecules[60]. At least two pathways are involved[61], one of which is for haem, and another for non-haem iron. Haem is taken up directly by the enterocyte. Iron is then released from the porphyrin ring by action of haem oxygenase and enters a common pathway for subsequent metabolism in the same manner as non-haem iron.

There is evidence that iron from lactoferrin is transported into the mucosal cell by a specific pathway. Receptors for lactoferrin have been isolated from brush-border membranes, but their functions have not yet been clarified[62].

All other forms of iron are transported into the enterocyte by a divalent metal transporter protein. This is known as DMT1 (divalent metal transporter) and is a proton symporter that can transport ferrous iron and other divalent metals. It is also known as Nramp2 and DCT1 (divalent cation transporter)[63]. The iron is bound to DMT1 on the luminal surface of the enterocyte and is transported across the membrane into the cell interior. DMT1 is also capable of transporting other divalent cations[64]. Though the transporter's preference in order of affinity is for Fe^{2+}, Zn^{2+}, Mn^{2+}, Co^{2+}, Cd^{2+}, Cu^{2+}, Ni^{2+} and Pb^{2+}, high doses of any one of the metals can interfere with this order[65]. This ability to recognise other divalent cations may also account for the finding that haemochromatosis patients accumulate other metals in addition to iron[66].

While the major route for dietary iron absorption probably depends on DMT1, there is evidence that several other factors are involved[67]. Of particular importance among these is the ability of the intestinal mucosa to reduce iron from the ferric to the ferrous state. While this is to a considerable extent achieved by enhancing factors in the diet, especially ascorbic acid, the intestinal mucosa itself has been shown to have ferrireductase activity in mice[68]. Little is known about the reductase enzymes responsible for this activity in mammals. In yeast, an iron-transporting enzyme with ferrireductase activity has been identified as a flavocytochrome. It is possible that a similar type of protein may be involved in the human intestinal brush border[69].

A caeruloplasmin-stimulated iron uptake mechanism that appears to be specific for ferric iron, as well as for other trivalent metals, has been characterised. However, the physiological relevance of the process is still uncertain[70].

Although the major route for iron absorption is most probably mediated by DMT1, this transporter is found only at the apical surface of enterocytes. This suggests that other transporters are involved in transfer across the intestinal epithelium. It is possible that transferrin, internalised by enterocytes from the basolateral surfaces, acquires iron imported from the apical brush border[71]. However, transferrin does not appear to regulate iron uptake across the duodenum, and transferrin receptors have not been identified in intestinal brush-border membranes[72].

2.4.3 Handling of iron within the intestinal enterocyte

Iron entering the cytoplasm of the mucosal cell cannot be allowed to exist freely in its ionic state once it is released from the transfer proteins. Because of its potential toxicity, it has to bound immediately to a protein already present, either transferrin, ferritin or another iron-binding protein. Most of the iron that enters the mucosal cells is rapidly exported to the blood in an initial rapid transfer stage, with transfer continuing at a much slower rate for up to 24 hours. This later transfer is probably of iron that was temporarily stored in ferritin. Iron that is not transferred to the plasma is stored in ferritin and is lost when the enterocyte is eventually shed. More than 50 years ago, Granick proposed his 'mucosal block' theory, according to which ferritin acts as an 'iron sink' and binds excessive iron that has been taken in from the intestinal lumen. This ferritin-bound iron is subsequently lost to the body when mucosal cells are shed[73]. However, while such a mechanism could, in theory, efficiently remove excess iron from the system, since the average life of an intestinal cell is only 3 days, regulation of iron uptake is far more complex than can be accounted for in this way.

2.4.4 Export of iron from the mucosal cells

There is a good deal of uncertainty about how iron is released from the intestinal enterocyte into the circulation. An iron-export protein, ferroportin-1, also known as Ireg-1 and MTP1, has been shown to be involved in transfer from the enterocyte to the plasma in the duodenum[74]. It is known that the iron transported in this way is bound to transferrin at the basolateral surface of the enterocyte, but how it is released to circulation is unclear. There is some evidence that the copper protein caeruloplasmin may be responsible for oxidation of the iron, which is necessary for its binding to transferrin at the membrane[75]. However, more recent findings suggest that it is not caeruloplasmin itself but its homologue, hephaestin, which is abundant in the small intestine, that is involved. Like caeruloplasmin, hephaestin is believed to have ferroxidase activity, but unlike the serum protein, it is anchored to the cell surface via a single transmembrane-spanning domain[76].

2.4.5 Regulation of iron absorption and transport

The absorption of iron from food is known to be related to the body's stores and to the amount of iron to which the intestinal mucosal cells have been exposed[77], as well as to physiological factors, such as the rate of erythropoiesis. There is evidence that as crypt cells mature into absorptive enterocytes, they are programmed via two independent regulators, the 'stores regulator', which transmits information about the body's iron stores, and the 'erythropoietic regulator', which communicates iron requirements for red cell production[78]. Although the latter is believed to have a greater impact on the net flux of iron in the body, the stores regulator appears to play an essential role in maintaining iron balance and preventing excess accumulation of iron[79]. It is not clear how the absorptive enterocyte is programmed to assimilate the correct amount of dietary iron. Recent studies have found evidence that a peptide, hepcidin, may play a key role as an iron-regulating hormone in modulating iron absorption to reflect the body's iron status[80]. Hepcidin is a small peptide, with antifungal and bactericidal activity. It has been purified from human urine and also identified in liver[81]. Hepcidin has been shown to have a potential role in iron metabolism in a number of studies using genetically modified mouse models[82].

There is still much that is not known about the mechanism possessed by crypt cells for accumulating iron and for their ability to sense body iron stores. Two pointers to the involvement of transferrin-bound iron uptake from blood are, first, the fact that the amount of iron absorbed from the intestine is inversely related to the degree of transferrin saturation in serum, and, second, that the transferrin receptor is expressed at high concentration in the crypt. It has been suggested that HFE protein, the gene for which is mutated in the common form of hereditary haemochromatosis, is also involved. This protein is expressed in the crypt cells of the mucosa and moves to the apex of the villus when iron absorption takes place. The protein forms a complex with the transferrin receptor on the cell surface, which alters its affinity for transferrin. It appears to be able to sense iron status and to programme the mucosal cell to absorb more iron if deficiency occurs. It may do this by increasing expression of DMT1 at the luminal surface of the cell[83].

While many questions about factors and mechanisms involved in iron absorption and utilisation remain unanswered, it is becoming ever more certain that iron homeostasis is maintained by a combination of sensory and regulatory networks that modulate the expression of proteins of iron metabolism at the transcriptional and/or post-transcriptional levels. Regulation of gene transcription provides critical development, cell cycle and cell-type-specific controls on iron metabolism. Post-transcriptional control is coordinated through the action of intracellular iron response proteins (IRPs). These are iron-sensing proteins that regulate iron homeostasis locally and bind to iron response elements in specific mRNAs encoding proteins involved in the uptake, storage and use of iron.

Multiple factors, including iron itself, nitric oxide, oxidative stress, phosphorylation and hypoxia/reoxygenation, influence IRP function[84].

As has been noted by one of the leading experts in the field in a recent review:

The enterocyte is unique in that it must not only respond to iron loading and deficiency through the regulatory function of IRPs, it must also serve as a gated channel to permit sufficient entry of iron into the body. In unicellular organisms like yeast, iron-responsive transcription factors are found to coordinate control of the genes involved in maintaining iron homeostasis. Although not yet identified, a similar regulatory mechanism can readily be envisioned for mammalian cells. It is also conceivable that posttranslational control mechanisms participate in the regulation of mammalian iron transport[85].

What is now required, the author continues, is for investigators to focus not only on the identification of molecules involved in mammalian cell iron transport, such as the ferroreductases and ferroxidases, but also on how the regulation of iron homeostasis is maintained via transcriptional, post-transcriptional, and/or post-translational control mechanisms.

2.5 Transport of iron in plasma

As with other aspects of iron metabolism, much still remains to be clarified about the steps involved in transfer of the element from the enterocyte to the various cells where it is required, as well as about the pathways it follows to intracellular sites. The iron binding protein transferrin is responsible for transfer from the basolateral surface of the enterocyte through the plasma to where it is required either to be used metabolically for the synthesis of iron-containing proteins or incorporated into the iron storage protein ferritin. Plasma concentration of transferrin in adults is normally about 2.4 g/l, each milligram of which can bind 1.4 μg of iron. Normally, about one-third of the transferrin-binding sites in plasma are iron-saturated.

Release of iron from transferrin and its delivery to reticulocytes, hepatocytes and other cell types are brought about by interaction with specific high-affinity transferrin receptors (TfRs) in the cell membrane, followed by receptor-mediated endocytosis and by removal of iron and release of apotransferritin (apoTf) within the cell. The freed iron is then pumped into the cytoplasm, possibly through the action of DMT1. The apoTf–TfR complex is returned to the cell surface, where the apoTf dissociates from the TfR and is free to pick up more iron elsewhere[86].

The extent of this transfer depends on the amount of iron taken up, as well as on the iron status and the metabolic needs of the cell. Iron-containing proteins are present in numerous locations within the cell, including the cytosol and a number of organelles. The mitochondrion, for instance, is the site of incorporation of iron into protoporphyrin IX to form haem. It is also where metal centres for haem and non-haem (e.g. iron–sulphur proteins) are assembled and inserted into proteins required for mitochondrial function. In liver and especially erythroid cells, much of the iron delivered to the cytoplasm is used for haem formation[87].

Iron not required for synthesis of iron-containing proteins is stored by being incorporated into the iron-storage protein ferritin within the cell. Such storage is important for maintenance of iron homeostasis. Ferritin provides a means for protecting cells from the toxic effects of iron by storing the element in a safe and available manner.

2.5.1 Iron turnover in plasma

Iron turnover in the plasma is a significant means of recycling iron in the body. It depends primarily on transferrin and is mediated mainly by the synthesis and breakdown of haemoglobin. At any one time, the plasma iron pool contains about 4 mg of transferrin-bound iron, though daily turnover is about 35 mg[88]. Most of the iron which leaves the plasma is taken up by erythroblasts in the bone marrow for incorporation into haem. It then re-enters the blood as haemoglobin in the erythrocytes. There is, in addition, a small exchange of iron between the plasma and other cells and tissues where the element is used for other metabolic functions.

Erythrocytes, which contain about 80% of the body's functional iron, have a life of approximately 120 days. At the end of this time, they become senescent and are catabolised in the reticuloendothelial system by Kupffer cells and spleen macrophages. After phagocytosis, the globin chain of haemoglobin is denatured, and haem is released. Iron is then released from the haem by the action of haem oxygenase and is returned to the plasma. About 85% of the iron derived from haemoglobin degradation is released to the body in the form of iron bound to transferrin or ferritin[89]. Each day, 0.66% of the body's total iron is recycled in this manner. Smaller contributions to turnover are made by the degradation of myoglobin and iron-containing enzymes.

2.6 Iron losses

Though the body does not have a mechanism for excreting iron, in contrast to other trace metals, iron losses do occur. Total loss in adult males is about 1 mg/d. Most of this is from the gastrointestinal tract, in shed enterocytes, extravasated erythrocytes, and biliary haem breakdown products. A smaller amount is lost in the urine and as shed skin cells[90]. In premenopausal adult females, loss of iron in menstrual blood is about 1.5 mg/d, but can be as high as 2.1 mg/d. Approximately 1 g of iron can be lost over the course of a pregnancy. This is made up of basal losses of 230 mg, increased maternal red cell mass of 450 mg, fetal needs of 270–300 mg, placenta, decidua and amniotic fluid content, totalling 50–90 mg[91].

Iron losses can also result from a number of clinical and pathological conditions, including haemorrhage, peptic ulcer, bowel cancer and ulcerative colitis. The use of aspirin and some anti-inflammatory drugs, as well as of corticosteroids, can also contribute to loss of iron as a result of internal bleeding[92]. In tropical countries, hookworm and other intestinal parasite infestations can be a major cause of iron deficiency, especially in children[93].

2.7 Iron status

The iron status of an individual can, depending on various circumstances, range from iron overload to extreme deficiency, with in between the extremes a normal level which allows the body to function efficiently and cope with the demands of life. This normal iron status is difficult to define, since it must account for levels of the body's functional as well its storage iron. Other factors, such as the presence of diseases, age, sex and race, as well as composition of the diet, may also be involved. It is for such reasons that, historically, many different methods have been used to assess the iron status of an individual, as any clinical laboratory handbook will confirm. In practice, no single method, or combination of methods, is suitable for all purposes[94].

2.7.1 Methods for assessing iron status

Table 2.2 lists methods which can be found among those described in laboratory handbooks. As the table indicates, body iron is considered as residing in two main compartments of storage and functional iron, a convenient, if not an absolutely accurate, division. Not all the methods listed are suitable in every situation. Some, for a variety of reasons, are no longer considered to be the methods of choice[95]. For example, not all those used in epidemiological studies and in field work are suitable for clinic and laboratory-based investigations, and vice versa. The technology is constantly evolving, and several procedures, which were formerly standard laboratory practice, have been replaced by modern methods such as enzyme-linked immunosorbent assay (ELISA) and radioimmunoassay (RIA).

2.7.1.1 Measuring body iron stores

The most practical way of measuring the size of the body's iron store in epidemiological studies is by determining serum ferritin[96]. Methods based on ELISA are available which are reliable and relatively simple to use, and require only a few microlitres of serum or

Table 2.2 Measurements of iron status.

- Iron stores
  - Quantitative phlebotomy
  - Tissue biopsy:
    - Liver
    - Bone marrow
  - Serum ferritin
- Functional iron
  - Haemoglobin concentration
  - Red cell indices:
    - Mean cell volume (MCV)
    - Mean cell haemoglobin (MCH)
    - Packed cell volume
- Tissue iron supply
  - Serum iron
  - Transferrin saturation
  - Red cell zinc protoporphyrin
  - Red cell ferritin
  - Serum transferrin receptor

plasma. Other methods, using both RIA (labelled ferritin) and IRMA (immunoradiometric assay with labelled antibody) are also used[97]. While more cumbersome methods such as quantitative phlebotomy, or more invasive methods such as bone marrow biopsy, are also available, they are far less commonly used and then usually as a means of validating the simpler serum ferritin assay[98].

Serum ferritin concentrations are normally in the range of 15–300 μg/l. In healthy subjects, 1 μg of ferritin per litre corresponds to about 10 mg of storage iron. Values are lower in children than in adults, and from puberty to middle age, levels are higher in men than in women[99]. However, ferritin levels do not necessarily reflect iron status, since a large number of disorders and other factors can affect them. Serum ferritin is an acute phase reactant, and its level is raised by acute and chronic infections, inflammatory diseases, malignancies and liver disorders. Repeated blood donations, alcohol consumption and diet also affect ferritin levels[100].

2.7.1.2 Measuring functional iron

A variety of different methods are used for identifying iron-deficient erythropoiesis. The iron transport variables, serum iron, total iron-binding capacity (TIBC) and transferrin saturation have been traditionally accepted indices of levels of functional iron, though today they are generally believed to be inadequate for this purpose[101]. Isolated serum iron measurements are of limited value because of diurnal variation. Though TIBC increases in iron deficiency, it has a low specificity and is at least as good an index of protein status as of iron lack. While the calculation of transferrin saturation (serum iron/TIBC) partly compensates for the limitations of individual measurements, it does not overcome the problem that plasma iron transport is affected by a wide range of disorders[102].

Measurement of erythrocyte protoporphyrin is widely used to evaluate the supply of iron to the bone marrow where it is used by developing erythrocytes. If this is low, zinc protoporphyrin (ZPP) replaces the excess or free protoporphyrin IX which accumulates in iron deficient erythrocytes. Levels of ZPP, as μmol/mol haemoglobin, are easily determined by measuring its fluorescence with a portable electronic haemofluorometer[103]. An advantage of the method is that only a few microlitres of blood are required for the test. However, the assay is also highly sensitive to environmental exposure to lead, which inhibits the action of a number of enzymes involved in haemoglobin synthesis, in particular δ-aminolaevulinic acid dehydrase (ALA-D)[104]. Since the amount of free protoporphyrin in blood varies inversely with lead levels, zinc protoporphyrin levels are often used as a test for lead poisoning[105].

Measurement of the average size of circulating erythrocytes, or mean corpuscular volume (MCV), is also used to detect iron deficient erythropoiesis. This is done using an automated electronic cell-counting instrument and fresh whole blood. Though widely used in clinical situations, the test lacks sensitivity. Moreover, low MCV values occur in anaemia secondary to inflammation, and in persons suffering from the hereditary condition of thalassaemia.

A relatively recently introduced method for determining levels of bone marrow erythropoiesis, which has been found to be a useful alternative to other methods, is measurement of serum transferrin receptors. The method was developed as a result of studies which found that uptake of transferrin-bound iron is carried out using a transmembrane receptor protein[106]. Raised serum transferrin receptor levels are the first indicator of depressed erythropoiesis and deficient iron stores, and occur even before there are any clinical signs of iron deficiency anaemia. They continue to rise in direct proportion to the severity of the deficiency[107]. A number of different methods, most based on ELISA, are used to measure the receptor levels.

2.7.2 Haemoglobin measurement

The usual laboratory method for determining haemoglobin levels depends on the conversion of the haemoglobin to cyanmethaemoglobin and determination of the absorbance at 540 nm. The analysis is relatively easily carried out in the laboratory using an electronic blood cell counter that can give immediate and accurate results[108]. It is also conveniently carried out in the field with a hand-held instrument. An international standard is available for calibration. The method is widely used in nutritional surveys[109]. Many clinicians have traditionally equated the prevalence of iron deficiency with the prevalence of anaemia, but in fact, since haemoglobin levels only identify anaemia, which can have many different causes, they should not be used as an indication of iron status[110].

2.7.3 Iron deficiency

Optimal iron nutrition has been defined by Cook as the normality of key laboratory indices of body iron status, such as normal haemoglobin levels showing absence of iron deficiency anaemia, normal serum transferrin which establishes adequate tissue iron supply and normal serum ferritin reflecting the presence of storage iron[111]. He notes that it has become common practice in recent years to define two levels of the severity of iron deficiency, depending on the presence or absence of anaemia. More advanced deficiency, which is referred to as iron deficiency anaemia (IDA), is accompanied by a reduced packed cell volume and haemoglobin concentration. Milder deficiency, unaccompanied by IDA, is referred to simply as iron deficiency (ID). It is difficult to demonstrate any significant liabilities of depressed iron stores in the absence of overt anaemia, since this is generally without effect on physiological function[112]. In clinical practice, it is customary to use the same criteria to define ID and IDA, with the exception that the haemoglobin concentration is normal in ID. However, this raises the question, especially in the general field of nutrition, whether this approach results in an excessive concentration on the treatment of anaemia at the expense of prevention of iron deficiency. In the affluent Western society, 10–20% of infants and children and premenstrual women are believed to be iron deficient, and about 3% have IDA[113]. In minority and poverty groups, and in many developing countries, the risk of IDA is significantly higher[114]. In both situations, the availability of methods which allow the easy determination of ID, independent of IDA, is highly desirable.

2.7.4 Iron deficiency anaemia (IDA)

Iron deficiency anaemia is the final stage of a progressive negative iron balance. The progression occurs in two stages prior to the depletion of functional iron: (1) depletion of iron stores in bone marrow, spleen and liver; (2) diminished erythropoiesis leading to anaemia and reduced activity of iron-dependent enzymes[115]. As a result of a negative iron balance, serum ferritin levels fall, as storage iron is taken up by plasma transferrin for delivery to iron-requiring tissues where it is used for synthesis of red cell haemoglobin and iron enzymes. As storage iron is used up, saturation of plasma transferrin is reduced below the 16% required for normal erythropoiesis. This is the point at which iron deficient erythropoiesis begins to develop, even though the total amount of circulating haemoglobin may still be above the threshold used to define anaemia[116]. The development of iron deficient erythropoiesis is accompanied by increased expression of serum transferrin receptors on the cell membranes of the iron deficient erythrocytes[117], accumulation of free erythrocyte protoporphyrin[118] and increased erythrocyte heterogenity. The final result is frank IDA.

2.7.4.1 Consequences of IDA

The consequences of full blown IDA after the depletion of iron stores are easily recognised clinically. Physical signs include pallor of the fingernails and mucous membranes in the mouth and under the eyelids, a rapid heart rate (tachycardia) and, in severe cases, oedema. Associated with these manifestations may be general fatigue, breathlessness on exertion, insomnia, giddiness, palpitation, anorexia and dyspepsia. There may also be paraesthesia with tingling and 'pins and needles' in the fingers and toes. Not all, however, of these manifestations are seen in all individuals or at all stages of the condition. They are not mutually exclusive events and do not occur independently of each other[119].

Any significant degree of anaemia will be associated with an inability to make a sustained physical effort. The endurance activity of workers can be reduced significantly as a result of defective oxidative production of cellular energy in skeletal muscle caused by a reduced iron-carrying capacity of the blood[120]. Supplementation with iron has been shown to bring about dramatic improvements in work productivity in several low iron status groups, such as tea pickers in Sri Lanka and rubber tappers in Indoncsia[121]. However, it is not clear whether the defect in work performance is due to anaemia itself or whether it reflects a defect in muscle function that is specific for iron lack.

Other effects associated with anaemia include depression of the mechanisms for combating infection, in particular those associated with cell-mediated immunity. There are also abnormalities in thermoregulation and in cognitive performance and behaviour. However, as with other liabilities of iron deficiency, there is no convincing evidence that iron supplementation in the absence of anaemia is of benefit[122].

Several other conditions of major consequence are found in association with IDA. These include defects in mental and motor development of children in the first years of life[123]. Anaemia is also associated with impaired scholastic performance and learning ability in later years[124]. There is evidence that significant anaemia in pregnant women predisposes to low birth weight and prematurity. However, the relation between maternal haemoglobin levels and birth weight is not clear. Though iron supplementation has been found to improve birth weight in certain low income populations[125], it has not been shown to do so in certain industrialised countries[126]. This uncertainty has resulted in a range of sometimes contradictory recommendations about iron supplementation during pregnancy[127].

2.7.4.2 *Anaemia of chronic disease (ACD)*

As has already been noted, there are many other kinds of anaemia besides IDA, and the symptoms and consequences may be shared in common between the different kinds. Various inflammatory or infectious disorders, referred to collectively as anaemia of chronic disease (ACD), are a common cause of defective erythropoiesis. In many developing countries, especially, anaemia can be due, not directly to dietary iron deficiency, but to malaria, thalassaemia, human immunodeficiency virus (HIV) or other infection. The different types of anaemia are not often identified separately in nutritional surveys, because of difficulties in distinguishing between them. However, with the introduction of the serum transferrin receptor as a laboratory criterion of IDA, it is now possible to distinguish between the different anaemias relatively easily[128].

2.7.5 Iron overload

Since we do not have a homeostatic mechanism for getting rid of excess iron, if too much is absorbed, it accumulates in the body, in some cases in quantities far greater than are required for metabolism or are found in normal stores. The consequences of such iron overload can be very serious.

Chronic iron overload is characterised by increased deposition of iron in liver, heart or other organs or generalised in tissues. A number of different names are used to describe the condition. Excess iron deposition identified by tissue examination is commonly termed *haemosiderosis*. The term *haemochromatosis* is used to describe excess iron deposition associated with tissue injury or when the total body iron estimate is >5 g[129].

2.7.5.1 *Haemochromatosis*

Haemochromatosis is an inherited disorder, characterised by abnormal absorption of iron from the gastrointestinal tract with progressive accumulation of the metal in various organs, especially the heart, endocrine organs and liver[130]. It is one of the commonest genetic diseases among Caucasians, occurring in about one in 300 men of north-west European descent, and at a somewhat lower rate in women, with one in nine being carriers[131]. It is an inherited autosomal recessive disorder, associated with two separate mutations in the HFE gene[132].

The disease does not manifest itself normally before middle age. If detected before clinical symptoms appear, its complications can be prevented by the use of therapeutic phlebotomy. If untreated, it can lead to serious consequences such as cirrhosis, liver cancer, diabetes, cardiomyopathy and arthritis. In its extreme stages, total iron levels in the body can rise to as much as 60 g[133].

2.7.5.2 *Non-genetic iron overload*

An excessive intake and storage of iron can be caused by a number of factors, other than hereditary iron overload. This occurs commonly in those suffering from intractable anaemias, such as thalassaemia, a hereditary abnormality resulting in impaired haemoglobinisation and chronic anaemia. Patients who require frequent blood transfusions, for example as a result of bone marrow failure, are also at risk of iron overload. The overload is the result of the increased turnover of red blood cells and an increased iron burden.

Iron overload is also associated, in certain cases, with high dietary intakes of the metal. One form of this dietary overload is known to occur most frequently among indigenous people living in parts of southern Africa who use iron cooking and food storage utensils. It was formerly referred to as 'Bantu siderosis'[134]. It occurs especially in men who consume large quantities of beer with a high iron content. It is unlikely that the resulting excess absorption of iron is the sole cause of the overload, and there is evidence that it is at least partly due to a genetic component. The gene involved appears to be distinct from that responsible for hereditary chromatosis, and its expression is probably dependent on exposure to a high oral iron intake[135].

Excessive alcohol intake, resulting in liver disease, also may lead to iron overload, with high levels of the metal stored in the liver. In many cases, alcoholic patients showing this condition are also homozygous for the haemochromatosis gene. The increased uptake of iron may be the result of the ability of alcohol to increase permeability of the intestinal mucosa to iron. In some cases, it may be the result of the high iron content of certain types of wine[136].

2.7.6 Iron and cellular oxidation

Iron is able to fulfil its key roles in living organisms because of its potent chemical properties. When iron is not available in sufficient amounts to perform these roles, serious problems can result. Yet, paradoxically, there are situations in which the human body seems to say that you can have too much of a good thing[137] and makes every effort to prevent the uptake of iron by its tissues. The reason for this rejection, as it is for its utilisation, is once more iron's chemical potency.

Iron is a redox-active transition metal which functions by oscillating between two oxidation states, the ferrous and the ferric, accepting electrons from, and donating an electron to, a variety of biological substances. It can also catalyse the generation of free radicals, such as superoxide (O_2^-) and hydroxyl radicals ($OH^\cdot$). Other transition metals can also catalyse the formation of such reactive oxygen species (ROS), but iron is believed to be the main metal responsible for their synthesis *in vivo*. There is considerable evidence that such free radicals are responsible for a variety of degenerative diseases, including some kinds of cancer, cardiovascular disease, cataracts and certain neurological disorders[138].

Though the body cannot do without iron, any less than the other essential trace metals, it must also be able to protect itself against the undesirable effects of free, ionic iron, in particular its ability to catalyse the formation of free radicals. It is for this reason that iron is transported and stored in bound, or safe, form. Most of the metal is incorporated into iron porphyrin forms, as haemoglobin in blood and myoglobin in muscle, and in a variety of iron enzymes in tissues. When being transported around the body, iron is bound into proteins such as caeruloplasmin, metallothionein, albumin and transferrin. During storage, iron is bound tightly into ferritin or, even more tightly for long-term storage, into haemosiderin. In all these bound forms, iron is very unreactive and is not available for catalysing free radical formation. A small amount of iron is found in low molecular weight complexes, such as iron citrate and iron-ATP. Ionic iron can also be released at metabolically active sites within cells, but its level in healthy individuals is believed to be minimised by the structural integrity of tissues and is unlikely to contribute to cell damage[139].

Though, under normal conditions, the availability of free iron is tightly controlled, this may not be the case as a result of iron overload. Though there is no direct evidence that the pool of ionic iron is increased under such conditions, it is likely that the flux of iron through the pool is enhanced, and the ratio of iron to transferrin and other iron complexing molecules is increased. However, this of itself does not mean that free radical generation is stimulated, since, for this to happen, the cell's antioxidant defence systems must also be overwhelmed[140]. These defences include the superoxide dismutases, which convert superoxide into hydrogen peroxide, as well as the two other enzymes catalase and glutathione peroxidase which convert the hydrogen peroxide to water. Vitamins E and C, certain carotenoids and bioflavonoids also carry out a variety of antioxidant activities, including scavenging of free radicals and chain stopping[141].

A secondary effect of disease is often disturbance in iron metabolism. This is seen, for example, in children suffering from kwashiorkhor, who often also suffer from malaria and other infectious diseases. Though they are usually anaemic, their plasma ferritin levels can be very high. This redistribution of body iron is apparently the body's way of depriving the invading pathogens of the iron they require if they are to thrive. Unfortunately, interventions intended to improve nutrition through iron supplementation can, therefore, have the undesired effect of providing the pathogens with iron and thus increasing morbidity[142].

Vitamin C is one of the principal antioxidants used by the body to protect itself against free radical damage. Yet, in the simultaneous presence of either iron (III) or copper (II), ascorbate can also promote generation of reactive oxygen species. The limiting factor for this to occur appears to be availability of the metal ions. There is, however, little evidence that the vitamin acts as a pro-oxidant under normal conditions, though, under conditions of iron overloading and those that facilitate the release of free iron from stores, ascorbate-mediated free radical damage may be promoted[143].

2.7.7 Iron, immunity and susceptibility to infection

There is much evidence that abnormalities in the iron status of the body can lead to impaired immune function. How this occurs, is, however, as yet far from clear[144]. The human immune system consists of a collection of tissues, cells and molecules whose prime physiological function is to maintain the internal environment by destroying infectious organisms[145]. It is a very complex network, whose activities are regulated in highly specific ways. Iron is believed to play a part in many different aspects of immune function, in both a positive and negative manner. To attempt to consider each of these roles would demand a specialist knowledge of immunology and go well beyond the scope of this book. For readers who wish to do so, several extensive reviews, such as those by Brock[146] and Jurado[147], are recommended. Here, the example of Brock and Mulero, in their recent review of molecular aspects of iron immunity[148], will be followed and attention given to just two of the components of the immune system, lymphocytes and macrophages.

Iron is known to be required for the proliferation phase of T-cell lymphocyte activation. The reason for this is that iron is essential for enzymes involved in DNA synthesis[149].

Depressed cell-mediated immunity is a frequently observed consequence of iron deficiency, with a failure in T-cell mitogen response. Activated lymphocytes normally obtain iron from transferrin by a mechanism involving interaction with cell surface transferrin receptors. The finding of low transferrin saturation in iron deficient experimental animals with a defective T-cell response has been interpreted as indicating an inadequate supply of iron to the activated lymphocytes, thus preventing optimal proliferation[150].

Macrophages, phagocytic cells found in all body tissues and which, together with the monocytes of the blood, make up the reticulo-endothelial system (or the monocyte–macrophage system), play a key role in iron metabolism. They are responsible for catabolising effete erythrocytes in the spleen and liver, and the release of iron to the circulation for subsequent binding by transferrin. This iron is then transferred to the erythroid bone marrow, where it is reincorporated into erythroid precursors.

Unlike most other cells that acquire iron for metabolic use from transferrin via the transferrin-receptor endocytotic route, macrophages take up large amounts of iron via phagocytosis of effete erythrocytes[151]. Though there is a considerable amount of uncertainty about the details, it appears that the macrophages are able to handle the stored iron in different ways, depending on conditions. Inflammatory macrophages, for instance, have been shown to release iron more slowly than resting macrophages, pointing to what is known as a 'reticulo-endothelial blockade' of iron recirculation in inflammation[152]. This sequestration of iron by the macrophages may be responsible for reducing its availability to microorganisms, especially in the early stages of infection. However, the subsequent development of an adaptive immune response requires that iron be unlocked to allow proper immune function. Apart from its role in ensuring optimal lymphocyte activation and proliferation, iron is also essential for the cytotoxic activity of the activated macrophages. The production of hydroxyl radicals, for instance, depends on the presence of adequate iron in the macrophages, and if levels fall, their cytotoxic activity is reduced[153]

2.7.7.1 Iron and infection

Though iron deficiency has been shown to lead to impaired cell immunity, evidence linking iron deficiency with increased susceptibility to infection is contradictory. While some earlier studies found that iron supplementation decreased the incidence of respiratory infection in children[154], others failed to do so[155]. Evidence from more recent studies has indicated a correlation between impaired immune response resulting from iron deficiency and incidence of gastrointestinal and respiratory infection in infants[156]. Yet, there is also some evidence that iron deficiency may actually decrease the incidence of infection, apparently due to reduced iron availability to invading microorganisms. It has been shown, for example, that dietary iron deficiency can reduce the level of mortality from *Salmonella typhimurium* infection in experimental mice[157]. In the case of humans, a number of studies have found evidence of a lower incidence of infection in iron deficient populations compared to controls, for example, from malaria[158] and certain other agents[159]. The interpretation of these findings has, however, been queried, and the question of whether iron deficiency can reduce infection remains unresolved[160].

There is some evidence that excessive use of iron supplements may increase the risk of infection. Several investigators have reported, for example, an increased incidence of neonatal sepsis in Polynesian infants[161], and malaria in Somali nomads[162], following iron supplementation. Though there is evidence that excess iron increases growth of bacteria *in vitro*, iron overload does not appear to have the same effect *in vivo*. Indeed, infection is an infrequent complication of hereditary chromatosis[163].

2.7.8 Iron and cancer

There are several reasons why it has been suggested that iron overload may cause cancer[164]. In addition to being an essential nutrient for tumour cells, iron catalyses the formation of hydroxyl and other free radicals capable of causing oxidative damage. It also has the potential to suppress cell immunity. Since the liver is the primary site of iron accumulation, it is believed that it may be at high risk of iron overload-induced oxidative stress and tissue damage[165]. An increased risk of liver cancer has been linked with hereditary chromatosis[166]. Excessive iron accumulation has also been found to enhance the development of liver tumours in rats treated with certain chemical carcinogens[167]. Nevertheless, apart from such extreme cases, there is little evidence that dietary iron plays any role in the aetiology of cancer in the general population[168]. Similarly, in the case of colorectal cancer (CRC), it has been suggested that iron overload in the lower intestine, resulting from unabsorbed dietary iron, may, in conjunction with gut bacteria, increase the production of free radicals at the mucosal surface. These may then enter the colonocytes and increase the risk of DNA damage leading to carcinoma[169]. Evidence in support of this hypothesis is not strong. In fact, a significant inverse relationship between serum ferritin and risk of colon cancer has been reported[170]. In a recent study, it has been shown that while moderate iron overload enhances lipid peroxidation in livers of rats, it does not significantly increase oxidative stress induced by a hepatocarcinogenic peroxisome proliferator[171].

2.7.9 Iron and coronary heart disease

There is some evidence that a low iron status may be protective against coronary heart disease (CHD). An early finding was of a reduced risk of the disease in premenopausal women, compared with men, which could at least partly be accounted for by their lower haematocrit levels[172]. This view was supported by the subsequent observation of a rapid increase in risk following menopause and a rise in stored iron levels[173]. Further support came from epidemiological studies that compared rates of CHD in different countries and found a correlation between iron stores and mortality rate from the disease[174].

Though a number of case-control studies, for example of some 500 Scottish men[175] and a larger group of US male physicians[176], failed to find any support for a significant relationship between iron status and CHD risk, evidence for a positive association has come from several other studies. A Finnish three-year follow-up study found that men with a serum ferritin of 200 $\mu g/l$ or above had a significantly higher risk of myocardial infarction than those with a lower level[177]. Results of a Canadian 17-year follow-up study indicated that there was an increased relative risk among subjects with abnormally high serum iron concentrations[178]. In contrast to these findings, several other studies have reported either a negative or total lack of association between iron status and CHD. Of particular importance are the conclusions from a reanalysis of the NHANES (National

Health and Nutrition Examination Surveys) data covering the years 1971–1987, which found significant reductions in risk of both myocardial infarctions and CHD with increases in serum iron and transferrin saturation[179].

In spite of these differing views, iron's role as a pro-oxidant, with its ability to promote the production of free radicals, makes it a likely participant in the development of CHD. This is because iron, especially in the presence of free radicals, has the potential to oxidise low-density lipoprotein (LDL) cholesterol, which has been implicated in the pathogenesis of the atherosclerotic plaque[180]. However, it is not clear how, in practice, iron would induce the oxidation of LDL to bring about this result[181].

Many questions about the role of iron in CHD remain to be answered. The situation is reflected in the decision of the US National Academy of Sciences (NAS), in its revision of the RDAs, not to exclude iron as a risk factor for CHD, in spite of concluding that currently available data do not provide convincing support for an association between high body-iron stores and increased risk of CHD[182].

2.8 Iron in the diet

Iron is the second most abundant metal, after aluminium, in the earth's crust and is found in all foods. In spite of this, as has been noted, iron deficiency is one of the most common of all nutritional problems, in the developed and developing world. Even the wide availability of fortified foods, to which iron is added to improve nutritional quality, has done little to improve the situation. Indeed, iron intake from foods in many countries, including the UK, has been falling in recent years[183].

2.8.1 Iron in foods and beverages

Iron levels in different foods can vary greatly, depending on the kind of food and the processing, if any, to which it has been exposed. A range of about 0.1 mg/kg or less to about 100 mg/kg can be expected in foods usually consumed in a mixed, meat and vegetable-type Western diet. This is seen in Table 2.3, which gives the mean concentrations determined in different food groups examined in the 1994 UK Total Diet Study (TDS)[184]. Similar results have been reported in other industrialised countries, including the US[185].

Animal offal, especially liver, is one of the foods with the highest concentrations of iron. Other animal products, in particular red meat, are also rich in iron. Shellfish are good sources, as are fish that are eaten whole, such as sardines and pilchards, but not most other types of fish. Most plant foods contain little, with some exceptions, such as certain dark green vegetables like spinach. Boiled spinach can contain on average 16 mg/kg, which is the same as levels found in roast beef[186]. Nuts are also a good source of iron. Levels of 25 mg/kg have been reported in Brazil nuts, 37 mg/kg in coconut and 62 mg/kg in cashews[187]. A surprisingly good source, though possibly in most cases not of any great significance in terms of total dietary intake, are certain types of spices and herbs. Curry powder, for instance, can contain as much as 580 mg/kg. Another possibly unexpected useful source of iron for certain consumers is chocolate, which can contain 24 mg/kg. Such sources are easily overlooked when estimating nutrient intakes in food surveys[188].

Table 2.3 Iron in UK foods.

Food group	Mean concentration (mg/kg fresh weight)
Bread	21
Miscellaneous cereals	32
Carcass meat	21
Offal	69
Meat products	23
Poultry	7.1
Fish	16
Oils and fats	0.5
Eggs	20
Sugar and preserves	9.4
Green vegetables	11
Potatoes	8.1
Other vegetables	7.5
Canned vegetables	12
Fresh fruit	2.7
Fruit products	3.2
Beverages	0.4
Milk	4.1
Dairy products	12
Nuts	34

Adapted from from Ysart, G., Miller, P., Crews, H. *et al.* (1999) Dietary exposure estimates of 30 elements from the UK Total Diet Study. *Food Additives and Contaminants,* **16**, 391–403.

Contrary to a widely held popular view, red wine, like other beverages, is not a rich source of iron, with less than 1 mg/kg[189].

As has been discussed in some detail in an earlier section, there is an important difference between the iron in animal and in plant foodstuffs. The former is organic iron, principally haemoglobin and myoglobin, while the iron in cereals, vegetables and other plant products is in the inorganic form. This difference can be of considerable nutritional significance. In fact, knowing only the total amount of iron, rather than the proportion of its different chemical forms in a food, is of little help in calculating how much that food can contribute to meeting the body's nutritional need for the element. Yet, in spite of this well-recognised truth, most official tables, such as those published by the UK's Food Standards Agency[190], still continue to provide data solely on total levels of iron. Until relatively recently, this practice could be justified on the grounds of analytical difficulties in determining the chemical forms of the element, but with the facilities now available, it should not be beyond the abilities of analysts to produce data on the proportions of organic and inorganic iron in foods.

2.8.2 Iron fortification of foods

The figures given in Table 2.3 for iron levels in the bread and miscellaneous cereals may be somewhat misleading if used to estimate iron intakes in countries other than the UK and a few other countries where flour used for breadmaking is required by law to be fortified with iron. As a consequence of fortification, brown and white wheaten flours, for example, contain 32 and 21 mg/kg of iron, respectively, in contrast to levels in unfortified flours of 15 and 15 mg/kg. Most breakfast cereals sold in the UK are also fortified with iron. Most contain about 60 mg/kg of iron, with some made from wheat bran containing more than 100 mg/kg, far higher than the levels of less than 10 mg/kg found in unfortified products[191].

As has been noted in an earlier section, the deliberate addition of iron to certain foodstuffs during processing was initially introduced in some countries as a health intervention to prevent iron deficiency as a result of wartime food restrictions. In 1941, legislation was introduced in the US which required the enrichment of flour and bread with iron, as well as with certain other nutrients, to the level found in whole wheat[192]. A similar legal requirement was introduced in the UK and certain other countries at about the same time. It is still in force in some countries, including the UK[193]. Under the UK's current *Bread and Flour Regulations,* flour other than wholemeal must contain not less than 1.65 mg of iron per 100 g as ferric ammonium citrate, ferrous sulphate or iron powder[194].

Several other foods besides flour and bread are required by UK law to be fortified with iron. Infant formulas must contain iron at a minimum of 0.12 mg per 100 kJ and a maximum of 0.36 mg per 100 kJ. Follow-on formulas must be fortified with iron to a minimum of 0.25 mg per 100 kJ and a maximum of 0.50 mg per 100 kJ[195]. Processed products used as substitutes for meat, officially described as 'foods that simulate meat', must also be fortified to a mean concentration of 20 mg per 100 g of protein. In addition, UK legislation allows for fortification with iron of several different types of processed foods, such as breakfast cereals, infant weaning foods, meal replacements and other diet foods. The amounts of iron that can be added are related to the RDIs, and range from 17 to 100% of the RDA[196].

When the requirement for fortification with iron was first made mandatory in the UK, white flour was chosen as the vehicle for its introduction into the general diet, because white bread provided up to one-third of food energy in poorer families. It was believed that the measure would reduce the high level of anaemia which was then common among this section of the population. This may no longer be the case, since bread and flour consumption has fallen considerably, in the UK as in other countries, with increasing prosperity and diversification of dietary patterns.

2.8.2.1 Bioavailability of iron added to foods

The original UK legislation approved three different forms of iron for use as fortificants in flour. Besides these officially sanctioned forms, several different forms have subsequently been proposed. There is considerable debate about their relative effectiveness in meeting the requirements of the legislation[197]. A major problem with all of them is their bioavailability, as shown in Table 2.4. Unfortunately, some of the more bioavailable forms, such as ferrous sulphate, can cause problems of food quality, including increased vitamin degradation, oxidative rancidity, colour changes, off-flavour and precipitates in the foods to which they are added. To avoid these problems, less well absorbed but less damaging forms of iron are normally used[198].

Table 2.4 Bioavailability of different forms of iron.

Form of iron	Relative bioavailability (%)
Ferrous sulphate	100
Ferrous lactate	106
Ferrous succinate	101
Ferrous gluconate	89
Ferrous citrate	74
Ferrous pyrophosphate	39
Haemoglobin iron	37–118
Ferric sulphate	34
Ferric citrate	31
Ferric orthophosphate	31
Iron (III) EDTA	30–290
Reduced elemental iron	13–90
Carbonyl iron	5–20

After Fairweather-Tait, S.J. (1997) Iron fortification in the UK: how necessary and effective is it? In: *Trace Elements in Man and Animals – TEMA9* (eds. P.W.P. Fischer, M.R. L'Abbé, K.A. Cockell & R.S. Gibson), pp. 392–6. NRC Research Press, Ottawa.

Not all nutritionists believe that iron fortification of staple foods is a good thing. Iron overload, which is a serious health problem for some people, may be exacerbated by increasing levels of iron in the diet through fortification[199]. It is also argued that, because of the use of some forms of iron with low bioavailability, fortification fails to produce any worthwhile result. Reduced iron powder, in particular, has been singled out for criticism, though the evidence for this has been challenged[200].

The problem of bioavailability of the different forms of iron and their suitability for use in food fortification, is not easily resolved. In the case of the absorption of reduced elemental iron, for instance, human studies have produced conflicting results Such variations can be related to a variety of different factors, including particle size, porosity, surface area and manufacturing processes[201]. When tested under carefully controlled conditions, using bread enriched with the stable isotope ^{58}Fe, it has been shown that hydrogen-reduced iron powder is soluble under gastric conditions and is available for uptake into the mucosal cells of the GI tract, to an extent comparable to that of iron(II) sulphate[202].

2.8.2.2 Levels of iron used in food fortification

The amounts of iron required to be added to fortified foods by legislation has caused controversy in some countries. When, in 1971, the USFDA proposed that levels in refined wheat products should be increased from 2.6 to 8.8 mg per 100 g, there was considerable opposition from some health professionals. It was argued that the increase could result in an excessive intake by some sections of the community, especially those who suffer from hereditary haemochromatosis. The proposal was withdrawn[203]. In Sweden, where an increase in levels of iron fortification up to 6.5 mg per 100 g had been approved in 1970, legislation requiring fortification of flour was totally withdrawn in 1995[204]. Other countries are currently considering whether they should follow the example of Sweden and remove the requirement for compulsory fortification with iron of bread and flour[205].

2.8.2.3 *Adventitious iron in food*

Apart from the iron naturally present in foods, as a result of uptake by plants from the soil or, in animals, consumption of iron-containing fodder, foods may also contain iron obtained from non-natural sources. Such adventitious iron can make a significant contribution to total iron intake, with both positive and negative effects on health[206].

Foods in metal cans and other containers normally have higher levels of iron, and certain other metals, than do fresh products. Particularly high levels are sometimes found in fruits and vegetables stored in tin-plated cans. Actual concentrations will depend on a number of factors, such as pH, whether or not nitrate is present, age of the can, and the standard of hygiene maintained in the canning plant. Some fruits, such as pawpaw (papaya), naturally contain such high levels of nitrate that they cannot be stored at all in cans without excessive iron uptake. With other types of fruit, high acidity also results in uptake of iron from the metal container. Iron levels of 5.5 mg/kg have been found in canned grapefruit, 5.0 mg/kg in canned pears and a massive 1300 mg/kg in canned blackcurrants[207].

With other types of food, as well as with acid foods, the age of the can and length of storage are also important in relation to iron uptake. Iron levels in a variety of canned foods have been shown to increase by an average of 34.8% after 280 days' storage and 42.8% after a full year. An extreme case was a can of anchovies which was found to contain 5800 mg/kg of iron after four years in storage. Today, the sale of such goods would be illegal since the introduction by most countries of a requirement that cans carry a 'use by' date when they must be removed from sale[208].

Unintentional iron fortification of foods can also occur through the use of iron cooking and processing equipment. The significance of this uptake can be considerable. An investigation of the incidence of IDA in Brazilian infants found that the use of iron cooking pots in the preparation of their food significantly improved their iron nutritional status[209]. Another study, in South Africa and Zimbabwe, found that the use of a traditional beverage, a low alcohol 'sweet' beer, which was prepared in iron vessels, helped to prevent IDA in women of childbearing age[210]. In contrast to these findings of the beneficial effects of the use of iron vessels to prepare foods and beverages, some earlier studies in southern Africa, found evidence that iron-enriched home-brewed beer was a contributing cause of iron overload[211].

2.8.3 *Dietary intake of iron*

Overall intake of iron in a country or region or in a particular population group will depend on the pattern of the diet normally consumed. For example, consumption of a mixed, Western-style diet can be expected to result in an intake by adults of between about 10 and 20 mg/day, as shown in Table 2.5. The relatively small variations in intakes between countries relate to differences in amounts of certain types of foodstuffs consumed. Thus, in Denmark, 50% of the intake comes from cereals, 19% from meat and

Table 2.5 Iron intakes in different countries.

	Intake (mg/d)		
Country	Males	Females	Reference
Denmark	18	13	1
France	10	8.1	2
Germany	11.6	(all adults)	3
Ireland	14.5	10.5	4
Italy	11 ± 0.19	9 ± 0.13	5
UK	14.0	12.3	6

1. Haraldsdóttir, J., Holm, L., Højmark-Jensen J. & Møller, A. (1986) *Dietary Habits of Danes in 1985. I. Main Results. Publication No. 136* (in Danish). Levenedsmiddelstyrelsen, Søborg.
2. Lamandm M., Tressol, J.C. & Bellanger, J. (1994) The mineral and trace element composition in French food items and intake levels in France. *Journal of Trace Elements and Electrolytes in Health and Disease,* **8**, 195–202.
3. Heseker, H., Adolf, T., Eberhardt, W. *et al.* (1992) Food and nutrient intakes in the German Federal Republic (in German). In: *VERA-Schriftenreihe,* Vol. 3, pp. 188–9 (eds. W. Kübler, H.J. Anders, W. Heeschen & M. Kohlmeier). Fleck Verlag, Niederkleen.
4. Irish Nutrition and Dietetic Institute (1990) *Irish National Nutrition Survey 1990.* INDI, Dublin.
5. Freudenheim, J.L., Krogh, V. & D'Amicis, A. *et al.* (1993) Food sources of nutrients in the diet of Italian elderly. 2. Micronutrients. *International Journal of Epidemiology,* **22**, 869–77.
6. Gregory, J., Foster, K., Tyler, H. & Wiseman, M. (1990) *The Dietary and Nutritional Survey of British Adults.* HMSO, London.

Adapted from Van Dokkum, W. (1995) The intake of selected minerals and trace elements in European countries. *Nutrition Research Reviews,* **8**, 271–302.

meat products, and 12% from vegetables. In Germany, cereals, including bread, contribute 26–28%, meat 12–13%, with another 5% from potatoes and, surprisingly, 10–11% from beverages, principally beer. In contrast, in Italy, the most important dietary sources of iron are wine (19%), pasta (8%), white bread (8%), and meat a low 7%[212]. In the UK, where cereals and cereal products contribute 48.3% of intake, 14.1% of the total is from breakfast cereals and 21% from bread, both types of food fortified with iron[213]. An earlier study estimated that 12% of the UK intake is in the form of haem iron[214].

In the US, where average dietary intakes of iron by adults is about 15 mg/day, the element comes from a wide range of foods, including meat, eggs, vegetables and cereals (especially fortified cereals)[215]. In a study of intake of young Americans, it was found that females obtained 31% of the total from meat, poultry and fish, with another 25% from iron added to cereals and other foods as fortification or enrichment. Haem iron represented 7–10% of intake of females and 8–12% of young males[216].

Intakes of iron from foods have been falling in several countries in recent decades, mainly because of a reduction in consumption of bread and other wheat products. In some cases, the fall can be attributed to a reduction in consumption of red meat and a growth in vegetarianism. In the UK, a long-term decline in the consumption of red meat has been observed, with, it has been estimated, a consequent reduction of up to 9% in average iron intake[217]. To some extent, this is compensated for by an increase in the use of iron supplements. In 1991, iron intake from food sources by women was reported to average 11.6 mg/d, while those taking supplements consumed an additional 7.5 mg/d[218]. In one group of free-living elderly people, dietary supplements were consumed by 33% of men and 41% of women, making an irregular and sizeable, though not easily quantified, contribution to intake of iron and other micronutrients[219].

A low meat intake, however, does not mean that intake of iron is necessarily restricted. The actual iron status of vegetarians, for example, depends on the overall composition of the diet, not least on the presence of ascorbic acid and other enhancers of iron absorption. However, some studies of the diet of vegans, who consume plant foods only, have raised concerns that they may not obtain an adequate intake of certain micronutrients from food alone and might need to take, in addition, dietary supplements[220]. This view is not supported by a study of a group of UK vegans which found that non-supplement-using vegans had a mean daily iron intake of 16.7 (range 1.4–35.7) mg, while for those using supplements, it was 17.9 (range 10.5–27.6) mg, both means well above the UK RNI of 8.7–14.8 mg/d[221]. Though, in other studies, vegetarians have been found to have lower iron stores than non-vegetarians, adverse health effects of lower iron absorption have not been demonstrated with varied plant-based diets[222].

2.9 Recommended intakes of iron

The determination of recommendations for intake of iron requires that a variety of factors affecting requirements be taken into consideration. In developing the current US DRI, for instance, the expert panel used factorial modelling, which included consideration of basal iron losses, menstrual losses, fetal requirements in pregnancy, increased requirements during growth for the expansion of blood volume and/or increased tissue and storage iron[223]. Another factor to be taken into account is bioavailability. The UK Panel on Dietary Reference Values assumed a value of 15% for iron absorption from the typical British diet[224]. In countries where cereal-based diets are normally consumed, iron availability from food is estimated to be 5–7%[225]. Such differences, as well as the absence of reliable data on availability from different foods, mean that official dietary reference values differ between countries. For these reasons, DRVs for iron should generally, when being applied in practical situations, be interpreted with caution[226].

Table 2.6 gives the DRVs for iron published by the UK Department of Health. They are broadly similar to those of other countries where a mixed, Western-style diet is consumed, and bioavailability of dietary iron is assumed to be 15%. However, as can be seen in Table 2.7, there are some interesting differences between the US and UK values. For example, while the US RDA for all age groups of men and postmenopausal women is 8 mg/d, close to the UK RNI, for premenopausal women it is 18 mg/d compared with the UK's 14.8 mg. Moreover, the UK DRVs do not specify additional iron for women during pregnancy and lactation, but simply note that the RNI may not meet their particular needs and that supplements may be required, whereas additional iron intakes are recommended in the US.

Dietary recommendations for iron in countries where Western-style diets are not consumed and where absorption from a high cereal and other plant food diet is estimated to be 10% or less are generally higher than in the UK and other Western countries. This is seen in Table 2.8, which summarises RDAs from a number of Southeast Asian countries.

Table 2.6 DRVs for iron in the UK.

Age	LNRI	EAR	RNI
0–3 months	0.9	1.3	1.7
4–6 months	2.3	3.3	4.3
7–12 months	4.2	6.0	7.8
1–3 years	3.7	5.3	6.9
4–6 years	3.3	4.7	6.1
7–10 years	4.7	6.7	8.7
Males			
11–14 years	6.1	8.7	11.3
15–18 years	6.1	8.7	11.3
19–50+ years	4.7	6.7	8.7
Females			
11–14 years	8.0	11.4	14.8
15–50 years	8.0	11.4	14.8
50+ years	4.7	6.7	8.7

Adapted from Department of Health (1996) *Dietary Reference Values for Food Energy and Nutrients for the UK*. Table 28.2, p. 163. HMSO, London.

2.10 Strategies to combat iron deficiency

In spite of all the efforts that have been made over the past half century and more, iron deficiency remains a chronic and apparently ineradicable problem worldwide. As was stated at a recent International Conference,

> *Iron deficiency is a global problem affecting the health, quality of life, and productivity of millions of people worldwide. It is the most prevalent micronutrient deficiency, impacting particularly on the health of infants, children and women of childbearing age, especially during pregnancy. Despite the widespread impact of this condition, little progress is being made towards effective prevention and control*[227].

Progress in combating iron deficiency has been mainly in industrialised countries of North America and Western Europe. In Sweden, for instance, the prevalence of IDA declined between 1963 and 1975 from 25 to 7% among women of reproductive age[228]. In the US, iron deficiency has been reported to have declined from 21 to 6% in young children, between 1974 and 1994[229]. These, and similar changes in certain other countries, cannot be attributed to any one cause, but rather to a range of different approaches that have come about as a result of both economic development and the implementation of specific policies, such as supplementation and food fortification[230]. In many less industrialised and economically developed countries, especially in the non-Western world, the implementation of similar policies to combat iron deficiency is of recent origin and, since the outcome of many of them takes time to become apparent, the iron problem continues to persist at an unacceptably high level. However, many national governments in these countries, in conjunction with WHO and other international agencies, have in recent

Table 2.7 DRIs in the US.

Life-stage group	RDA (μg/d)	UL*
Infants		
0–6 months	0.27 (AI†)	40
7–12 months	11	40
Children		
1–3 years	7	40
4–8 years	10	40
Males		
9–13 years	8	40
14–18 years	11	45
19–30 years	8	45
31–50 years	8	45
50–70 years	8	45
>70 years	8	45
Females		
9–13 years	8	40
14–18 years	15	45
19–30 years	18	45
31–50 years	18	45
50–70 years	8	45
>70 years	8	45
Pregnancy		
≤18 years	27	45
19–30 years	27	45
31–50 years	27	45
Lactation		
≤ 18 years	10	45
19–30 years	9	45
31–50 years	9	45

*UL: tolerable upper levels intakes.
†AI = adequate intakes.
Adapted from Food and Nutrition Board (2002) *Dietary Reference Intakes – Minerals.* http://www4.nationalacademies.org/IOM/IOMHome.net/pages/Food+and+Nutrition+Board

years begun to implement public health measures that are proving effective in improving the iron status, especially of women and children.

2.10.1 Iron fortification of dietary staples

Iron fortification of foods was identified by the Pan American Health Organization as one of the important strategies for control of iron deficiency, and it is currently implemented widely in Central and South America[231]. Fortification of wheat flour was introduced in Chile by legislation in the early 1950s. Voluntary fortification was later practised by millers in a number of other Latin American countries[232]. In the 1990s, all countries in the

Table 2.8 RDAs for iron in some Southeast Asian countries.

Age	Country				
	Indonesia	Malaysia	Philippines	Thailand	Vietnam
Children					
0–1 years	3–5	10	10–15	6–8	10–11
1–9 years	8–10	10	9–12	10	6–12
Boys					
10–19 years	14–23	10–18	16–18	10–12	11–12
Girls					
10–19 years	14–25	10–28	17–25	15	12–24
Men					
20≥	13	9	12	10	11
Women					
20≥	14–26	9–28	11–26	10–15	9–24
Pregnancy	+30	+0	+41	+30	+6
Lactation	+2	+0	+23	+0	+0

Adapted from Tee, E-S. (1998) Current status of Recommended Dietary Allowances in Southeast Asia: a regional overview. *Nutrition Reviews*, **56**, S10–8.

region, apart from Argentina and Uruguay, introduced mandatory wheat flour fortification. In Venezuela, a national fortification of maize flour was introduced. It has also been proposed in Mexico and some other countries of Central America where maize is commonly consumed. Technical problems have been experienced, however, since corn is rich in phytic acid, and calcium is added when cooking maize flour for consumption, both of which result in lower iron bioavailability[233].

Fortification with iron of other kinds of widely consumed food is being undertaken in several countries. In the Philippines, iron is added to rice, which is sold at low cost to low income families. In Vietnam, fortification of fish sauce, and in China of soy sauce, has been introduced. In all cases, there is evidence that these developments have contributed to a reduction of iron deficiency in sections of the population[234]. In Chile, fortification of powdered milk used in infant formulae, to which ascorbic acid was also added, is reported to have resulted in a reduction of the incidence of anaemia in infants from 27 to 8.8%[235].

While fortification of staple foods can be a useful means of ensuring an adequate iron intake for the general population, it is less effective in doing so for particular subgroups. The practice could also expose some people whose requirements may be less than average, or who have a hereditary tendency to iron overload, to unsafe levels of intake. It was because of this that proposals to increase levels of iron fortification of bread and flour were rejected in the US, and fortification of flour with iron was halted in Denmark and several other Scandinavian countries in the late 1980s[236].

In the UK in 1981, the Committee on Medical Aspects of Food Policy recommended that fortification of flour was no longer necessary and stated, moreover, that iron fortification failed to achieve its primary purpose of improving the iron status of the population. The principal reason for this view was that bread was no longer eaten in anything like the quantity it had been when the legislation was first introduced in the 1940s. In addition, the overall nutritional quality of the British diet had improved, leading to improvements in iron status[237]. The Committee's recommendation was not, however, acted upon by the Department of Health, and the fortification requirement remained in force.

2.10.2 Use of iron supplements

It has been claimed that iron supplementation is probably the best available option for effectively addressing iron deficiency in pregnant women and young children, mainly because it can be targeted specifically to these high-risk groups[238]. Medically prescribed and over-the-counter iron supplements are widely used in many countries. In the UK, it is estimated that about 1% of the population, predominantly women, take them on prescription from their physicians for anaemia, and another 4% as non-prescribed supplements[239]. In the US, where the use of dietary supplements is also widespread, at least 36 brand names of iron supplements are marketed. Among the most common forms used are ferrous fumarate, ferrous gluconate, ferrous sulphate, ferrous glycine sulphate and iron polysaccharides, as well as many kinds of multimineral mixtures[240]. Whether the use of such supplements has an impact on the iron status of a normally adequately nourished Western population is questionable[241], but there is good evidence that, in a well designed intervention, they can achieve desirable results where nutritional deficiency is endemic.

Though there are still questions to be resolved about the role of supplementation as a treatment for existing anaemia or as a preventive measure to reduce the risk of acquiring it[242], supplements are increasingly used in large- and small-scale public health programmes in developing countries for this purpose[243]. The results of these interventions, using different forms of supplement, different means of delivery and a variety of strategies, have varied. They have been especially effective when targeted at specific groups, such as pregnant women. However, there has also been frequent lack of effectiveness of large-scale programmes, especially when used for the treatment and prevention of IDA in children[244]. A major problem with many of them is sustainability, without which long-term benefits will not be obtained. To achieve this, the supplement must have a low production cost, distribution must be simple, it must be easy to administer and ingest, and it must have few, if any, undesirable side effects. These are not simply pharmaceutical problems but also involve inadequacies in knowledge, of providers as well as of recipients of the supplements[245]. It is also important for planners of any programme that encourages the sustained use of supplements to take into consideration the fact that iron interacts with another essential trace metal, zinc, and that an excessive intake of iron may inhibit zinc absorption, and vice versa[246]. This could have serious health implications, especially among women and children whose trace metal nutritional status is marginal[247].

Steps to address difficulties, such as those discussed here, have been taken in a number of developing countries, with good results. The problems of administration and ingestion found, for example with large, unpalatable tablets, have been tackled in a number of ways. Drops and syrups have been found to be a successful substitute for tablets. They have, however, certain disadvantages, not least storage and cost. In trials in Ghana and in India, 'sprinklers' (powdered microencapsulated ferrous fumarate) which can be added directly to food, have been found to be as effective as iron drops for the treatment of anaemia[248]. However, as with drops, cost and the need for sophisticated manufacturing skills would seem to limit the ready availability of such preparations, especially among the very poor.

Technical improvements in the form and production of iron supplements in themselves will not guarantee the success of efforts to overcome iron deficiency. This can only be done, especially in developing countries, through effective information, education and communication (IEC) programmes. Considerable success has been achieved in Indonesia, where a well designed IEC programme has been implemented. This involved the dissemination of specific messages to the community, including community leaders, the commercial sector, traditional birth attendants and community volunteers. Training of health workers in communication skills, as well as in development, and distribution of IEC materials were also undertaken[249].

Among the conclusions which emerged from a recent international conference devoted to the question of iron deficiency was the view that while iron supplementation is a key strategy for reaching target groups, large-scale programmes cannot be effective unless supply and demand constraints are addressed in an integrated way. Among critical issues pinpointed was the need to increase demand for and access to high quality iron tablets, as part of an improved quality of service to secure a continued supply of iron at distribution points. Development of effective management and monitoring systems, and the need to enhance compliance through IEC, were also stressed[250].

2.10.3 The effect of changing dietary habits on iron status

It is unlikely that any individual intervention, such as fortification of staple foods or use of supplements, will have its intended effect of bringing about a sustained improvement in the iron status of a whole population or of specific targeted groups, unless it is accompanied by other interventions and, especially, by an overall improvement in the general diet. This is how adequate intakes of iron have been achieved in several countries, following improved food intakes and a replacement of cereal-based with mixed diets, assisted by the use of fortified foods and dietary supplements[251]. The importance of economic development, leading to a better and more plentiful diet, richer in iron as well as in ascorbic acid and other enhancers of iron absorption, has, it is believed, contributed significantly to a decline in iron deficiency in the US since the 1970s[252]. Better economic conditions in developing countries can also be expected to bring about an improvement in iron status, as well as in general health. Unfortunately, this does not occur in some countries because of socio-economic and political problems[253]. In such circumstances, iron deficiency remains at unacceptably high levels of incidence, especially among women and children.

Methods for improving the diets of vulnerable sections of the population, even though resources are limited, have been proposed by a number of investigators. These low cost proposals range from encouraging women to increase their consumption of cereal-based fermented foods and gooseberry juice[254], to the development of iron-rich cereals and other food staples through plant breeding, by selection as well as by genetic engineering[255]. However, useful though these and other similar strategies may be in certain cases, the problem of iron deficiency is unlikely to be resolved, especially in many of the poorer countries, without sustained economic improvement backed by an even-handed and socially responsible political will.

References

1. Buttriss, J. (2001) The mysteries of iron metabolism: magnetic attractions. *Nutrition Bulletin*, **26**, 271–2.
2. Chrisitan, H.A. (1903) History of chlorosis treatment with iron. *Medical Library and Historical Journal*, **1**, 176, as cited in McCay, C.M. (1973) *Notes on the History of Nutrition Research*. H. Huber, Berne.
3. McCay, C.M. (1973) *Notes on the History of Nutrition Research*. H. Huber, Berne.
4. Berzelius, J.J. (1814) *Zusammensetzung der tierischen Flüssigkeiten*, Nuremberg.
5. Beard, J.L., Dawson, H. & Piñero, D.J. (1996) Iron metabolism: a comprehensive review. *Nutrition Reviews*, **54**, 295–317.
6. McCay, C.M. (1973) *Notes on the History of Nutrition Research*. H. Huber, Berne.
7. Boussingault, J.B. (1872) Du fer contenu dans le sang et dans les aliments. *Comptes Rendus des Académies Scientifiques de Paris*, **74**, 1353–9.
8. Rickard, D., Butler, I.B. & Oldroyd, A. (2001) A novel iron sulphide mineral switch and its implications for Earth and planetary science. *Earth and Planetary Science Letters*, **189**, 85–91.
9. Looker, A.C., Dallman, P.R., Carroll, M.D., Gunter, E.W. & Johnson, C.L. (1997) Prevalence of iron deficiency in the United States. *Journal of the American Medical Association*, **227**, 973–6.
10. Cammack, R., Wriggleworth J.M. & Baum, H. (1990) Iron-dependent enzymes in mammalian systems. In *Iron Transport and Metabolism* (ed. P. Ponka). CRC Press, Boca Raton, FL.
11. Wilkins, P.C. & Wilkins, R.G. (1997) *Inorganic Chemistry in Biology*. Oxford University Press, Oxford.
12. Shriver, D.F. & Atkins, P.W. (1999) *Inorganic Chemistry*, 3rd ed. Oxford University Press, Oxford.
13. Cowan, J.A. (1997) *Inorganic Biochemistry*. Wiley, New York.
14. Beard, J.L., Dawson H. & Piñero, D.J. (1996) Iron metabolism: a comprehensive review. *Nutrition Reviews*, **54**, 295–317.
15. Perutz, M.F. (1990) *Mechanism of Cooperativity and Allosteric Regulation in Proteins*. Cambridge University Press, Cambridge.
16. Moore, G.R. & Pettigrew, G.W. (1990) *Cytochrome c: Structural and Physicochemical Aspects*. Springer, Berlin.
17. Moore, G.R. & Pettigrew, G.W. (1990) *Cytochrome c: Structural and Physicochemical Aspects*. Springer, Berlin.
18. Keilin, D. (1966) *The History of Cell Respiration and Cytochromes*. Cambridge University Press, Cambridge.
19. Nerbert, D.W., Nelson, D.R., Coon, M.J. *et al.* (1991) The P450 superfamily: update on new sequences, gene mapping, and recommended nomenclature. *DNA Cellular Biology*, **10**, 1–33.
20. Shriver, D.F. & Atkins, P.W. (1999) *Inorganic Chemistry*, 3rd ed. Oxford University Press, Oxford.
21. Princiotto, J.V. & Zapolski, F.J. (1976) Functional heterogeneity and pH dependent dissociation properties of human transferrin. *Biochimica et Biophysica Acta*, **428**, 766–71.
22. Aschner, M. & Aschner, J.L. (1990) Manganese transport across the blood brain barrier: relationship to iron homeostasis. *Brain Research Bulletin*, **24**, 857–60.
23. Bothwell, T.H., Charlton, R.W., Cook, J.D. & Finch, C.A. (1979) *Iron Metabolism in Man*. Blackwell, Oxford.
24. Iacopetta, B.J., Morgan, E.H. & Yeoh, G.C.T. (1982) Transferrin receptors and iron uptake during erythroid cell development. *Biochimica et Biophysica Acta*, **687**, 204–10.
25. British Nutrition Foundation (1995) *Iron, Nutritional and Physiological Significance*. Chapman & Hall, London.

26. Thiel, E.C. (1987) Ferritin structure, gene regulation, and cellular function in animals, plants and microorganisms. *Annual Review of Biochemistry*, **56**, 289–315.
27. Crichton, R. & Ward, R.J. (1992) Iron metabolism – new perspectives in view. *Biochemistry*, **31**, 11255–64.
28. Levi, S., Yewdall, S.J., Harrison, P.M. *et al.* (1992) Evidence that H- and L-chains have cooperative roles in the iron-uptake mechanisms of human ferritin. *Biochemical Journal*, **288**, 591–6.
29. De Silva, D. & Aust, S.D. (1992) Stoichiometry of Fe(II) oxidation during caeruloplasmin-catalysed loading of ferritin. *Archives of Biochemistry and Biophysics*, **298**, 259–64.
30. Zahringer J., Baliga, B.S. & Munro, H.N. (1976) Novel mechanism for translational control in regulation of ferritin synthesis by iron. *Proceedings of the National Academy of Sciences*, **73**, 857–61.
31. Wesling-Resnick, M. (2000) Iron transport. *Annual Reviews of Nutrition*, **20**, 129–51.
32. Pietrangelo, A. (1998) Hemochromatosis 1998: is one gene enough? *Journal of Hepatology*, **29**, 502–9.
33. Carpenter, C.E. & Mahoney, A.W. (1992) Contributions of heme and nonheme iron to human nutrition. *Critical Reviews of Food Science and Nutrition*, **31**, 333–67.
34. Raja, K.B., Simpson, R.J. & Peters, T.J. (1987) Comparison of $^{59}Fe^{3+}$ uptake *in vitro* and *in vivo* by mouse duodenum. *Biochimica et Biophysica Acta*, **901**, 52–60.
35. Hastings-Wilson, T. (1962) *Intestinal Absorption*. Saunders, Philadelphia.
36. Conrad, M.E., Umbreit, J.N. & Moore, E.G. (1994) Iron absorption and cellular uptake of iron. *Advances in Experimental Medicine and Biology*, **356**, 69–79.
37. Roughead, Z.K., Zito, C.A. & Hunt, J.R. (2002) Initial uptake and absorption of nonheme iron and absorption of heme iron in humans are unaffected by the addition of calcium as cheese to a meal with high iron bioavailability. *American Journal of Clinical Nutrition*, **76**, 419–25.
38. Lynch, S.R., Dassenko, S.A., Morck, T.A. Beard, J.L. & Cook, J.D. (1985) Soy protein products and heme iron absorption in humans. *American Journal of Clinical Nutrition*, **41**, 13–20.
39. FAO/WHO (1988) Report of a Joint Expert Group: Requirements of Vitamin A, Iron, Folate and Vitamin B_{12}: expert consultation. In: *FAO Food and Nutrition Series No. 23*. Food and Agriculture Organisation, Rome.
40. Simpson, K.M., Morris, E.R., & Cook, J.D. (1981) The inhibitory effect of bran on iron absorption in humans. *American Journal of Clinical Nutrition*, **34**, 1469–78.
41. Baig, M.M., Burgin, C.W. & Cerda, J.J. (1983) Effect of dietary pectin on iron absorption and turnover in the rat. *Journal of Nutrition*, **113**, 2615–22.
42. Brune, M., Rossander-Hulthén, L., Hallerberg, L., Gleerup, A. & Sandberg, A. (1992) Iron absorption from bread in humans: inhibiting effects of cereal, fibre, phytate and inositol phosphates with different numbers of phosphate groups. *Journal of Nutrition*, **122**, 442–9.
43. Brune, M., Rossander, L. & Hallberg, L. (1989) Iron absorption and phenolic compounds: importance of different phenolic structures. *European Journal of Clinical Nutrition*, **43**, 547–58.
44. Schäfer, S.G., & Förth, W. (1982) The influence of tin, nickel, and cadmium on the intestinal absorption of iron. *Ecotoxicological and Environmental Safety*, **7**, 87–95.
45. Roughead, Z.F., Zito, C.A. & Hunt, J.R. (2002) Initial uptake and absorption of nonheme iron and absorption of heme iron in humans are unaffected by the addition of calcium as cheese to a meal with high iron bioavailability. *American Journal of Clinical Nutrition*, **76**, 419–25.
46. Solomons, N.W. & Jacob, R.A. (1981) Studies on the bioavailability of zinc in humans IV: effects of heme and nonheme iron on the absorption of zinc. *American Journal of Clinical Nutrition*, **34**, 475–82.
47. Reilly, C. & Henry, J. (2000) Geophagia: why do humans consume soil? *British Nutrition Foundation Nutrition Bulletin*, **25**, 141–4.

48. Hooda, P.S., Henry, C.J.K., Seyoum, T.A., Armstrong, L.D.M. & Fowler, M.B. (2002) The potential impact of geophagia on the bioavailability of iron, zinc and calcium in human nutrition. *Environmental Geochemistry and Health*, **24**, 305–19.
49. Zhang, D., Hendricks, D.G., Mahoney, A.W. & Yu, Y. (1988) Effect of tea on dietary iron bioavailability in anaemic and healthy rats. *Nutrition Reports International*, **37**, 1225–35.
50. Zijp, I.M., Korver, O. & Tijburg, B.M. (2000) Effect of tea and other dietary factors on iron absorption. *Critical Reviews in Food Science and Nutrition*, **40**, 371–98.
51. Lynch, S.R. & Cook, J.D. (1980) Interaction of vitamin C and iron. *Annals of the New York Academy of Science*, **355**, 32–43.
52. Skikne, B. & Baynes, R.D. (1994) Iron absorption. In: *Iron Metabolism in Health and Disease* (eds. J.H. Brock, J.W. Halliday, M.J. Pippard & L.W. Powell). Saunders, London.
53. Baynes, R.D., Bothwell, T.H., Bezwoda, W.R. *et al.* (1987) Relationship between absorption of inorganic and food iron in field studies. *Annals of Nutrition and Metabolism*, **31**, 109–16.
54. Fairweather-Tait, S.J. (1986) Iron availability – the implications of short-term regulation. *British Nutrition Foundation Nutrition Bulletin*, **11**, 174–80.
55. Whittaker, P.G., Lind, T. & Williams, J.G. (1991) Iron absorption during normal human pregnancy: a study using stable isotopes. *British Journal of Nutrition*, **65**, 457–63.
56. Skikne, B.S., Lynch, S.R. & Cook, J.D. (1981) Role of gastric acid in food iron absorption. *Gastroenterology*, **81**, 1068–70.
57. Skikne, R.S. & Cook, J.D. (1992) Effect of enhanced erythropoiesis on iron absorption. *Journal of Laboratory and Clinical Medicine*, **20**, 746–51.
58. Skikne & Baynes (1994) Iron absorption. In: *Iron Metabolism in Health and Disease* (eds. J.H. Brock, J.W. Halliday, M.J. Pippard & L.W. Powell). Saunders, London.
59. Bothwell, T.H., Charlton, R.W., Cook, J.D. & Finch, C.A. (1979) *Iron Metabolism in Man*. Blackwell, Oxford.
60. Wessling-Resnick, M. (2000) Iron transport. *Annual Review of Nutrition*, **20**, 129–51.
61. Skikne, B. & Baynes, R.D. (1994) Iron absorption. In: *Iron Metabolism in Health and Disease* (eds. J.H. Brock, J.W. Halliday, M.J. Pippard, & L.W. Powell). Saunders, London.
62. Cox, T.M., Mazurier, J., Spik, G. *et al.* (1979) Iron binding proteins and influx of iron across the duodenal brush border: evidence for specific lactoferrin receptors in the human intestine. *Biochimica et Biophysica Acta*, **588**, 120–8.
63. Roy, C.N. & Enns, C.A. (2000) Iron homeostasis: new tales from the crypt. *Blood*, **96**, 4020–7.
64. Gushin, H., Mackenzie, B., Berger, U.V. *et al.* (1997) Cloning and characterization of a mammalian proton-coupled metal-ion transporter. *Nature*, **388**, 482–8.
65. Ituri, S. & Nunez, M.T. (1998) Effect of copper, cadmium, mercury, manganese and lead on Fe^{2+} and Fe^{3+} absorption in perfused mouse intestine. *Digestion*, **59**, 671–5.
66. Nichols, G.M. & Bacon, B.R. (1989) Hereditary hemochromatosis: pathogenesis and clinical features of a common disease. *American Journal of Gastroenterology*, **84**, 851–62.
67. Canonne, F., Gruenheid, S., Ponka, P. & Gros, P. (1999) Cellular and subcellular localization of the Nramp2 iron transporter in the intestinal brush border and regulation by dietary iron. *Blood*, **93**, 4406–17.
68. Raja, K.B., Simpson, R.J. & Peters, P.J. (1992) Investigation of a role for reduction in ferric iron uptake by mouse duodenum. *Biochimica et Biophysica Acta*, **1135**, 141–6.
69. Gunshi, H., Mackenzie, B., Berger, U.V. *et al.* (1997) Cloning and characterization of a mammalian proton-coupled metal-ion transporter. *Nature*, **388**, 482–8.
70. Attieh, Z.K., Mukhopadhyay, C.K., Seshadri, V. *et al.* (1999) Ceruloplasmin ferroxidase activity stimulates cellular iron uptake by a trivalent cation-specific transport mechanism. *Journal of Biological Chemistry*, **274**, 1116–23.

71. Nunez, M.T. & Tapia, V. (1999) Transferrin stimulates iron absorption, exocytosis, and secretion in cultured intestinal cells. *American Journal of Physiology*, **276**, C1085–90.
72. Simpson, R.J., Lombard, M., Raja, K.B. *et al.* (1986) Studies on the role of transferrin and endocytosis in the uptake of Fe^{3+} from Fe-nitriloacetate by mouse duodenum. *Biochimica et Biophysica Acta*, **884**, 166–71.
73. Granick, S. (1946) Protein apoferritin in iron feeding and absorption. *Science*, **103**, 107–13.
74. McKie, A.T., Marciani, P., Rolfs, A. *et al.* (2000) A novel duodenal iron-regulated transporter, IREG1, implicated in basolateral transfer of iron to the circulation. *Molecular Cell*, **5**, 299–309.
75. Osaki, S., Johnson, D.A. & Freiden, E. (1966) The possible significance of the ferrous oxidase activity of caeruloplasmin in normal human serum. *Journal of Biological Chemistry*, **241**, 2746–8.
76. Vulpe, C.D., Kuo, Y.M. & Murphy, T.L. *et al.* (1999) Hephaestin, a caeruloplasmin homologue implicated in intestinal iron transport, is defective in the sla mouse. *Nature Genetics*, **21**, 195–9.
77. Bothwell, T.H., Charlton, R.W., Cook, J.D. & Finch, C.A. (1979) *Iron Metabolism in Man*. Blackwell, Oxford.
78. Roy, C.N. & Enns, C.A. (2000) Iron homeostasis: new tales from the crypt. *Blood*, **96**, 4020–7.
79. Eisenstein, R. & Blemings, K. (1998) Iron regulatory proteins, iron responsive elements and iron homeostasis. *Journal of Nutrition*, **128**, 2295–8.
80. Wessling-Resnick, M. (2002) A possible link between hepcidin and regulation of dietary iron absorption. *Nutrition Reviews*, **60**, 371–4.
81. Park, C.H., Valore, E.V., Waring, A.J. & Ganz, T. (2001) Hepcidin, a urinary antimicrobial peptide synthesized in the liver. *Journal of Biological Chemistry*, **276**, 7806–10.
82. Pigeon, C., Ilyin, G., Courslaud, B. *et al.* A new mouse liver-specific gene, encoding a protein homologous to human antimicrobial peptide hepcidin, is overexpressed during iron overload. *Journal of Biological Chemistry*, **276**, 7811–9.
83. Kelly, C. (2002) Can excess iron increase the risk of coronary heart disease and cancer? *British Nutrition Foundation Nutrition Bulletin*, **27**, 165–79.
84. Wessling-Resnick, M. (2000) Iron transport. *Annual Review of Nutrition*, **20**, 129–51.
85. Wessling-Resnick, M. (2000) Iron transport. *Annual Review of Nutrition*, **20**, 129–51.
86. Levy, J.E., Jin, O., Fujiwara, Y., Kuo, F. & Andrews, N.C. (1999) Transferrin receptor is necessary for development of erythrocytes and the nervous system. *Nature Genetics*, **21**, 396–9.
87. Eisenstein, R.S. (2000) Iron regulatory proteins and the molecular control of mammalian iron metabolism. *Annual Review of Nutrition*, **20**, 627–62.
88. Finch, C.A., Deubelbliss, K., Cook, J.D. *et al.* (1970) Ferrokinetics in man. *Medicine* **49**, 17–53.
89. Jacobs, A. & Worwood, M. (1980) Iron metabolism, iron deficiency and iron overload. In: *Blood and its Disorders* (eds. R.M. Hardisty & D.J. Weatherall), 149–97. Blackwell, Oxford.
90. Green, R., Charlton, R., Seftel, H. *et al.* (1968) Body iron excretion in man. A collaborative study. *American Journal of Medicine*, **45**, 336–53.
91. Cole, S.K., Billewicz, W.Z. & Thomson, A.M. (1971) Sources of variation in menstrual blood loss. *Journal of Obstetrics and Gynaecology*, **78**, 933–9.
92. Beard, J.L., Dawson H. & Piñero, D.J. (1996) Iron metabolism: a comprehensive review. *Nutrition Reviews*, **54**, 295–317.
93. Layrisse, M., Chaves, J.F., Mendez-Castellano, E. *et al.* (1996) Early response to the effect of iron fortification in the Venezuelan population. *American Journal of Clinical Nutrition*, **64**, 903–7.
94. Cook, J.D. (1999) Defining optimal body iron. *Proceedings of the Nutrition Society*, **58**, 489–95.
95. Cook, J.D. (1999) Defining optimal body iron. *Proceedings of the Nutrition Society*, **58**, 489–95.
96. Addison, G.M., Beamish, M.R., Hales, C.N. *et al.* (1972) An immunoradiometric assay for ferritin in the serum of normal subjects and patients with iron deficiency and iron overload. *Journal of Clinical Pathology*, **25**, 326–9.

97. Worwood, M. (1980) Serum ferritin. In: *Methods in Haemotology*, (ed. J.D. Cook), Vol. 1, pp. 59–89. Churchill Livingstone, Edinburgh.
98. Walters, G.O, Miller, F.M. & Worwood, M. (1973) Serum ferritin concentration and iron stores in normal subjects. *Journal of Clinical Pathology*, **26**, 770–2.
99. Worwood, M. (1982) Ferritin in human tissues and serum. *Clinics in Haematology*, **11**, 275–307.
100. Leggett, B.A., Brown, N.N., Bryant, S.J. *et al.* (1990) Factors affecting the concentrations of ferritin in serum in a healthy Australian population. *Clinical Chemistry*, **36**, 1350–5.
101. International Committee for Standardisation in Haematology (1990) Revised recommendations for the measurements of serum iron in human blood. *British Journal of Haematology*, **75**, 615–6.
102. Cook, J.D. (1999) Defining optimal body iron. *Proceedings of the Nutrition Society*, **58**, 489–95.
103. Labbé, R.F. & Rettmer, R.L. (1989) Zinc protoporphyrin: a product of iron-deficient erythropoiesis. *Seminars in Hematology*, **26**, 40–6.
104. Reilly, C. (2002) *Metal Contamination of Food*. Blackwell, Oxford.
105. Looker, A.C., Dallman, P.R., Carroll, M.D. *et al.* (1997) Prevalence of iron deficiency in the United States. *Journal of the American Medical Association*, **277**, 973–6.
106. Shih, Y.J., Baynes, R.D., Hudson, B.G. *et al.* (1990) Serum transferrin receptor is a truncated form of tissue receptor. *Journal of Biological Chemistry*, **265**, 19077–81.
107. Skikne, B.S., Flowers, C.H. & Cook, D.J. (1990) Serum transferrin receptors: a quantitative measure of tissue iron deficiency. *Blood*, **75**, 1870–6.
108. Dacie, J.V. & Lewis, S.M. (1991) *Practical Haematology*. Churchill Livingstone, Edinburgh.
109. Beard, J.L. & Finch, C.A. (1985) Iron deficiency. In: *Iron Fortification of Foods* (eds. F. Clydesdale & K.L. Weimer), 3–16. Academic Press, New York.
110. Lipschitz, D.A. (1990) The anaemia of chronic disease. *Journal of the American Geriatric Society*, **38**, 1258–64.
111. Cook, J.D. (1999) Defining optimal body iron. *Proceedings of the Nutrition Society*, **58**, 489–95.
112. Tucker, D.M., Sandstead, H.H., Swenson, R.A., Sawler, B.G., & Pentland, J.G. (1982) Longitudinal study of brain function and depletion of iron stores in individual subjects. *Physiology of Behaviour*, **29**, 737–40.
113. Gibson, S. (1999) Iron intake and iron status of preschool children: associations with breakfast cereals, vitamin C and meat. *Public Health Nutrition*, **2**, 521–8.
114. Looker, A.C., Dallman, P.R., Carroll, M.D., Gunter, E.W. & Johnson, C.L. (1997) Prevalence of iron deficiency in the United States. *Journal of the American Medical Association*, **277**, 973–6.
115. Beard, J.L., Dawson H. & Piñero, D.J. (1996) Iron metabolism: a comprehensive review. *Nutrition Reviews*, **54**, 295–317.
116. British Nutrition Foundation (1995) *Iron, Nutritional and Physiological Significance*. Chapman & Hall, London.
117. Skikne, B.S., Flowers, C.H. & Cook, J.D. (1990) Serum transferrin receptor: a quantitative measure of tissue iron deficiency. *Blood*, **75**, 1870–6.
118. Bessman, J.D., Gilmer, P.R. & Gardner, C.W. (1983) Improved classification of anemias by MCV and RDW. *American Journal of Clinical Pathology*, **80**, 322–36.
119. Scrimshaw, N.S. (1984) Functional consequences of iron deficiency in human populations. *Journal of Nutritional Science and Vitaminology*, **30**, 47–63.
120. Davies, K.J.A., Donovan, C.M., Refino, C.J. *et al.* (1984) Distinguishing effects of anemia and muscle iron deficiency on exercise bioenergetics in the rat. *American Journal of Physiology*, **246**, E535–43.

121. Basta, S.S., Soekirman, M.S., Karyadi, D. & Scrimshaw, N.S. (1979) Iron deficiency anaemia and the productivity of adult males in Indonesia. *American Journal of Clinical Nutrition*, **32**, 916–25.
122. Cook, J.D. (1999) Defining optimal body iron. *Proceedings of the Nutrition Society*, **58**, 489–95.
123. De Andraca, I., Castillo, M. & Walter,T. (1997) Psychomotor development and behaviour in iron-deficient anemic infants. *Nutrition Reviews*, **55**, 125–32.
124. Pollitt, E., Hathirat, P., Kotchabhakdi, N.J., Missell, L. & Valyasevi, A. (1989) Iron deficiency and educational achievement in Thailand. *American Journal of Clinical Nutrition*, **50**, 687–97.
125. Scholl, T.O., Hedigere, M.L., Fischer, R.L. & Shearer, J.W. (1992) Anemia vs iron deficiency: increased risk of preterm delivery in a prospective study. *American Journal of Clinical Nutrition*, **55**, 985–8.
126. Doyle, W., Crawford, M.A., Wynn, A.H.A. & Wynn, S.W. (1990) The association between maternal diet and birth dimensions. *Journal of Nutrition in Medicine*, **1**, 9–17.
127. Allen, L.H. (1997) Pregnancy and iron deficiency: unresolved issues. *Nutrition Reviews*, **55**, 91–101.
128. Ferguson, B.J., Skikne, B.S., Simpson, K.M., Baynes, R.D. & Cook, J.D. (1992) Serum transferrin receptor distinguished the anemia of chronic disease from iron deficiency anemia. *Journal of Laboratory and Clinical Medicine*, **119**, 385–90.
129. Kelly, C. (2002) Can excess iron increase the risk of coronary heart disease and cancer? *British Nutrition Foundation Nutrition Bulletin*, **27**, 165–79.
130. Edwards, C., Griffin, L., Goldgar, D. *et al.* (1988) Prevalence of hemochromatosis among 11 065 presumably healthy blood donors. *New England Journal of Medicine*, **318**, 1355–62.
131. McLaren, C.E., Gordeuk, V.R., Looker, A.C. *et al.* (1995) Prevalence of heterozygotes for hemochromatosis in the white population of the United States. *Blood*, **86**, 2021–7.
132. Hanson, E., Imperatore, G. & Burke, W. (2001) HFE gene and hereditary hemochromatosis: a HuGE review. *American Journal of Epidemiology*, **154**, 193–206.
133. Kelly, C. (2002) Can excess iron increase the risk of coronary heart disease and cancer? *British Nutrition Foundation Nutrition Bulletin*, **27**, 165–79.
134. Walker, A.R.P. & Arvidsson, U.B. (1953) Iron 'overload' in the South African Bantu. *Transactions of the Royal Society of Tropical Medicine and Hygiene*, **47**, 536–48.
135. Gordeuk, V., Mukiibi, J., Hasstedt, S.J. *et al.* (1992) Iron overload in Africa. Interaction between a gene and dietary iron content. *New England Journal of Medicine*, **326**, 95–100.
136. Conrad, M.E. & Barton, J.C. (1980) Anaemia and iron kinetics in anaemia. *Seminars in Hematology*, **17**, 149–63.
137. Buttriss, J. (2001) The mysteries of iron metabolism: magnetic attractions. *British Nutrition Foundation Nutrition Bulletin*, **26**, 271–2.
138. Bacon, B.R. & Britton, R.S. (1990) The pathology of hepatic iron overload: a free radical-mediated process. *Hepatology*, **11**, 127–37.
139. Dormandy, T.L. (1983) An approach to free radicals. *Lancet*, **ii**, 1010–4.
140. Kelly, C. (2002) Can excess iron increase the risk of coronary heart disease and cancer? *British Nutrition Foundation Nutrition Bulletin*, **27**, 165–79.
141. Thurnham, D.I. (1994) β-Carotene, are we misreading the signals in risk groups? Some analogies with vitamin C. *Proceedings of the Nutrition Society*, **53**, 557–69.
142. Oppenheimer, S.J., Gibson, F.D., Macfarlane, S.B. *et al.* (1987) Iron supplementation increases prevalence and effects of malaria: report on clinical studies in Papua New Guinea. *Transactions of the Royal Society of Tropical Medicine and Hygiene*, **80**, 603–12.
143. Stadman, E.R. (1991) Ascorbic acid and oxidative inactivation of proteins. *American Journal of Clinical Nutrition*, **54**, 1125S–8S.
144. Walter, T., Olivares, M., Pizarro, F. & Muñoz, C. (1997) Iron, anaemia, and infection. *Nutrition Reviews*, **55**, 111–24.

145. Staines, N., Brostoff, J. & James, K. (1994) *Introducing Immunology*, 2nd ed. Mosby, St. Louis, MO.
146. Brock, J.H. (1993) Iron and immunity. *Journal of Nutritional Immunology*, **2**, 47–106.
147. Jurado, R.L. (1997) Iron, infections, and anemia of inflammation. *Clinical Infectious Diseases*, **25**, 888–95.
148. Brock, J.H. & Mulero, V. (2000) Cellular and molecular aspects of iron and immune function. *Proceedings of the Nutrition Society*, **59**, 537–40.
149. Liberman, H.M., Cohen, A., Lee, J.W.W. *et al.* (1984) Deferoxamine: a reversible S-phase inhibitor of lymphocyte proliferation. *Blood*, **64**, 748–53.
150. Mainou-Fowler, T. & Brock, J.H. (1985) Effect of iron deficiency on the response of mouse lymphocytes to concanavalin A: the importance of transferrin-bound iron. *Immunology*, **54**, 325–32.
151. Brock, J.H. & Mulero, V. (2000) Cellular and molecular aspects of iron and immune function. *Proceedings of the Nutrition Society*, **59**, 537–40.
152. Konijn, A.M. & Hershko, C. (1977) Ferritin synthesis in inflammation. I Pathogenesis of impaired iron release. *British Journal of Haematology*, **37**, 7–16.
153. Alford, C.E., King, T.E. & Campbell, P.A. (1991) Role of transferrin, transferrin receptors, and iron in macrophage listericidal activity. *Journal of Experimental Medicine*, **174**, 459–66.
154. Andleman, M.B. & Sered, B.R. (1966) Utilization of dietary iron by term infants: a study of 1048 infants from a low socioeconomic population. *American Journal of Diseases of Childhood*, **111**, 45–55.
155. Burman, D. (1972) Haemoglobin levels in normal infants aged 3–24 months and the effect of iron. *Archives of the Diseases of Childhood*, **47**, 261–71.
156. Berger, J., Schneider, D., Dyck, J.L. *et al.* (1992) Iron deficiency, cell-mediated immunity and infection among 6–36 month old children living in rural Togo. *Nutrition Research*, **12**, 39–49.
157. Puschmann, M. & Ganzoni, A.M. (1977) Increased resistance of iron-deficient mice to *Salmonella* infection. *Infection and Immunity*, **17**, 663–4.
158. Murray, M.J., Murray, A.B., Murray, N.J. & Murray, M.B. (1975) Refeeding malaria and hyperferraemia. *Lancet*, **I**, 653–4.
159. Murray, M.J., Murray, A.B., Murray, M.B. & Murray, C.J. (1978) The adverse effect of iron repletion on the course of certain infections. *British Medical Journal*, **2**, 1113–5.
160. Hershko, C., Peto, T.E.A. & Weatherall, D.J. (1988) Iron and infection. *British Medical Journal*, **296**, 660–4.
161. Barry, D.M.J. & Reeve, A.W. (1976) Iron and neonatal infection – the Hawkes Bay experience. *New Zealand Journal of Medicine*, **84**, 287.
162. Murray, M.J., Murray, A.B., Murray, M.B., & Murray, C.J. (1978) The adverse effect of iron repletion on the course of certain infections. *British Medical Journal*, **2**, 1113–5.
163. Higginson, J., Gerritsen, T. & Walker, A.R.P. (1953) Siderosis in the Bantu of South Africa. *American Journal of Pathology*, **29**, 779–815.
164. Haliwell, B. & Gutteridge, J.M.C. (1999) *Free Radical Biology and Medicine*, 3rd ed. Oxford University Press, Oxford.
165. Toyokuni, S. (1996) Iron-induced carcinogenesis: the role of redox regulation. *Free Radical Biology and Medicine*, **20**, 553–66.
166. Bacon, B.R. & Britton, R.S. (1990) The pathology of hepatic iron overload: a free radical-mediated process? *Hepatology*, **11**, 127–37.
167. Smith, A.G., Carthew, P., Francis, J.E., Cabral, J.R.P. & Manson, M.M. (1993) Enhancement by iron of hepatic neoplasia in rats caused by hexachlorobenzene. *Carcinogenesis*, **14**, 1381–7.
168. Kelly, C. (2002) Can excess iron increase the risk of coronary heart disease and cancer? *British Nutrition Foundation Nutrition Bulletin*, **27**, 165–79.
169. Babbs, C. (1990) Free radicals and the etiology of colon cancer. *Free Radical Biology and Medicine*, **8**, 191–200.

170. Kato, I., Dnistrian, A., Schwartz, M. *et al.* (1999) Iron intake, body iron stores and colorectal cancer risk in women: a nested case-control study. *International Journal of Cancer*, **80**, 693–8.
171. Fischer, J.G., Glauert, H.P., Yin, T. *et al.* (2002) Moderate iron overload enhances lipid peroxidation in liver of rats, but does not affect NF-κB activation induced by the peroxisome proliferator, Wy-14,643. *Journal of Nutrition*, **132**, 2525–31.
172. Stokes, J. (1962) Haematological factors as related to the sex difference in coronary-artery disease. *Lancet*, **ii**, 25.
173. Sullivan, J.L. (1981) Iron and the sex difference in heart disease. *Lancet*, **i**, 1293–4.
174. Lauffer, R.B. (1991) Iron stores and the international variation in mortality from coronary artery disease. *Medical Hypotheses*, **35**, 96–102.
175. Riemersma, R.A., Wood, D.A., MacIntyre, C.C.A. *et al.* (1991) Anti-oxidants and pro-oxidants in coronary heart disease. *Lancet*, **337**, 677.
176. Stampfer, M.J., Grodstein, F., Rosenberg, L. *et al.* (1993) A prospective study of plasma ferritin and risk of myocardial infarction of US physicians [Abstract]. *Circulation*, **87**, 688.
177. Salonen, J.T., Salonen, R., Nyyssonen, K. & Korpela, H. (1992) Iron sufficiency is associated with hypertension and excess risk of myocardial infarction. The Kuopio ischaemic heart disease risk factor study. *Circulation*, **85**, 864.
178. Morrison, H.I., Semenoiw, R.M., Mao, Y. & Wigle, D.T. (1994) Serum iron and risk of fatal acute myocardial infarction. *Epidemiology*, **5**, 243–6.
179. Cooper, R.S. & Liao, Y. (1993) Iron stores and coronary heart disease: negative findings in the NHANES 1 epidemiologic follow-up study [Abstract]. *Circulation*, **87**, 686.
180. Kelly, C. (2002) Can excess iron increase the risk of coronary heart disease and cancer? *British Nutrition Foundation Nutrition Bulletin*, **27**, 165–79.
181. Burt, M., Halliday, J. & Powell, L. (1993) Iron and coronary heart disease. Iron's role is undecided. *British Medical Journal*, **307**, 575–6.
182. National Academy of Sciences (2001) *Dietary Reference Intakes. Vitamin A, Vitamin K, Arsenic, Boron, Chromium, Copper, Iodine, Iron, Manganese, Molybdenum, Nickel, Silicon, Vanadium and Zinc.* http://www.nap.edu/books/0309072794/html.
183. British Nutrition Foundation (1995) *Iron, Nutritional and Physiological Significance*. Chapman & Hall, London.
184. Ysart, G., Miller, P., Crews, H. *et al.* (1999) Dietary exposure estimates of 30 elements from the UK Total Diet Study. *Food Additives and Contaminants*, **16**, 391–403.
185. Pennington, J.A.T. & Schoen, S.A. (1996) Total Diet Study: estimated dietary intakes of nutritional elements, 1982–1991. *International Journal of Vitamin and Nutrition Research*, **66**, 350–62.
186. British Nutrition Foundation (1995) *Iron, Nutritional and Physiological Significance.* Chapman & Hall, London.
187. Food Standards Agency (2002) *McCance and Widdowson's The Composition of Foods*, 6th Summary Edition. Royal Society of Chemistry/Food Standards Agency, London.
188. Holland, B., Welch, A.A., Unwin, I.D. *et al.* (1991) *The Composition of Foods*, 5th ed. Royal Society of Chemistry, Cambridge.
189. British Nutrition Foundation (1995) *Iron, Nutritional and Physiological Significance.* Chapman & Hall, London.
190. Food Standards Agency (2002) *McCance and Widdowson's The Composition of Foods*, 6th Summary Edition. Royal Society of Chemistry/Food Standards Agency, London.
191. Food Standards Agency (2002) *McCance and Widdowson's The Composition of Foods*, 6th Summary Edition. Royal Society of Chemistry/Food Standards Agency, London.
192. Monson, E.R. (1971) The need for iron fortification. *Journal of Nutrition Education*, **2**, 152–5.

193. Brady, M.C. (1996) Addition of nutrients. Current practice in the UK. *British Food Journal*, **98**, 12–9.
194. Statutory Instrument (1995a) No. 3202. *Bread and Flour Regulations*. HMSO, London.
195. Statutory Instrument (1995b) No. 77. *The Infant formula and Follow-on Formula Regulations*. HMSO, London.
196. Fairweather-Tait, S.J. (1997) Iron fortification in the UK: how necessary and effective is it? In: *Trace Elements in Man and Animals – 9: Proceedings of the Ninth International Symposium on Trace Elements in Man and Animals* (eds. P.W.P. Fischer, M.R. L'Abbé, K.A. Cockell & R.S. Gibson), pp. 392–6. National Research Council Research Press, Ottawa.
197. Hurrell, R.F. (1985) Non-elemental sources. In: *Iron Fortification of Foods* (eds. F.M. Clydesdale & K.L. Wiemer), pp. 39–53. Academic Press, London.
198. Fairweather-Tait, S.J. (1997) Iron fortification in the UK: how necessary and effective is it? In: *Trace Elements in Man and Animals – 9: Proceedings of the Ninth International Symposium on Trace Elements in Man and Animals* (eds. P.W.P. Fischer, M.R. L'Abbé, K.A. Cockell & R.S. Gibson), pp. 392–6. National Research Council Research Press, Ottawa.
199. Powell, I.W., Halliday, J.W. & Bassett, M.C. (1982) The case against iron supplementation. In: *The Biochemistry and Physiology of Iron* (eds. P. Saltmann & J. Hegenauer), pp. 811–43. Elsevier, New York.
200. Roe, M.A. & Fairweather-Tait, J. (1999) High bioavailability of reduced iron added to UK flour. *Lancet*, **353**, 1938–9.
201. Hurrell, R.F. (1977) Preventing iron deficiency through iron fortification. *Nutrition Reviews*, **55**, 210–22.
202. Roe, M.A. & Fairweather-Tait, J. (1999) High bioavailability of reduced iron added to UK flour. *Lancet*, **353**, 1938–9.
203. Crosby, W.H. (1977) Current concepts in nutrition: who needs iron? *New England Journal of Medicine*, **297**, 255–68.
204. Arens, U. (1996) Iron nutrition in health and disease. *British Nutrition Foundation Nutrition Bulletin*, **21**, 71–3.
205. Reilly, C. (1996) Too much of a good thing? The problem of trace element fortification of foods. *Trends in Food Science and Technology*, **7**, 139–42.
206. Reilly, C. (2002) *Metal Contamination of Food*, pp. 50–6. Blackwell, Oxford.
207. Crosby, N.T. (1977) Determination of heavy metals in food. *Proceedings of the Institute of Food Science and Technology*, **10**, 65–70.
208. Biffoli, R., Chiti, F., Mocchi, M. & Pinzauti, S. (1980) Contamination of canned foods with metals. *Rivista Società Italiano Scienza Alimentazione*, **27**, 11–16.
209. Boirgiato, E.V.M. & Martinez, F.E. (1998) Iron nutritional status is improved in Brazilian preterm infants fed food cooked in iron pots. *Journal of Nutrition*, **128**, 855–9.
210. Mandishona, E.M., Moyo, V.M., Gordeuk, V.R. *et al.* (1999) A traditional beverage prevents iron deficiency in African women of childbearing age. *European Journal of Clinical Nutrition*, **53**, 722–5.
211. Walker, A.R.P. (1999) Iron overload in Sub-Saharan Africa: to what extent is it a public health problem? *British Journal of Nutrition*, **81**, 427–34.
212. Van Dokkum, W. (1995) The intake of selected minerals and trace elements in European countries. *Nutrition Research Reviews*, **8**, 271–302.
213. Ministry of Agriculture, Fisheries and Food (1994) *National Food Survey 1993*. HMSO, London.
214. Bull, N.L. & Buss, D.H. (1980) Haem and non-haem iron in British household diets. *Journal of Human Nutrition*, **34**, 141–5.

215. Life Sciences Research Office (1985). Summary of a report on assessment of the iron nutritional status of the United States population. *American Journal of Clinical Nutrition*, **42**, 1032–45.
216. Raper, N.R., Rosenthal, J.C. & Wotcki, C.F. (1984) Estimates of available iron in diets of individuals 1 year old and older in the Nationwide Food Consumption Survey. *Journal of the American Dietetics Association*, **84**, 783–7.
217. Gibson, S. & Ashwell, M. (2000) Implications of reduced red and processed meat consumption for iron intakes among British women. *Proceedings of the Nutrition Society*, **60**, 60A.
218. Ministry of Agriculture, Fisheries and Food (1991) *Report of the Working Group on Dietary Supplements and Health Foods*. HMSO, London.
219. Saini, N., Maxwell, S.M., Dugdill, L. & Miller, A.M. (2000) Micronutrient intake of free-living elderly people. *Proceedings of the Nutrition Society*, **60**, 41A.
220. Draper, A., Lewis, J., Malhorta, N. & Wheeler, E. (1993) The energy and nutrient intakes of different types of vegetarians: a case for supplements? *British Journal of Nutrition*, **69**, 3–19.
221. Lightowler, H.J. & Davies, G.J. (2000) Micronutrient intakes in a group of UK vegans and the contribution of self-selected dietary supplements. *Journal of the Royal Society for the Promotion of Health*, **120**, 117–24.
222. Hunt, J.R. (2002) Moving towards a plant-based diet: are iron and zinc at risk? *Nutrition Reviews*, **60**, 127–34.
223. National Academy of Sciences (2001) *Dietary Reference Intakes. Vitamin A, Vitamin K, Arsenic, Boron, Chromium, Copper, Iodine, Iron, Manganese, Molybdenum, Nickel, Silicon, Vanadium and Zinc*. http://www.nap.edu/books/0309072794/html
224. Department of Health (1996) *Dietary Reference Values for Food Energy and Nutrients in the United Kingdom*. HMSO, London.
225. Muhilal (1998) Indonesian recommended dietary allowance. *Nutrition Reviews*, **56**, S19–S20.
226. British Nutrition Foundation (1995) *Iron, Nutritional and Physiological Significance*. Chapman & Hall, London.
227. Martorell, R. & Trowbridge, F. (2002) Foreword: Forging effective strategies to combat iron deficiency. Proceedings of the 6th Biennial International Conference on Health Promotion, 2–7 May 2001, Atlanta, GA. *Journal of Nutrition*, **132**, 789S.
228. Hallberg, L., Bengtsson, C., Garby, L. *et al.* (1979) An analysis of factors leading to a reduction in iron deficiency in Swedish women. *Bulletin of the World Health Organisation*, **57**, 947–54.
229. US Department of Health and Human Services (2000) *Healthy People 2010; Understanding and Improving Health and Objectives for Improving Health*. DHHS, Washington, DC.
230. Ramakrishnan, U. & Yip, R. (2002) Experiences and challenges in industrialised countries: control of iron deficiency in industrialised countries. *Journal of Nutrition*, **132**, 820S–4S.
231. Pan American Health Organization (2001) *Iron Fortification: Guidelines and Recommendations for Latin America and the Caribbean*. Pan American Health Organization, Washington, DC.
232. Hertrampf, E. (2002) Iron fortification in the Americas. *Nutrition Reviews*, **60**, S22–5.
233. Uauy, R., Hertrampf, E. & Reddy, M. (2002) Iron fortification of foods: overcoming technical and practical barriers. *Journal of Nutrition*, **132**, 849S–52S.
234. Mannar, V. & Gallego, E.B. (2002) Iron fortification: country level experiences and lessons learned. *Journal of Nutrition*, **132**, 856S–8S.
235. Walter, T., Olivares, M. & Hertramp, E. (1990) Field trials of food fortification with iron: the experience of Chile. In: *Iron Metabolism in Infants* (ed. B. Lonnerdal). CRC Press, Boca Raton, FL.

236. Osler, M., Milman, N. & Heitmann, B.L. (1999) Consequences of removing iron fortification of flour on iron status among Danish adults: some longitudinal observations between 1987 and 1994. *Preventive Medicine*, **29**, 32–6.
237. Department of Health and Social Security (1981) *Nutritional Aspects of Bread and Flour.* Report on Health and Social Subjects No. 23. HMSO, London.
238. Mora, J.O. (2002) Iron supplements: overcoming technical and practical barriers. *Journal of Nutrition*, **132**, 853S–5S.
239. Gregory, J.R., Foster, K., Tyler, H. & Wiseman, M. (1990) *The Dietary and Nutritional Survey of British Adults.* HMSO, London.
240. Dawson, E.B., Dawson, R., Behrens, J., DeVora, M.A. & McGanity, W.J. (1998). Iron in prenatal multivitamin/multimineral supplements. *Journal of Reproductive Medicine*, **43**, 133–40.
241. Elmstahl, S., Wallstrom, P., Janzon, L. & Johansson, U. (1996) The prevalence of anaemia and mineral supplement use in a Swedish middle-aged population. Results from the Malmo Diet and Cancer Study. *European Journal of Clinical Nutrition*, **50**, 450–5.
242. Allen, L.H. (2002) Iron supplements: scientific issues concerning efficacy and implications for research and programs. *Journal of Nutrition*, **132**, 813S–9S.
243. United Nations Administrative Committee on Coordination, Subcommittee on Nutrition (1991) *Controlling Iron Deficiency. ACC/SCN State of the Art Series: Nutrition Policy Discussion Paper 9.* United Nations Administrative Committee on Coordination, Subcommittee on Nutrition, Geneva.
244. Mora, J.O. (2002) Iron supplements: overcoming technical and practical barriers. *Journal of Nutrition*, **132**, 853S–5S.
245. Yip, R. & Ramakrishnan, U. (2002) Experiences and challenges in developing countries. *Journal of Nutrition*, **132**, 827S–30.
246. Solomons, N.W. (1986) Competitive interaction of iron and zinc in the diet: consequences for human nutrition. *Journal of Nutrition*, **116**, 927–35.
247. Donangelo, C.M., Woodhouse, L.R., King, S.H., Viteri, F.E. & King, J.C. (2002) Supplemental zinc lowers measures of iron status in young women with low iron reserves. *Journal of Nutrition*, **132**, 1860–4.
248. Mora, J.O. (2002) Iron supplements: overcoming technical and practical barriers. *Journal of Nutrition*, **132**, 853S–5.
249. Politt, E., Durnin, J.V.G.A., Husaini, M. & Jahari, A. (2000) Effects of an energy and micronutrient supplement on growth and development in undernourished children in Indonesia: methods. *European Journal of Clinical Nutrition*, **54**(Supplement), S16–20.
250. Mora, J.O. (2002) Iron supplements: overcoming technical and practical barriers. *Journal of Nutrition*, **132**, 853S–5S.
251. Ramakrishnan, U. & Yip, R. (2002) Experiences and challenges in industrialised countries: control of iron deficiency in industrialised countries. *Journal of Nutrition*, **132**, 820S–4S.
252. US Department of Health and Human Services (2000*) Healthy People 2010; Understanding and Improving Health and Objectives for Improving Health.* DHHS, Washington, DC.
253. Borgiato, E.V.M. & Martinez, F.E. (1998) Iron nutritional status is improved in Brazilian preterm infants fed food cooked in iron pots. *Journal of Nutrition*, **128**, 855–9.
254. Gopaldas, T. (2002) Iron-deficiency anaemia in young working women can be reduced by increasing the consumption of cereal-based fermented foods or gooseberry juice at the workplace. *Food and Nutrition Bulletin*, **23**, 94–7.
255. Bouis, H. (1996) Enrichment of food staples through plant breeding: a new strategy for fighting micronutrient malnutrition. *Nutrition Reviews*, **54**, 131–7.

Chapter 3
Zinc

3.1 Introduction

It was possible, not so many decades ago, to refer to zinc as the 'unassuming nutrient'[1]. Though the metal had been shown to be essential for the growth of the mould *Aspergillus niger* as early as 1869[2], it was another 50 years before it was recognised as essential, also, for animals. This was shown in the case of rats in 1934[3], and, shortly afterwards, the practical importance of zinc deficiency in farm animals was established[4]. By the 1950s, there was increasing evidence that zinc was required by humans and that certain metabolic abnormalities were related to zinc deficiency. There was some doubt, however, whether zinc deficiency could be of any real nutritional significance, since the element was so widely and abundantly distributed in the environment and was present in all diets. Then, in 1961, there was a major breakthrough in understanding of the role and essentiality of zinc when the syndrome of 'adolescent nutritional dwarfism' was identified in certain Middle Eastern countries and was shown to be related to zinc deficiency[5]. There was an immediate surge in interest in the element among investigators, though some still questioned whether zinc deficiency was of any relevance to prosperous industrialised countries that did not share the nutritional problems and restricted diets of the Middle East. By the mid-1970s, however, zinc deficiency was recognised even in industrialised countries. The condition, *acrodermatitis enteropathica* (AE), a rare autosomal recessively inherited disorder in which there is a defect in the body's ability to absorb zinc from the gut, had been identified[6]. Iatrogenic zinc deficiency was increasingly found to be a consequence of inadequate zinc in intravenous fluids used in total parenteral nutrition (TPN). Growth-limiting zinc deficiency has also been shown to occur in young urban children from socially deprived areas in the US[7].

In spite of this early interest in zinc and human nutrition, enthusiasm among investigators subsequently declined. There were a number of reasons for this, not least of which was the difficulty of determining zinc status in humans. That situation gradually changed, and by the end of the twentieth century, interest once more increased to such an extent that zinc had become one of the most widely investigated of the trace metal nutrients, not far behind iron in the number of papers in the scientific literature. Now, rather than the handful of research reports that would normally have been presented at scientific meetings a few decades earlier, whole conferences were devoted to the element. An international workshop held at the US National Institutes of Health in 1998, for instance, focused totally on what had become key areas of zinc research, including zinc nutrition; zinc and the GI tract and immune system; antioxidant defence functions of zinc; zinc and cellular mechanisms; zinc and the central nervous system; and zinc in growth and specific disease entities[8]. At a more recent conference, almost a third of the 300 presentations made were on zinc[9], 10 times more than were presented at a similar meeting some 15 years earlier[10].

3.2 Zinc distribution in the environment

Though not as abundant as iron, zinc is very widely distributed in the environment. Its concentration in soil ranges from less than 5 to about 3000 mg/kg[11]. In household dust, levels of more than 2 mg/kg have been recorded[12], while sewage sludge can contain 700–49 000 mg/kg[13]. Zinc is present in all foods, with 1 mg/kg or less in fruits to as much as 1 g/kg in oysters.

Zinc ores are widely distributed throughout the world. The principal commercially exploited ores are sphalerite or zinc blende (ZnS), calamine ($ZnCO_3$) and zincite (ZnO). Zinc frequently occurs in ores in association with other metals, such as lead, copper and cadmium, as well as arsenic.

Zinc is widely used commercially, both as the metal itself and as its compounds. Its principal use for many centuries was in brass, an alloy of 60–82% copper and 18–40% zinc. Today, its major use is in galvanising, the application of a layer of zinc to iron and other structural metals as a protection against corrosion. Zinc compounds are used in paints, plastics, pharmaceutical and domestic products, including ointments, nutritional supplements, detergents and other products. It is this widescale use that accounts for the high level of environmental contamination by zinc.

3.3 Zinc chemistry

Zinc is element number 30 of the periodic table. Its atomic weight of 65.37 is a consequence of its mixture of five stable isotopes: ^{64}Zn, ^{66}Zn, ^{67}Zn, ^{68}Zn and ^{70}Zn. It also has two radioisotopes, ^{65}Zn and ^{69}Zn. As we shall see, the availability of these isotopes has allowed considerable advances to be made in our understanding of its nutritional role.

Zinc has a density of 7.14, making it one of the 'heavy metals'. It is a bluish white, lustrous metal but tarnishes in air as a coat of zinc carbonate [$Zn_2(OH)_2CO_3$] develops. This forms a tough adhering layer and is one of the reasons why zinc is used to 'galvanise' other less resistant metals. Zinc has a low melting point of 420°C and is ductile and malleable when heated to 100°C.

Zinc belongs to Group 12/IIB of the Periodic Table, along with cadmium and mercury, and like them, its electronic structure has two electrons in its outer shell and 18 in its underlying shell. It is thus, strictly speaking, a *representative* metal, with a +2 oxidation state. It does, however, have certain characteristics similar to those of the first-row *transition* metals that are its neighbours in Period 4. For this reason, zinc is often treated in the literature as one of the transition metals[14], even though it does not have their variable valency and therefore cannot function directly in redox reactions[15].

Zinc is a chemically reactive element. It combines readily with non-oxidising acids, releasing hydrogen and forming salts. It also dissolves in strong acids to form zincate ions

(ZnO_2^{2-}). It reacts with oxygen, especially at high temperatures, to form zinc oxide (ZnO). It also reacts directly with halogens, sulphur and other non-metals. Zinc forms alloys with other metals. One of these is brass, made of copper, zinc and other metals; zinc is also added to the copper and tin alloy, bronze.

Fraústo da Silva and Williams, in their insightful study of bio-inorganic chemistry[16], ask the question: why was zinc, rather than another metal, such as one of the transition elements, selected during the course of evolution for its unique role in life processes? The answer they give is because zinc has highly distinctive chemical properties that make it more suitable than other elements for this purpose. It is not any one property that accounts for this selection, but rather a combination of several characteristics, that enables zinc to perform roles for which other elements are less well suited. These characteristics include the small size of the zinc ion that gives it a highly concentrated charge and strong electrostatic binding capacity. Its high affinity for electrons makes zinc a strong Lewis acid enabling it to form a bond with a base by accepting from it a lone pair of electrons. These properties are not unique to zinc. Copper and nickel, for example, also have strong electrostatic binding and can attach themselves as firmly to donors, such as thiolates and amines, as can zinc. But, unlike them, zinc does not show variable valence and oxidation state change, and consequently does not introduce the risk of free-radical oxidative damage when used in biological compartments. Cadmium, its closely related non-transition neighbour in Group 12, does have similar properties and is known to be able to substitute for zinc in several enzymes. However, cadmium is a much rarer element and is less readily available, two reasons why zinc, rather than cadmium, is used in life processes.

3.4 The biology of zinc

Zinc is ubiquitous in cellular metabolism. It is an essential component of the catalytic site of at least one enzyme in each of the six classes listed by IUPAC[17], as indicated in Table 3.1. More than 200 zinc enzymes are known, of which more than 50 play metabolic roles in animals. The metal also has other vital functions, including the provision of structural integrity to many metabolically important proteins, including enzymes. This extraordinary

Table 3.1 Examples of zinc metalloenzymes.

Enzyme	Number of Zn ions in enzyme	Enzyme class
Alcohol dehydrogenase	Two	Oxidoreductase
RNA polymerase	Two	Transferase
Alkaline phosphatase	Two	Hydrolase
Carbonic anhydrase	One	Lyase
Aldolase	One	Isomerase
t-RNA synthetase	One or two	Ligase

Adapted from Rink, L. & Gabriel, P. (2000) Zinc and the immune system. *Proceedings of the Nutrition Society,* **59**, 541–52.

usefulness in biological systems is accounted for by a combination of chemical properties. Not least of these is the exceptional ability of the zinc atom to participate in strong but readily exchangeable ligand binding, together with considerable flexibility of its coordination chemistry[18]. Because its *d*-shell orbital is filled, the zinc atom has a ligand-field stabilisation energy of zero in all liganding geometries, and hence no geometry is inherently more stable than another. This lack of an energy barrier to a multiplicity of equally accessible coordination geometries can be used by zinc metalloenzymes to alter the reactivity of the metal ion and may be an important factor in its ability to catalyse transformations accompanied by changes in the metal coordination geometry[19]. The activity of the catalytic sites in many zinc metalloenzymes is enhanced by the slightly distorted condition of the metal geometry imposed by proximity of the atom to the protein side chains adjacent to the site[20].

3.4.1 Zinc enzymes

The zinc ion can have three different roles in enzymes: catalytic, co-catalytic or structural[21]. In a catalytic site, the ion is located at the active centre of an enzyme and participates directly in the catalytic mechanism, interacting with the substrate molecule in a bond-making or -breaking step. In multimetal enzymes, two or more zinc, or other metal, atoms operate in concert in a co-catalytic role. Examples are the enzyme alkaline phosphatase, which has two zinc and one magnesium ion, and leucine aminopeptidase, with two zinc ions[22]. In structural sites, the function of the zinc ion is to stabilise the tertiary structure of the metalloenzyme. The zinc ion is coordinated by four amino acids in a tetrahedral geometry which provides both local and overall stability analagous to that provided by disulphides[23].

3.4.2 Zinc finger proteins

Zinc atoms have structural roles also in many other proteins. These are ubiquitous and of considerable importance in cellular and subcellular metabolism, especially in a regulatory role[24]. One of these, of considerable current interest, is the zinc finger motif which is the most common recurring motif for those transcription factors that link with the double helix of DNA[25]. The configuration of a finger, which determines its binding to DNA, is dependent on a single zinc atom at its base. The linking of zinc fingers to corresponding sites on DNA initiates the transcription process and gene expression. Similar motifs have been identified in the tertiary structure of nuclear hormone receptors, such as those for oestrogen, testosterone and vitamin D. The large number of zinc finger proteins that have been identified points to a major role for zinc in gene expression[26]. There is growing evidence that the expression of a number of genes is modulated by the quantity of zinc ingested and absorbed[27].

The many zinc-dependent metabolic and other functions that occur in the body provide an explanation why the consequences of zinc deficiency are so many and so varied, and also why they are so non-specific. The multiple roles of zinc in cellular growth and development also underline the element's importance during periods of rapid pre- and postnatal growth, as well as for the immune system, in which cells have such rapid turnover[28].

3.5 Absorption and metabolism of zinc

Though zinc is widely distributed in both plant and animal foodstuffs, the amounts in different kinds of foods show a wide variation, from less than 1 mg/kg in some fruits to more than 1000 mg/kg in certain shellfish[29]. Consequently, uptake of the element from different diets will vary, depending on the actual mixture of different foods consumed. However, it is not simply the total amount of zinc present that accounts for the amount taken in by the body. This will be determined, partly by the chemical form of the element and, to a much greater extent, by the presence or absence of other components of the food which either inhibit or enhance uptake. In addition, several other factors, such as the zinc status of the consumer, are of importance in determining how much of the zinc present in the foods ingested is actually absorbed. Depending on the composition of the diet, and other factors, intestinal zinc absorption in humans is between 20 and 40% of intake[30]. A range of 1–58% of the total ingested has been estimated for most animal species, including man[31].

3.5.1 *Chemical forms of zinc in food*

Little information has been published on the different chemical forms of zinc that occur in foods. It is clear that much of the element in plants and animals used as food is incorporated into organic compounds, in zinc metalloenzymes and other zinc-containing proteins. Some zinc may also be present in an inorganic form, especially in plant foodstuffs[32]. As has been seen in the case of iron, it can be expected that organically bound zinc is more readily bioavailable than inorganic zinc, though there is no evidence that there are separate pathways for absorption of the two forms, as there is for haem and inorganic iron. Different inorganic chemical species of zinc, which are used as dietary supplements, have been shown to differ in their bioavailability. For example, though zinc oxide is widely used as a supplement in animal husbandry, it is considerably less bioavailable than either zinc sulphate or zinc acetate. Zinc carbonate is also poorly absorbed, compared with the sulphate or acetate[33]. Organically bound zinc, including zinc methionine and zinc proteinates, also used as dietary supplements for farm animals, has been shown to be more readily absorbed and more effective than inorganic forms[34].

3.5.2 *Promoters and inhibitors of zinc absorption*

Several naturally occurring components of the diet can have a considerable effect on zinc absorption. Protein has a positive effect, and the presence of even modest amounts of animal protein (meat, poultry, fish) has been shown to enhance uptake, while at the same time increasing the absolute amount of zinc in the meal[35]. Uptake is also enhanced by the presence of low molecular weight organic substances, including the sulphur-containing amino acids methionine and cysteine, and hydroxy acids such as citric and lactic acid[36].

While there is interest, especially from a public health point of view, among nutritionists, in promoters of zinc absorption, this is considerably less than the level of interest shown in inhibitors of the process, at least to judge by the number of publications on the subject in recent years. Several naturally occurring inhibitors of zinc absorption are widespread in foods and occur in sufficient quantities to have significant consequences for the nutritional status of large numbers of people.

Phytates, which are phosphorylated forms of inositol (inositol hexaphosphates) and phytic acid (inositol pentaphosphate) are the most important of the naturally occurring inhibitors of zinc absorption. Both occur in different amounts in different foodstuffs, with the highest concentrations in cereals and legumes.

Fractional absorption of zinc is inversely related to the phytate content of a meal[37]. As we shall see later, the high phytate-to-zinc molar ratio of many plant-based diets is a major factor contributing to zinc deficiency on a worldwide basis[38]. Absorption of zinc can also be significantly affected by the presence of other metals in the diet. Uptake is inhibited by the divalent cations, including calcium, cadmium, iron, copper, nickel, magnesium and tin[39]. The negative effect of iron on zinc uptake is of some concern because of the use of iron supplements, especially by women during pregnancy. A reduction in their plasma zinc levels following iron supplementation, with possible adverse effects on the fetus, has been demonstrated[40]. A similar problem may result from the use of iron supplements, especially in nutritional rehabilitation programmes in situations where populations may be at risk of deficiencies of both iron and zinc. This is of particular concern in the case of infants and young children[41]. Calcium, especially in the presence of phytate, can also limit zinc uptake from food. However, whether calcium supplementation has an adverse effect on zinc homeostasis is still to be clarified[42].

3.5.3 Relation of zinc uptake to physiological state

During periods of active growth and in physiological states, such as infancy, pregnancy and lactation, when zinc requirements are high, there is a corresponding increase in the fractional absorption of zinc. In breast-fed infants, for instance, fractional absorption of zinc can be as high as 55%[43]. Fractional absorption has also been found to increase during gestation, though the level of increase may depend on the pre-existing zinc status of the pregnant women[44]. A significant increase in zinc absorption has been reported to occur during the early stages of human lactation[45].

3.6 Zinc homeostasis

Zinc is absorbed into the body throughout the gut, but, since there is a large enteropancreatic circulation of the element, net intestinal absorption occurs in the distal small intestine[46]. The total body zinc content of adult humans ranges from about 1.5 to 2.5 mg, most of which is found intracellularly, primarily in muscle, bone, liver and other organs[47], as indicated in Table 3.2. Less than 0.2% of the total body zinc content circulates in plasma, at a concentration of about 1 mg/l. It has been demonstrated in experimental animals that the body is able to maintain a relatively constant level of zinc in the whole body, even though dietary zinc intake varies by as much as 10-fold.[48] The same appears to be the case with humans. The mechanisms involved in maintaining this constancy of zinc levels are complex and not yet fully understood.

The body's zinc is divided between two separate pools or series of pools of unequal size. As much as 90% is contained in slowly exchanging pools located principally in

Table 3.2 Zinc content of some human organs.

	Zinc content	
Organ	μg/g dry weight	% whole body Zn
Muscle	51	57.0
Bone	100	29.0
Skin	32	6.0
Liver	58	5.0
Brain	11	1.5
Kidneys	55	0.7
Heart	23	0.4

Adapted from Mills, C.F. (1989) *Zinc in Human Biology: Human Nutrition Reviews*, p. 19. Springer, London.

muscle and bone. This pool appears to be important especially for total body zinc homeostasis[49]. The other 10% of the body's zinc is located in a combination of pools in the liver, pancreas, gastrointestinal tract and other viscera. This zinc exchanges rapidly with zinc in plasma and is particularly sensitive to the quantity of zinc ingested and absorbed[50].

The ability of the body to maintain a constant internal state in the face of varying external conditions is refereed to as *homeostasis*, when the nutrient flow is within an open system, and *homeorhesis*, when continual retention occurs in the form of growth, reproduction or production of products, such as milk and eggs. The body adapts to a variable dietary supply of zinc, as well as of other trace elements, by controlling absorption, excretion and secretion, as well as by transient changes in the trace element content of storage tissues.

3.6.1 Zinc absorption in the gastrointestinal tract

Zinc homeostasis involves adjustment of both zinc absorption and endogenous excretion into the faeces and urine. The gastrointestinal tract plays a predominant role in maintaining total body homeostasis. In addition to providing partial regulation of absorption of exogenous dietary zinc, the gut is the major route for excretion of endogenous zinc. After a meal, large quantities of zinc are secreted into the gut lumen, most of which is subsequently reabsorbed[51].

Endogenous excretion of trace elements is made up of two components and takes place primarily via the faeces and urine. One consists of inevitable, or obligatory, losses, which are attributable to the maintenance of metabolism and account for the total trace element excretion, if the dietary supply is deficient or just adequate. The other is an additional excretion that starts as soon as the absorbed amount of the element exceeds requirements. Which regulatory excretion pathway (faeces or urine) is given preference depends on the type of the trace element in question. In the case of zinc, urinary excretion is relatively unimportant compared with the endogenous excretion[52].

In balance studies using rats, it has been shown that the efficiency of zinc absorption can decrease from nearly 100% when a zinc-free diet is fed, to approximately 55% when intake is significantly increased, while endogenous faecal zinc (EFZ) varies as much as 30-fold over the same range of intake[53]. EFZ represents the main portion of the total zinc in faeces. Its excretion is of major importance in maintaining zinc balance just above and below optimal intakes.

Use of the isotope dilution technique, in which the body's zinc pool is labelled with a stable isotope and zinc concentration measured in faeces and in blood once a steady state relative to total excretion has been reached, has allowed calculation of levels of endogenous excretion in response to differing intakes. Such studies have shown that there is a pronounced homeostatic regulation of absorption, which responds to the ratio of dietary supply to intermediate requirement and declines with increasing dietary intake[54].

Adjustments in fractional zinc absorption in response to levels of dietary intake can be considerable. In a study of the effect of reduction of zinc intake to a very low level by healthy adult men, fractional zinc absorption increased from 25 to 93%. In contrast, a doubling of zinc intake reduced fractional intake to 21%[55]. In general, the lower the intake, the higher the rate of fractional zinc absorption. Increases in fractional zinc absorption can be used as a gross indicator of the amount of zinc consumed. However, since it also varies sufficiently within a group of individuals consuming the same amount of zinc, it is impossible to predict zinc intakes from the efficiency of absorption measured at a single time[56].

3.6.1.1 Transfer of zinc across the mucosal membrane

How zinc is carried across the mucosal membrane, or any other cell membrane, and on to sites for storage or utilisation, or how it is re-exported from absorptive cells, is still far from fully understood. Earlier studies found evidence of a saturable, energy-dependent process in which low-molecular-weight zinc-binding ligands in the intestinal lumen and metallothionein within the mucosal cells played major roles. How exactly the zinc was translocated from the lumen across the cell membrane was unclear[57]. It is now recognised that zinc is moved in and out of cells by a series of transport proteins. A considerable amount of research is currently being carried out to clarify the nature and specific roles of these transporters.

3.6.1.2 Zinc transporters

A picture of a far more complex transport network than was initially expected is now appearing. It is becoming clear that an array of transporter proteins are involved from at least two gene families[58]. Though their functions often overlap, their locations, tissue specificities and responses to dietary zinc are different[59].

What is known as the ZnT family of transporters consists of four intergral membrane proteins that have specific groups for attaching and moving zinc. The proteins have six transmembrane domains that anchor the protein to the membrane and are positioned to assure unidirectional movement out of the cytosol. A histidine-rich loop extends from the protein into the cytosol and is believed to bind zinc destined for export from the cell. The zinc ions are transported through pores that are opened up in the cell membrane by interaction between neighbouring transport proteins. It is believed that the ZnT family mainly exports zinc ions from the cell or into cytosolic compartments, to prevent build up of free ions[60].

The four different ZnTs appear to have related, but biologically different, properties. They do not all occur in the same tissues or, where they are present in the same tissue, are not at the same concentration. The highest concentration of ZnT-1, for instance, occurs in placenta, kidney, adipose and upper intestine, mostly excretory tissues involved in transmural movement of zinc. ZnT-2 is also present in intestine and kidney, but with much less in placenta, and is virtually absent from adipose tissue. There are also differences between concentrations of the other two ZnTs in these tissues. Investigation of the levels of expression of mRNAs of the ZnTs has indicated that there are important differences between the transporters in their response to zinc, pointing to their different roles in relation to overall maintenance of zinc homeostasis[61]. While, for instance, ZnT-1 and ZnT-2 respond to zinc, ZnT-4 mRNA is not influenced by the presence of the metal, suggesting that, unlike the other two, it has a constitutive, as opposed to regulatory, capacity with regard to zinc. Interestingly, ZnT-4 appears to have a special role of its own. Its mRNA has been found to be highest in early mammary gland but declines with age, suggesting a link to lactation. In addition, ZnT-4 is known to be associated with the toxic milk mouse, a disorder characterised by the failure of pups to survive weaning because of a failure of zinc to pass into the milk of the dam[62]. An additional member of the group, ZnT-5, has recently been identified with a role in osteoblast maturation and cardiac electrical conductance[63].

This very complex picture of control of zinc homeostatis, as has been noted in a recent review on which much of the foregoing discussion is based, is only half the story[64]. Another important group of carriers, the ZIP family, is required for zinc influx and complements the efflux functions of the ZnT family. In addition to zinc, the ZIP family can transport iron, manganese, cadmium and other divalent cations into cells[65]. One member of the family has been shown to mediate zinc uptake in transfected human erythroleukaemic cells and to be located on the cell wall and not intracellularly[66]. Moreover, zinc transport is stimulated by bicarbonate (HCO_3^-) in the medium, suggesting that one of the ZIP transporters is the genetically impaired factor responsible for the disorder, AE, which is characterised by a lack of a bicarbonate-stimulated zinc transport mechanism[67].

The ZIP family is not the only type of transporter that brings zinc into cells. Another is the divalent metal transporter DMT1, also known as DCT-1 and Nramp2, which we have met when discussing uptake of iron by erythrocytes and other cells. In addition to iron, DMT1 has the capacity to transport zinc, manganese, cobalt, cadmium, copper, nickel and lead, in that order of affinity[68]. DMT1 is present in the gastrointestinal tract, bone marrow and other tissues, but little is known about its particular role in regard to zinc, especially its selectivity for zinc, rather than iron[69]. What is clear is that zinc transporters differ in tissue specificity, location in cells, outward or inward movement, regulated or constitutive expression, and sensitivity to zinc[70].

3.6.2 Regulation of zinc homeostasis at different levels of dietary intake

There is some evidence that zinc homeostasis is maintained differently in people with adequate zinc intakes compared with those who are deficient. Endogenous faecal zinc levels have been shown to be affected both by whole body zinc status and by current dietary intake[71], whereas fractional zinc absorption is only affected by current intake. Thus, the effect on EFZ losses of an increase in intake of dietary zinc by a population in marginal zinc status is not the same as it would be if their normal zinc status had been high. A study of long-term low zinc intakes in men found that under these conditions, fractional intake increased by 48%, while total absorption declined by 44% and EFZ losses by 27%. Over the six-month period of the study, fractional and total zinc absorption remained relatively constant, but EFZ continued to decline. The overall effect was that the men achieved a positive crude zinc balance on a very low zinc intake, though over a prolonged period[72].

Several other studies have also produced evidence that EFZ excretion is directly related to the total amount of zinc absorbed after a state of equilibrium has been established on the level of intake. One of these, a study of two groups of Chinese women, one rural, with a low dietary zinc intake, the other urban with a zinc-adequate diet, found that the increased amount of zinc absorbed by the urban women was nearly balanced by an increase in EFZ losses, while the rural women achieved balance by reducing EFZ losses[73].

While it is clear that zinc balance can be established, even if dietary intake is very low, by reducing endogenous zinc losses, this adjustment in zinc homeostasis may not be enough to replace zinc losses in the integument and, in the case of males, semen[74]. Moreover, when tissue demands for zinc are increased, the relationship between zinc absorption and EFZ losses is likely to change. During lactation, for example, fractional zinc absorption increases, while EFZ losses remain unchanged[75].

3.6.3 Effect of changes in zinc intake on renal losses

Renal losses of zinc are low compared with losses from the GI tract. They also tend to remain relatively constant over a wide range of dietary intake. When zinc intakes are very low, however, losses of zinc in urine decline. The fall in urinary zinc precedes any change in plasma zinc levels of fractional zinc absorption. How such regulation of urinary zinc excretion occurs is not well understood. Hormonal changes and adjustments in renal tubular zinc transport may be involved.

Compared with the effects of decreases in EFZ losses, changes in urinary zinc levels with a very low dietary zinc intake have little impact on zinc conservation. However, in combination with the rapid changes in EFZ levels, urinary losses help to limit a drop in plasma zinc levels following a decrease in dietary zinc intake. As a result, plasma zinc levels change very slowly, if at all, with changes in zinc intake. It is for this reason that measurement of plasma zinc levels is only of limited value as a means of assessing zinc status[76].

3.6.4 Other sources of zinc loss

Zinc is lost to the body by several other routes, in addition to the intestine and the kidneys. These include integumental losses, in sweat, skin and other surface tissues, seminal emissions in men and menstrual in women, as well as through hair and nail growth. Whole body surface losses of about 0.5 mg/d on an adequate diet have been estimated.

Surface losses of zinc are reduced when dietary intakes fall and increase with high intakes. Growth of nail and hair accounts for only a small proportion of overall surface losses, at about 0.03 mg/d[77]. These adjustments in surface losses can occur, even though plasma zinc levels remain in the normal range[78].

Levels of zinc in semen are normally high. Losses can be significant, at about 0.6 mg in each ejaculation. Semen zinc losses decline with zinc depletion. If this is severe, there can be a reduction of 50% in the amount of zinc per ejaculation. The reduction, however, seems to be due not to a reduction in zinc concentration but to a decrease in semen volume[79].

3.7 Effects of changes in dietary zinc intakes on tissue levels

A negative zinc balance can arise with an inadequate dietary intake, especially if this is prolonged. Under such circumstances, the body's homeostatic control may be unable to replace zinc losses. It has been shown, in rats on a low zinc diet, that total body zinc is reduced to about 30% of levels in controls. The loss does not come equally from all tissues: hair, skin, heart and skeletal levels remain constant, while blood plasma, bone and testes levels are significantly decreased. Similar changes have been observed in humans[80].

The reason for such differential retention and loss of zinc from different body tissues is a subject of debate at the present time. It has been suggested that the drop in plasma zinc levels after the initiation of a severely low-zinc diet signals certain tissues to retain their zinc and others to release it[81]. About 90% of the body's zinc is contained in slowly exchanging pools, mainly in bone and muscle. Though these pools are important to the organ systems in which they occur, as well as to total body homeostasis, it is the other 10% of body zinc that responds particularly to changes in dietary zinc levels. This is the rapidly exchangeable zinc pool and includes zinc found in liver, pancreas and other viscera[82].

3.7.1 Zinc in bone

Bone contains about one-third of the total zinc in the body. Bone can, apparently, accumulate zinc when dietary intake is high. However, it is not, strictly speaking, a zinc store, since release of the metal is not enhanced during dietary insufficiency. Nevertheless, bone plays an important part in ensuring a supply of endogenous zinc to the body. The fall in its levels of zinc may reflect, at least partially, a reduction in uptake in response to a fall in plasma zinc, rather than to increased release. The zinc released from bone has been shown to come primarily from a rapidly turning over pool that makes up 10–20% of total bone zinc. A second pool has a low turnover and releases zinc more slowly[83]. Thus, bone appears to function as a passive reserve of zinc that is released, but not replaced, when dietary intake is low. Normal bone turnover, rather than any specific mechanism, seems to be responsible for the release of zinc when plasma levels are reduced. This is in contrast to muscle, the other major store of slowly exchanging zinc in the body. In that tissue, zinc deposition is maintained at a rate that preserves the normal concentration[84].

3.7.2 Zinc in plasma

Plasma contains about 0.1% of the body's zinc, a total of about 3.5 mg at an average concentration of 1 mg/l. The metal is bound mainly to albumin, with smaller amounts attached to α_2-macroglobulin and oligopeptides[85]. Because of its high mobility and its immunological importance, plasma, though only a minor zinc pool compared, for example, with liver and muscle, is of major significance to health[86]. However, since zinc concentrations in these other tissues are as much as 50% higher than in blood, small differences in uptake or release of zinc from these sites can have a considerable effect on plasma zinc levels. For this reason, plasma zinc concentrations are not a reliable measure of total body stores under all circumstances. Even when dietary zinc intake is extremely low, for example as a result of starvation, catabolism of muscle can release sufficient zinc to cause an elevation of plasma levels[87]. In contrast, plasma zinc levels may fall, following consumption of a meal, even when dietary intake and tissue reserves are adequate[88]. Plasma levels can also be affected by a number of non-dietary factors, such as intestinal disease[89], infection[90], surgery[91] and strenuous physical exercise[92], all of which can affect transport and/or absorption of the metal.

3.8 Effects of zinc deficiency

Since zinc plays many important roles in a great variety of metabolic activities and is found so widely distributed in tissues and in every cell of the body, dietary zinc deficiency can be expected to have a wide range of consequences. What all these are, however, is not easy to pinpoint, mainly because so many of them overlap with the effects of deficiencies of other nutrients and are non-specific. This is especially true of mild zinc deficiency. In severe deficiency, the consequences of an inadequate uptake can be recognised more easily, though even then, there can be uncertainties.

3.8.1 Severe zinc deficiency

Observation of the effects of severe zinc deficiency in adolescent males in Egypt and Iran[93], and in children with AE[94], provided evidence that organ systems affected included the epidermal, gastrointestinal, central nervous, immune, skeletal and reproductive[95]. Clinical features seen in cases of AE include bullous pustular dermatitis and other epidermal lesions, especially prominent skin lesions primarily around the body orifices and at the extremities, as well as alopecia, diarrhoea and failure to thrive. Before the use of oral zinc supplements to treat the disease was introduced, its victims typically died in late infancy[96]. A wide variety and severity of immune defects, with corresponding vulnerability to infection[97], as well as defects in the central nervous system are also commonly identified in cases of AE[98].

3.8.2 Mild zinc deficiency

Many of the features of severe zinc deficiency are reproduced, but normally in a much less aggressive form, in milder zinc deficiency. Much of the information on the clinical effects of such deficiency has been obtained through observation of the results of randomised intervention studies with dietary zinc supplements. These have confirmed in particular the role played by zinc deficiency in impaired physical and neurophysiological development and the prevalence of gastrointestinal and respiratory infections among populations with a chronically low zinc intake[99].

3.8.3 Zinc deficiency and growth in children

There is a close connection between zinc deficiency and impairment of physical growth. Many studies carried out in different countries have shown that modest dietary zinc supplementation can lead to an increase in growth velocity and height in infants and young children whose normal zinc intake is low[100].

3.8.3.1 Zinc deficiency and diarrhoea in children

Zinc deficiency is commonly associated with acute and persistent diarrhoea, especially in children. This is a very serious and widespread problem in many poorer communities, of the developing as well as the developed world. The effectiveness of zinc supplementation in reducing the duration and severity of diarrhoea has been found in many studies[101]. A concurrent effect of zinc supplementation of children at a community level has been shown to be an increase in growth velocity. Whether these effects are due to improvements in immune response and the intestinal mucosal cell transport mechanisms[102] or simply to a correction of a zinc deficiency state that is the cause of, or contributing to, the diarrhoea is unclear. In populations in which these beneficial effects of zinc supplementation have been observed, habitual intake of dietary zinc is usually deficient. Moreover, losses of zinc via the intestine are likely to be increased by diarrhoea, contributing to the deficiency and thus involving a vicious cycle[103].

3.8.3.2 Zinc deficiency and infection in children

There is evidence of a connection between mild zinc deficiency and the incidence of various infections in children. There have been reports of reductions in the incidence of pneumonia, as well as of malaria and some other infections by the use of zinc supplements[104].

3.8.3.3 Zinc deficiency and neurophysiological behaviour

Zinc supplementation of young children in poor communities in certain developing countries has also, apparently, brought about improvements in neurophysiological performance[105], as well as of brain development[106]. A number of behavioural abnormalities which appear to respond favourably to zinc supplementation have been described in humans. These include mood changes, emotional lability, anorexia, dysfunction of taste and smell, irritability and depression[107]. There is uncertainty about the mechanisms by which zinc deprivation induces such behavioural responses. In the case of zinc deficiency-induced anorexia, for instance, it is not clear whether the deficiency is an initiating cause or an accelerating or exacerbating factor that may deepen the pathology of the condition[108].

3.9 Zinc and the immune system

The importance of zinc for host immunity has been recognised for several decades, but it is only relatively recently that the underlying mechanisms whereby the metal exerts its effects on immune function have begun to be understood[109]. Though many gaps still remain in out knowledge, the overall pattern can now be discerned. It is a very complex picture, parts of which are still obscure. It will not be considered in detail here, but for readers who have an adequate background in molecular and cell biology and want to learn more about the details of zinc immunobiology, a number of excellent reviews are available. Particularly recommended are those by Walsh *et al.*[110], and Zalewski[111], which, though written nearly a decade ago are still very informative. More up-to-date information is provided in the study by Shankar and Prasad[112], on which much of the present section is based, and by the review by Rink and Gabriel[113], also cited above.

Zinc is involved critically at many different levels of the immune system, from the protective barrier of the skin to gene regulation within lymphocytes. An adequate supply of the metal is essential for normal development and function of neutrophils and natural killer (NK) and other cells that mediate non-specific immunity. Key immunological mediators of acquired immunity are also dependent on zinc. Zinc deficiency prevents the outgrowth and some other functions of T-lymphocytes. B-lymphocyte development and antibody production are also compromised. There is also an adverse effect on macrophages, with consequent disruption of such immunological activities as intracellular killing, cytokine production and phagocytosis. These many effects of zinc deficiency have their origin in the multiple and varied role of the metal in cellular function, such as DNA replication, RNA transcription, cell division and activation[114].

3.9.1 Zinc and thymulin activity

Thymulin, a peptide composed of nine amino acids, which is secreted by thymic epithelial cells, promotes T-lymphocyte maturation, cytotoxicity, and IL-2 production. The peptide requires zinc for its biological activity. The metal is bound to the thymulin via the side chains of asparagine and the hydroxyl groups of two serines, in a 1:1 stoichiometry. The binding produces a conformational change in the peptide that is necessary for its activity. Thymulin can be detected in the plasma of zinc-deficient patients, but until zinc levels are increased, it remains inactive. For this reason, the assay of serum thymulin has been suggested as a sensitive method for detecting zinc deficiency in humans[115].

3.9.2 Zinc and the epidermal barriers to infection

The epidermal cells of the skin and the linings of the gastrointestinal and pulmonary tracts are important components of non-specific innate immunity. Zinc deficiency damages these cells and results, for example, in the characteristic lesions of AE[116]. This damage may also contribute to incidents of diarrhoea and diphtheria in zinc-deficient children[117].

3.9.3 Zinc and apoptosis

Apoptosis, the so-called cell suicide process, also known as gene-directed cell death or, less correctly, programmed cell death[118] is a normal physiological process involved in a number of important physiological processes, from epithelial turnover to T- and B-lymphocyte development[119]. Without apoptosis, cell development is not maintained, the exclusion of autoimmune T-cells and B-cells is lost, and the killing activity of cytotoxic T-cells and NK cells decreases. Apoptosis is regulated by zinc. On the one hand, zinc deficiency inhibits the process; on the other hand, the presence of zinc can protect cells against undergoing apoptosis. Zinc deficiency causes enhanced spontaneous and toxin-induced apoptosis in many different cell types, including thymocytes, macrophages and T-lymphocytes[120].

The protective action of zinc against apoptosis has been reported in relation to almost all apoptosis-inducing factors, including tumour necrosis factor-α, cytotoxic T-cells, cold shock, hyperthermia and γ-irradiation[121]. The mechanism involved in this inhibition of apoptosis is unclear, but it is likely that zinc has various independent anti-apoptotic effects[122]. There is evidence that the zinc/calcium balance in tissues is important in regulating the activity of Ca/Mg DNA endonuclease activity, which is correlated with inhibition of apoptotic DNA fragmentation[123]. It may also be that the zinc-dependent enzyme nucleoside phosphorylase may inhibit apoptosis by preventing accumulation of toxic nucleotides[124]. A major redistribution of zinc can be observed in cells undergoing apoptosis. Cytoplasmic zinc increases significantly, with a release of free zinc from intracellular pools and metalloenzymes[125].

3.9.4 Effects of high zinc intake on the immune system

There is evidence that a high intake of zinc may, in some cases, have a negative effect on immune function. Impairment of lymphocyte proliferative reponses and a reduction in chemotaxis and phagocytosis of circulating polymorphonuclear leukocytes have been reported in healthy adults given a zinc intake 10–20 times the recommended intake[126]. An adverse effect of excess zinc on neonate immunity has also been observed.[127] Anaemia, growth retardation, copper deficiency and immunosuppression have also been reported to occur as a result of excessive intake by both children and adults. Such adverse effects point to the need for caution when large zinc supplements are taken for prolonged periods of time[128].

3.9.5 Effect of zinc on immunity in the elderly

The immune response is often compromised in the elderly, with increased vulnerability to respiratory infections and greater morbidity. It is possible that these adverse developments may, in part, be related to zinc deficiency, which is also common in the elderly[129]. The use of zinc supplements has been shown to bring about a significant improvement in thymic function and antibody response in elderly subjects[130].

3.10 The antioxidant role of zinc

Zinc-deprived animals are known to be more sensitive than are zinc-replete animals to a variety of oxidative stresses[131]. The antioxidant properties of the metal have also been demonstrated[132]. How zinc functions in this way, however, is far from clear. Its antioxidant properties appear to be independent of its metalloenzyme activity. In strict chemical terms, zinc is not an antioxidant and cannot interact directly with antioxidant species. However, it is able to perform the role of antioxidant, which it does efficiently and in numerous locations in the body, in an indirect manner. A number of different mechanisms appear to be involved, but the biochemical bases of their antioxidant roles are not clear. In the short term, zinc may preserve the integrity of proteins against oxidative damage either by stabilisation of their sulphydryl groups or by causing steric hindrance or a conformational change by binding to a site adjacent to the sulphydryl groups. It may also be able to prevent the formation of oxygen radicals from hydrogen peroxide produced during immune activation by antagonising redox-active transition metals, such as iron and copper that can catalyse lipid peroxidation[133].

3.10.1 Zinc metallothionein

Zinc can also act as an antioxidant by inducing the formation of some other substance that will then function as the ultimate antioxidant. It is known, for example, that zinc regulates the expression in lymphocytes of metallothionein and metallothionein-like proteins that have antioxidant activity, and there is increasing evidence that metallothionein provides the crucial link between zinc and the cell's redox state[134].

The metallothioneins (MTs) are a family of low molecular weight proteins with at least 17 gene products[135]. They have strong metal-binding abilities, especially to zinc, as well as to cadmium, copper and other heavy metals. The MTs are known to play a role in the regulation of zinc and copper homeostasis and are also involved in protection against toxic metals[136], as well as in cellular defences against oxygen and nitrogen free radical species[137].

Each MT molecule contains 60–80 amino acids, of which 15–27% are cysteine, with no aromatic residues or disulphide bonds. MT can contain 5–7 g of zinc per mole bound to cysteine residues in two domains. The protein envelops the zinc in a zinc/sulphur network that shields it from external ligands. The metal is bound more tightly and is at a higher concentration than in most other zinc proteins. MT is believed to act as a thermodynamic 'sink' for zinc, and makes up 5–10% of the total zinc in a human hepatocyte. Release of the zinc appears to require a conformational change in the protein molecule[138].

It is not clear how this zinc-MT operates as an antioxidant. It is believed that the association of the zinc with the cysteine sulphur ligands in a sulphur-cluster structure is central to the molecular mechanisms involved. This allows the cysteine sulphur ligands to be oxidised and reduced with concomitant release and binding of the otherwise redox-inert zinc. In this way, MT becomes a redox protein, in which the redox chemistry originates not from the metal atom but from its coordination environment[139].

Because of the low redox potential of these zinc/sulphur clusters, MT is readily oxidised by a number of mild cellular oxidants, which results in the release of the Zn^{2+} ion. This allows biochemical coupling of reactions between zinc/sulphur centres and redox-active compounds, and thus the coordination states of zinc become part of the redox environment of the cell[140]. Evidence has been produced which indicates that certain sulphur compounds, including glutathione disulphide (GSSG) and other biological disulphides, as well as certain low molecular weight selenium compounds and seleno-enzymes, act as releasing factors for MT-bound zinc[141]. This would account for the part played by metallothionein in zinc homeostasis[142] and also for a possible role of selenium in the maintenance of zinc status[143].

3.10.2 Nitric oxide and zinc release from MT

Nitric oxide (NO) has also been shown to play a role in releasing zinc from metallothionein. NO is a metabolic intermediate involved in the regulation of critical physiological functions, including blood vessel homeostasis, neuronal transmission and host response to infection. It acts as a ubiquitous messenger which allows cells to communicate with each other through redox signalling[144]. It is known that NO is capable of increasing labile zinc levels in several different cells, including brain and vascular cells. There is evidence from *in vitro* studies that zinc/sulphur clusters of MT are involved in NO signalling in the vascular cell walls[145].

3.11 Zinc requirements

It has not proved easy for expert committees on dietary standards to estimate zinc requirements and to set recommended allowances. A particular impediment to their efforts has been the continuing absence of a sensitive indicator of zinc status. The difficulty is increased by the fact that there is strong homeostatic control over zinc absorption and excretion which maintains zinc balance, even when intakes are lower than real requirements in the long term. A number of other difficult-to-quantify factors can also obfuscate the issue. Of particular importance among these is the health status, since fluctuations in zinc excretion are associated with inflammation and a variety of diseases[146]. In addition, the availability of zinc in foods consumed, which, in its turn, is dependent on the overall composition of the diet, has to be taken into account when estimating zinc requirements. As might be expected, expert committees have differed in their interpretations of the significance of these factors in relation to requirements and, as a consequence, have produced recommendations that differ between countries. Even in the same country, dietary recommendations have not always remained the same, as national committees changed their mind about the best methods of estimating recommendations. Thus, for example in Australia, the National Health and Medical Research Council (NHMRC) set an RDI for zinc of 15 mg/d in 1980, changed it two years later to 12–16 mg/d, and in 1989 brought it back down to a maximum of 12 mg/d. It has since been changed once more[147].

3.11.1 WHO estimates of zinc requirements

How the different factors that affect zinc requirements are taken into account can be seen in the steps followed by the WHO Expert Committee on Trace Elements[148]. The Committee estimated the physiological zinc requirements of an adult to be the sum of the amounts needed to meet tissue growth, maintenance, metabolism and replacement of endogenous losses. Because zinc status affects zinc absorption and excretion, two separate estimates of requirements, namely *basal requirements*, for those fully adjusted to low dietary zinc intakes, and *normative requirements*, for those who are not adapted to a low intake, were developed. The Committee also took into account the estimated percentage zinc absorption from the diet and established population recommended intakes for those consuming diets with different levels of zinc bioavailability. These recommendations are summarised in Table 3.3.

Table 3.3 World Health Organisation: recommended zinc intakes.

	Dietary zinc bioavailability		
Population (group/years)	High	Medium	Low
Infants			
0–0.5	–	–	–
0.5–1	3.3	5.6	11.1
Children			
1–3	3.3	5.5	11.0
3–6	3.9	6.5	12.9
6–1	4.5	7.5	15.0
Males			
10–12	5.6	9.3	18.7
12–15	7.3	12.1	24.3
15–18	7.8	13.1	26.2
18–60	5.6	9.4	18.7
Females			
10–12	5.0	8.4	16.8
12–15	6.1	10.3	20.6
15–18	6.2	10.2	20.6
18–60	4.0	6.5	13.1
Pregnant	6.0	10.0	20.0
Lactating:			
0.5 month	7.3	12.2	24.3
≥ 6 months	5.8	9.6	19.2

Adapted from World Health Organisation (1996) *Trace Elements in Human Nutrition and Health*. WHO, Geneva.

3.11.2 Recommended intakes for zinc in the US and the UK

A similar factorial approach to that of the WHO Committee has been adopted in several other countries. The US National Research Council based its recommendations, as shown in Table 3.4, on the assumption that these could be established by measuring endogenous losses, with adjustments allowing for percentage zinc absorption from the diet. They took a mixed diet, with 20% zinc absorption as the basis for their estimations[149]. The UK Expert Panel on Dietary Reference Values applied a similar conceptual framework[150].

Table 3.4 Dietary Reference Intakes for Zinc for the US.

Life stage/group	RDA* (mg/d)	UL† (mg/d)
Infants		
0–6 months	2‡	4
7–12 months	3	5
Children		
1–3 years	3	7
4–8 years	5	12
Males		
9–13 years	8	23
14–18 years	11	34
19–30 years	11	40
31–50 years	11	40
50–70 years	11	40
>70 years	11	40
Females		
9–13 years	8	23
14–18 years	9	34
19–30 years	8	40
31–50 years	8	40
50–70 years	8	40
>70 years	8	40
Pregnancy		
≤18 years	12	34
19–30 years	11	40
31–50 years	11	40
Lactation		
≤18 years	13	34
19–30 years	12	40
31–50 years	12	40

*Recommended Dietary Allowance.
†Tolerable Upper Intake Level.
‡Adequate Intake.
Data from Food and Nutrition Board, National Academy of Sciences (2003) *Dietary Reference Values: Elements.* http://www4.nationalacademies.org/10M/10Mhome.nst/pages/Food+and+Nutrition+Board

Table 3.5 Dietary Reference Values for zinc in the UK (mg/d).

Age	LNRI*	EAR†	RNI‡
0–3 months	2.6	3.3	4.0
4–6 months	2.6	3.3	4.0
7–9 months	3.0	3.8	5.0
10–12 months	3.0	3.8	5.0
1–3 years	3.0	3.8	5.0
4–6 years	4.0	5.0	6.5
7–10 years	4.0	5.4	7.0
Males			
11–14 years	5.3	7.0	9.0
15–18 years	5.5	7.3	9.5
19–50 years	5.5	7.3	9.5
50+ years	5.5	7.3	9.5
Females			
11–14 years	5.3	7.0	9.0
15–18 years	4.0	5.5	7.0
19–50 years	4.0	5.5	7.0
50+ years	4.0	5.5	7.0
Pregnancy	No increment		
Lactation:			
0–4 months			+6.0
4+ months			+2.5

*Lower Reference Nutrient Intake.
†Estimated Average Requirement.
‡Reference Nutrient Intake.
Data from Department of Health (1991) *Dietary Reference Values for Food Energy and Nutrients for the United Kingdom,* p. 168. HMSO, London.

The assessment was based on the determination of basal losses during metabolic studies of deprivation, the turnover of radio-labelled endogenous zinc pools, deductions from studies of patients receiving TPN and factorial analysis. A 30% absorption rate of zinc from a mixed diet was assumed. The UK values are shown in Table 3.5.

3.12 High intakes of zinc

Zinc is not considered to be a very toxic element, but there is evidence that regular consumption of more than the recommended intake can have adverse effects. Acute toxicity can be caused by consumption of 1 g or more and results in nausea, vomiting, diarrhoea, fever and lethargy. Chronic ingestion of high levels of 75–300 mg/d, in the form of dietary supplements, has resulted in interference with the absorption of other trace elements, especially copper and iron. A fall in levels of the enzyme copper-zinc superoxide dismutase in erythrocytes has been observed after about six weeks of consumption of 50-mg zinc supplements daily[151]. Other effects of high chronic zinc intake include microcytic anaemia, changes in immune function and lipoprotein metabolism[152].

Advisory bodies in several countries set guidelines on upper limits of intake of zinc, as of other trace elements. In the US, an Upper Limit (UL), the maximum level of daily intake that is likely to pose no risk of adverse effects, has been set for each age group. This ranges from 4 mg for infants to 40 mg for adults.

3.13 Assessment of zinc status

The need to develop more reliable means of assessing zinc status was highlighted by the UK's Panel on Dietary Reference Values in 1991 as a major research need[153]. More than 10 years later, in spite of considerable effort on the part of investigators, our ability to diagnose zinc deficiency and excess is still inadequate, and there is no universally acceptable method of adequate specificity or sensitivity for assessing zinc status[154]. A major reason for this is the absence of any generally accepted and reliable biomarkers of individual zinc status.

3.13.1 An index of suspicion of zinc deficiency

In the absence of severe deficiency, when clinical symptoms of the condition become apparent, and changes in tissue concentrations of the metal can often be detected, diagnosis of zinc deficiency is sometimes based on what has been called 'a high index of suspicion'[155]. This suspicion is founded on observations of consumption of a diet low in zinc and/or high in phytates and other components that decrease zinc bioavailability, as well as of several different clinical signs in the community, such as growth retardation, delayed sexual development, dermatitis and other characteristics known to be associated with an inadequate intake. The suspicion may be confirmed by the results of a therapeutic trial in which a functional response to zinc supplementation is observed. Unfortunately, because of the time necessary for such procedures, they are not of great practical use in the clinical assessment of zinc status.

3.13.2 Assessment of zinc status using plasma and serum levels

As has been noted earlier, less than 0.1% of the body's zinc is present in blood, and the concentration is normally under strict homeostatic control. Moreover, plasma zinc levels can be affected by several factors not directly related to zinc status. For these reasons, plasma zinc content is generally considered a poor measure, especially of marginal zinc deficiency[156]. Nevertheless, despite difficulties in interpreting the significance of blood zinc levels in individual subjects, the most commonly used measurement of zinc status is plasma or serum zinc. Its main advantage is its convenience. It is especially useful for epidemiological investigations, provided there are facilities for the proper collection and processing of blood from a representative sample of the population, and there is access to analytical facilities[157].

3.13.3 Assessment of zinc status from dietary intake data

The results of dietary assessment have been used with good effect to determine the adequacy of dietary intakes of zinc, especially in developing countries. A manual describing a field-applicable method has been prepared by Gibson and Ferguson[158]. Problems can be caused by difficulties in obtaining a representative sample of the subject population, as well as by inadequacies of local food composition tables, nevertheless, the method is widely used to estimate the prevalence of zinc deficiency in low-income and some other countries[159].

3.13.4 Use of zinc-dependent enzymes to assess zinc status

In theory, since zinc plays a key role in many enzymes, it should be possible to use changes in the activities of these enzymes as a marker of zinc status. Unfortunately, this has not proved to be the case, and a reliable zinc-dependent enzyme marker of deficiency has not been identified. Among enzymes investigated, those that showed some promise included plasma ribonuclease and plasma alkaline phosphatase. However, conflicting results have been obtained in depletion studies, and though measurement of alkaline phosphatase activity, in particular, is widely used clinically, the method cannot be considered to be reliable on its own[160].

3.13.5 Other biomarkers for assessing zinc status

Several other biomarkers have been investigated in recent years, some of which appear to meet the criteria for a reliable and universally applicable index of zinc status. Measurement of thymulin activity has been shown to have considerable potential[161]. It is now being used in a number of laboratories as the method of choice for assessing zinc status. However, the current standard assay procedure is labour-intensive, which restricts its wider use[162].

The use of plasma or red cell metallothionein levels is also promising as an indicator of zinc status. In animal experiments, levels of plasma and erythrocyte metallothionein have been found to respond as predicted to changes in zinc status. Metallothionein levels in the blood of adult men have been reported to fall on a low zinc diet and to increase again when a zinc supplement is consumed[163]. Monocyte metallothionein mRNA also shows promise as a measure of zinc status. Supplementation with zinc causes a rapid increase in the mRNA above control levels, which declines on discontinuation of the supplementation[164]. A sensitive method using the competitive reverse transcriptase–polymerase chain reaction has been developed to quantify levels of metallothionein mRNA in human monocytes. Though there is some doubt about the specificity of the assay, measurement of mRNA in monocytes seems likely to be widely adopted in clinical practice for assessing zinc nutriture[165].

The use of certain protein cellular zinc transporters also shows possibilities as a specific marker for zinc status[166]. Levels of ZnT-1 mRNA in mouse intestine and liver have been found to respond to zinc loading[167]. Levels of ZnT-1 mRNA and protein increased modestly when rats were fed on a high zinc diet[168].

3.14 Dietary sources and bioavailability of zinc

A calculation, based on the food balance sheets of the Food and Agriculture Organisation (FAO), shows that, on a global basis, dietary intake of zinc is 10 ± 2.0 mg/d, with daily intake ranging from 12.4 ± 1.3 mg in Western Europe to 7.6 ± 0.6 mg in Vietnam. In between these extremes are countries of the Western Pacific with 11.8 mg, 9.3 mg in Sub-Saharan Africa and 9.0 in South Asia[169]. These intakes are strongly associated with the total food energy and the percentage of it that is provided by animal-based foodstuffs. In the richer countries, such as the US, Canada and western European nations, more than half the dietary zinc comes from animal sources compared with 15–25% in the poorer countries[170].

Not only do the poorer countries consume less meat and other animal products, and thus have a lower total zinc intake than do the industrialised countries, but their largely plant-based diet contains a much higher level of inhibitors of zinc absorption, especially phytate, than do foods normally consumed elsewhere. Thus, in Western Europe and North America, the daily phytate intake is approximately 1500 mg, compared with intakes of up to 2500 mg in some of the poorer countries. The phytate:zinc (P:Z) ratio, which can be used to estimate the amount of zinc potentially available for absorption from a diet[171], also shows major differences between the richer and the poorer countries, ranging from 13.2 ± 4.8 in Western Europe to 26.9 ± 3.7 in sub-Saharan Africa. It has been estimated that the normal diet consumed in Western Europe and North America can provide about 150% of the daily zinc requirements compared with as little as 50% in some of the poorer countries. Though these calculations are based on what are admittedly inadequate data, especially for many of the poorer countries, it is possible to interpret them as indicating that nearly half the world's population may be at risk of low zinc intake and consequent zinc deficiency[172].

Solomons and Shrimpton, in a study of zinc nutriture in tropical countries, have proposed a classification of different foods into 'zinc categories', from 'very poor' to 'very rich', based on nutrient-energy density[173]. Their table, reproduced here, in modified form, as Table 3.6, pinpoints some of the difficulties encountered in attempting to design a

Table 3.6 Classification of foods based on zinc-energy density.

Zinc category	mgZn/1000 kcal	Foods
Very poor	0–2	Fats, oils, butter, cream cheese, confectionery, soft/alcoholic drinks, sugar, preserves
Poor	1–5	Fish, fruit, refined cereal products, biscuits, cakes, tubers, sausage
Rich	4–12	Whole grains, pork, poultry, milk, low-fat cheese, yoghurt, eggs, nuts
Very rich	12–882	Lamb, leafy and root vegetables, crustaceans, beef kidney, liver, heart, molluscs

Adapted from Solomons, N.W. (2001) Dietary sources of zinc and factors affecting its bioavailability. *Food and Nutrition Bulletin*, **22**, 138–54.

realistic diet that would ensure an adequate intake of zinc, especially for poorer sections of a population. However, as Solomons notes elsewhere, 'assigning a bioavailability classification to a cuisine is more of an art than a science'. Nevertheless, what is clear is that very few, if any, of the 'very rich', or even 'rich' sources of zinc are economically available to developing country populations. Foods like oysters, lobster, ready-to-eat cereals, beef and lamb may be expensive, uncommon or perishable and are unlikely to be available to the most zinc-deficient vulnerable sectors of the population[174].

3.14.1 Dietary intake of zinc in the UK

Levels of zinc in foods consumed in the UK where, like other industrialised countries, the diet provides an adequate intake of zinc, are listed in Table 3.7. Similar levels have been reported in foods consumed in other European countries, such as Sweden[175], and in North America[176]. A typical mixed animal and plant product diet in such countries can be expected to provide a daily zinc intake of between 10 and 15 mg, enough to meet normal daily requirements. Where, however, a less traditional diet is consumed, zinc intakes can be considerably lower[177]. For example, a group of UK vegans, whose diet consisted of plant foods only, had a mean daily zinc intake of 7.9 mg with a range of 0.5–15.5 mg. When dietary supplements were also consumed by vegans, their daily zinc intake increased to 24.5 mg (range 5.0–150.6)[178].

Table 3.7 Zinc in UK foods.

Food group	Mean concentration (mg/kg fresh weight)
Bread	9.0
Miscellaneous cereals	8.6
Carcass meat	51.0
Offal	43.0
Meat products	25.0
Poultry	16.0
Fish	9.1
Oils and fats	0.6
Eggs	11.0
Sugar and preserves	3.8
Green vegetables	3.4
Potatoes	4.5
Other vegetables	2.6
Canned vegetables	3.9
Fresh fruit	0.8
Fruit products	0.7
Beverages	0.3
Milk	3.5
Dairy products	14.0
Nuts	31.0

Adapted from Ysart, G., Miller, P., Crews, H. *et al.* (1999) Dietary exposure estimates of 30 elements from the UK Total Diet Study. *Food Additives and Contaminants,* **16**, 391–403.

People whose diet contains less meat than is traditionally consumed in Britain and are, if not vegetarians, at least moving towards a plant-based diet, may also have a zinc intake that falls below the RNI. Current tendencies to reduce consumption of red and other meats, and to increase consumption of vegetables and fruit, may, in fact, be responsible for the findings of two recent surveys that 12.4% of 18–35-year-old males and 19.2% of females of the same age had zinc intakes below the EAR[179]. In another study of a group of free-living elderly people, zinc intakes of 46% of the men and 51% of the women were below the RNI[180].

3.15 Interventions to increase dietary zinc intake

Because of concern that zinc intakes may be insufficient to meet dietary requirements, an increasing number of interventions are being undertaken to improve zinc nutriture, especially in poorer countries where staple diets are predominantly plant-based, and consumption of animal products is low. Three of these strategies, based on programmes used with varying success to combat deficiencies of vitamin A, iron and iodine, are supplementation, food fortification and dietary diversification and/or modification[181].

3.15.1 Zinc supplementation of the diet

Dietary supplementation has been shown to be an effective method of improving zinc status, over a relatively short period, in at-risk communities. However, supplementation programmes can be costly and may put an unacceptable strain on an often overloaded health service. Their effectiveness is dependent on several factors, including successful communication of the health message, good compliance by those who consume the supplement and real commitment to the programme on the part of local, and national, health authorities. They are only appropriate when requirements cannot be met from habitual dietary sources, especially in acute situations such as children with acute and persistent diarrhoea[182]. Moreover, there is still uncertainty about the most appropriate chemical form of zinc for supplementary use. Not all zinc salts are equally bioavailable and side effect-free. Among the most widely used are zinc sulphate, zinc acetate and zinc gluconate, as well as zinc–amino acid chelates,[183].

As can be seen from published reports, some of the population interventions in which zinc supplements have been used have produced contradictory results. One programme, for example, in which 5 mg of elemental zinc, as zinc acetate, was provided daily over a five-week period to infants from very poor families in Bangladesh found improvements in growth rate and a reduced incidence of acute respiratory infection in infants who were initially zinc deficient, but not in those with normal serum zinc concentrations[184]. In several other interventions, zinc supplementation in populations has been shown to be generally beneficial in reducing the incidence of diarrhoea and pneumonia[185].

There have been conflicting reports on the effectiveness of zinc supplementation in reducing the incidence of other illnesses, besides diarrhoea and pneumonia. In Papua New Guinea, a reduction of malaria morbidity, as evidenced by a 38% fall in malaria-attributable health centre visits, has been reported[186]. However, a more recent report concludes that zinc supplementation does not appear to provide any beneficial effect in the treatment of acute, uncomplicated falciparum malaria in preschool children[187].

However, in spite of a certain level of uncertainty about the effectiveness of the use of zinc supplements on a population basis, there is sufficient evidence to justify the practice in particular circumstances. For example, a supplement of 25 mg of zinc as zinc sulphate given to otherwise healthy African-American pregnant women whose initial plasma zinc levels were below average resulted in significant improvements in both birth weight and head circumference in their infants. This and similar findings in other studies suggest that routine zinc supplementation may be advisable in early adolescence in countries where zinc deficiency is likely to be endemic, to ensure that women enter pregnancy with optimal zinc nutriture[188]. In the case of children with protein-energy malnutrition and persistent diarrhoea, preventive doses of supplemental zinc have been shown to reduce dramatically stool volume and diarrhoea duration[189], and at the same time improve intestinal permeability[190].

3.15.2 Zinc fortification of foods

Fortification of staple foodstuffs has the potential to be a cost-effective and sustainable method for improving dietary zinc intakes on a national level in countries where zinc deficiency is endemic. The procedure can be expected to be acceptable to consumers, since it can be introduced without changes in existing food consumption practices. Moreover, costs can be spread between food manufacturers and consumers and, with some government subsidy, could be kept at an acceptable level. This has been the case with iron fortification of foods in several countries. However, in the case of zinc, fortification programmes are still a long way from wide acceptance, even in countries where the presence of zinc deficiency is likely to be widespread.

There are a number of reasons why this is the case. A major problem is selection of a suitable food vehicle which is centrally processed, commonly used and contains a minimum of components which could interfere with zinc bioavailability. Meeting these criteria is difficult, especially in countries where largely plant-based diets contain a high proportion of phytates.

Availability of an appropritate form of zinc as a fortificant is another problem. It must be a relatively easily absorbed compound, with no undesirable organoleptic qualities, and must also be low cost. In a number of current fortification programmes, zinc oxide is used. It is a cheap white powder with no effect on taste or colour of the carrier food, but unfortunately, its bioavailability is low[191]. Hydrated zinc sulphate is better absorbed than the oxide, but its cost is considerably greater[192]. It can also cause unacceptable flavour changes in food[193]. Zinc sulphate has, however, been used successfully in a micronutrient premix to be added to cereal and pulse-based diets in supplementary feeding programmes[194]. Another micronutrient premix used for treating severely malnourished children in refugee camps contains zinc gluconate[195]. Various other compounds of zinc, including zinc-EDTA, have also been used in fortification trials. A combined iron and zinc fortified flour, using zinc oxide, has been shown to improve both iron and zinc status in Indonesian children[196].

3.15.3 Dietary diversification and modification to increase zinc intake

A programme of dietary diversification and/or modification is probably the most sustainable, feasible, culturally acceptable and nutritionally effective way of improving the zinc status, in spite of being a long-term undertaking. While increased use of zinc-rich animal-based foodstuffs is an obvious and effective way of increasing intake, this can only be done by those whose economic means allow them to purchase meat and are not deterred from doing so for cultural or religious reasons. A more practical approach, especially in poorer countries where the diet is largely plant-based, is to improve the zinc content of foods normally consumed. This can be done by fortification but, as has been seen above, not without problems. A more effective and less costly way is the introduction of improved cereal varieties, with higher zinc contents than those traditionally grown. Several of these new varieties also contain lower levels of phytates and have higher levels of sulphur-containing amino acids which may increase zinc absorption. These new strains are being developed through applications of traditional plant breeding as well as by genetic engineering. An added advantage which could encourage the use of such zinc-rich and phytate-poor cereals by farmers is that many of them are more disease resistant, drought tolerant and higher yielding than older varieties[197].

Even without the introduction of new zinc-rich varieties of cereals, zinc nutriture of a population can be improved in certain cases by making better use of foods already available, but underused. An example of a programme of dietary modification which relied on traditional foods is that successfully undertaken by Gibson and her colleagues in Malawi[198]. It consisted of a number of steps that were implemented at household level. Most important was the encouragement of increased consumption of locally available foods with a high zinc content, including several species of fish from Lake Malawi, as well as home-produced chicken and goats. Another readily available source of zinc used was groundnut flour added to maize porridge, a staple of the diet. The use of easily performed processing to increase the bioavailability of zinc from cereal-based foods, including soaking, germination and fermentation to induce hydrolysis of phytates, was also encouraged. The success of the scheme owed much to the enthusiastic cooperation of local authority figures, as well as to its adoption by a variety of local health groups and clubs and to support from volunteers in the villages.

3.15.4 An integrated approach to improving zinc nutriture in populations

None of the above interventions aimed at increasing dietary zinc consumption, especially in poorer countries where diets are predominantly plant-based, and intake of meat and other animal-based foods is low, will necessarily be successful on its own. What is required, as noted by Gibson and Ferguson, is an integrated approach employing targeted supplementation, fortification and dietary strategies. To maximise the likelihood of eliminating zinc deficiency at a national level, these strategies must be integrated also with ongoing national food, nutrition and health education programmes to enhance their effectiveness and sustainability, and implemented using nutrition education and social marketing techniques.[199]

References

1. Reilly, C. (1978) Zinc, the unassuming nutrient. In: *Getting the Most Out Of Food*, Vol. **13**, pp. 47–69. Van den Berg & Jurgens, London.
2. Raulin, J. (1869) Etudes chimiques sur la végétation. *Annales des Sciences Naturelles Botanique et Biologie Végétale*, **11**, 293–9.
3. Todd, W.K., Elvelym, A. & Hart, E.B. (1934) Zinc in the nutriture of the rat. *American Journal of Physiology*, **107**, 146–56.
4. Hambidge, M. (2000) Human zinc deficiency. *Journal of Nutrition*, **130**, 1344S–9S.
5. Prasad, A.S., Halsted, J.A. & Nadimi, M. (1961) Syndrome of iron deficiency anemia, hepatosplenomegaly, hypogonadism, dwarfism and geophagia. *American Journal of Medicine*, **31**, 532–44.
6. Moynahan, E.J. (1974) Acrodermatitis enteropathica: a lethal inherited human zinc-deficiency disorder. *Lancet*, **ii**, 399–400.
7. Walravens, P.A., Krebs, N.F. & Hambidge, K.M. (1983) Linear growth of low income preschool children receiving a zinc supplement. *American Journal of Clinical Nutrition*, **38**, 195–201.
8. Hambidge, M., Cousins, R.J. & Costello, R.B. (2000) Zinc and health: current status and future directions. *Journal of Nutrition*, **130**, 1341S–3S.
9. 11th International Symposium on Trace Elements in Man and Animals – TEMA 11. Berkeley, CA, 2–6 June 2002.
10. Guthrie, H.A. (1975) *Introductory Nutrition*, p. 171. Mosby, St. Louis, MO.
11. Sparks, D.L. (1995) *Environmental Soil Chemistry*, p. 24. Academic Press, New York.
12. Tong, S.T.Y. & Lam, K.C. (2000) Home sweet home? A case study of household dust contamination in Hong Kong. *Science of the Total Environment*, **256**, 115–23.
13. Pike, E.R., Graham, L.C. & Fogden, M.W. (1975) Metals in crops grown on sewage-enriched soil. *Journal of the American Pedilogy Association*, **13**, 19–33.
14. Brown, K.H., Wuehler, S.E. & Peerson, J.M. (2001) The importance of zinc in human nutrition and estimation of the global prevalence of zinc deficiency. *Food and Nutrition Bulletin*, **22**, 113–25.
15. McCall, K.A., Chin-chin, H. & Fierke, C.A. (2000) Function and mechanism of zinc metalloenzymes. *Journal of Nutrition*, **130**, 1437S–46S.
16. Fraústo da Silva, J.J.R. & Williams, R.J.P. (2001) *The Biological Chemistry of the Elements. The Inorganic Chemistry of Life*, p. 317. Oxford University Press, Oxford.
17. Fierke, C. (2000) Function and mechanism of zinc. *Journal of Nutrition*, **130**, 1437S–46S.
18. Williams, R.J.P. (1989) An introduction to the biochemistry of zinc. In: *Zinc in Human Biology* (ed. C.F. Mills), pp.15–31. Springer, Berlin.
19. McCall, K.A., Chin-chin, H. & Fierke, C.A. (2000) Function and mechanism of zinc metalloenzymes. *Journal of Nutrition*, **130**, 1437S–46S.
20. Hambidge, M. (2000) Human zinc deficiency. *Journal of Nutrition*, **130**, 1344S–9S.
21. McCall, K.A., Chin-chin, H. & Fierke, C.A. (2000) Function and mechanism of zinc metalloenzymes. *Journal of Nutrition*, **130**, 1437S–46S.
22. Vallee, B.L. & Auld, D.S. (1993) New perspectives on zinc biochemistry: cocatalytic sites in multi-zinc enzymes. *Biochemistry*, **32**, 6493–500.
23. Vallee, B.L. & Auld, D.S. (1992) Active zinc binding sites of zinc metalloenzymes. *Matrix Supplement*, **1**, 5–19.
24. Hambidge, M. (2000) Human zinc deficiency. *Journal of Nutrition*, **130**, 1344S–9S.
25. Berg, J.M. & Shi, Y. (1996) The galvanization of biology: a growing appreciation for the roles of zinc. *Science*, **271**, 1081–5.

26. Cousins, R.J. (2000) Integrative aspects of zinc metabolism and function. In: *Trace Elements in Man and Animals – TEMA 10* (eds. A.M. Roussel, R.A. Anderson & A.E. Favier), pp. 1–7. Kluwer/Plenum, New York.
27. Cousins, R.J. (1998) A role of zinc in the regulation of gene expression. *Proceedings of the Nutrition Society*, **57**, 307–11.
28. Hambidge, M. & Krebs, N.F. (2001) Zinc metabolism and requirements. *Food and Nutrition Bulletin*, **22**, 126–32.
29. Favier, A. & Favier, M. (1990) Conséquences des déficits en zinc durant la grossesse pour la mère et le nouveau-né. *Revue Française de Gynécologie et d'Obstetrique*, **85**, 13–27.
30. Mills, C.F. (1989) *Zinc in Human Biology. Human Nutrition Reviews*. Springer, London.
31. Sandstead, H.H. (1979) Zinc nutrition in the United States. *American Journal of Clinical Nutrition*, **26**, 1251–8.
32. Allen, J. (1998) Zinc and micronutrient supplements for children. *American Journal of Clinical Nutrition*, **68**, 495S–8S.
33. Hill, G.M., Cromwell, G.L., Crenshaw, T.D. *et al.* (1996) Impact of pharmacological intakes of zinc and (or) copper on performances of weanling pigs. *Journal of Animal Science*, **74**, Supplement 1, 181 (Abstract).
34. Harmon, R.J. & Torre, P.M. (1997) Economic implications of copper and zinc proteinates: role in mastitis control. In: *Biotechnology in the Feed Industry* (eds. T.P. Lyons & K.A. Jacques), pp. 419–30. Nottingham University Press, Nottingham, U.K.
35. Sandstrom, B., Arvidsson, B., Cederblad, A. & Bjorn-Rasmussen, E. (1980) Zinc absorption from composite meals. I. The significance of wheat extraction rate, zinc, calcium, and protein content in meals based on bread. *American Journal of Clinical Nutrition*, **33**, 739–45.
36. Lonnerdahl, B. (1989) Intestinal absorption of zinc. In: *Zinc in Human Biology* (ed. C.F. Mills), pp. 79–93. Springer, London.
37. Sandstrom, B. & Lonnerdal, B. (1989) Promotors and antagonists of zinc absorption. In: *Zinc in Human Biology* (ed. C.F. Mills), pp. 57–78. Springer, London.
38. Gibson, R.S. (1994) Zinc nutrition in developing countries. *Nutrition Research Reviews*, **7**, 18–27.
39. Valberg, L.S., Flanagan, P.R. & Chamberlain, M.J. (1984) Effect of iron, tin and copper on zinc absorption in humans. *American Journal of Clinical Nutrition*, **40**, 536–41.
40. Breskin, W., Worthington-Roberts, B.S., Knopp, R.H. *et al.* (1983) First trimester serum zinc concentrations in pregnancy. *American Journal of Clinical Nutrition*, **38**, 943–53.
41. Whittaker, P. (1998) Iron and zinc interactions in humans. *American Journal of Clinical Nutrition*, **68**, 442S–6S.
42. Wood, R.J. & Zheng, J.J. (1997) High dietary calcium intakes reduce zinc absorption and balance in humans. *American Journal of Clinical Nutrition*, **65**, 1803–9.
43. Krebs, N.F., Reidinger, C.J., Miller, L.V. & Hambidge, K.M. (1996) Zinc homeostasis in breastfed infants. *Pediatric Research*, **39**, 661–5.
44. Swanson, C.A. & King, J.C. (1987) Zinc and pregnancy outcome. *American Journal of Clinical Nutrition*, **46**, 763–71.
45. Moser-Veillon, P.B., Patterson, K.Y. & Veillon, C. (1996) Zinc absorption is enhanced during lactation. *Federation of American Societies for Experimental Biology (FASEB) Journal*, **10**, A729 (Abstract).
46. Taylor, C.M., Bacon, J.R., Aggett, P.J. & Bremner, I. (1991) The homeostatic regulation of zinc absorption and endogenous zinc losses in zinc deprived man. *American Journal of Clinical Nutrition*, **53**, 755–63.
47. Jackson, M.J. (1989) Physiology of zinc: general aspects. In: *Zinc in Human Biology* (ed. C.F. Mills), pp. 1–14. Springer, London.

48. King, J.C., Shames, D.M. & Woodhouse, L.R. (2000) Zinc homeostasis in humans. *Journal of Nutrition*, **130**, 1360S–6S.
49. Wastney, M.E., Aamodt, R.L., Rumble, W.F. & Henkin, R.I. (1986) Kinetic analysis of zinc metabolism and its regulation in normal humans. *American Journal of Physiology*, **251**, R398–408.
50. Chesters, J.K. (1982) Metabolism and biochemistry of zinc. In: *Clinical, Biochemical, and Nutritional Aspects of Trace Elements* (ed. A.S. Prasad), pp. 221–38. Liss, New York.
51. Matseshe, J.W., Phillips, S.F., Malagelada, J.R. & McCall, J.T. (1980) Recovery of dietary iron and zinc from the proximal intestine of healthy man: studies of different meals and supplements. *American Journal of Clinical Nutrition*, **33**, 1946–53.
52. Kirchgessner, M. (1993) Homeostasis and homeorhesis in trace element metabolism. In: *Trace Elements in Man and Animals – TEMA 8* (eds. M. Anke, C.F. Mills & D. Meissner), pp. 4–21. Verlag Media Touristik, Gersdorf, Germany.
53. Weigand, E. & Kirchgessner, M. (1978) Homeostatic adjustments in zinc digestion to widely varying dietary zinc intake. *Nutrition and Metabolism*, **22**, 101–12.
54. Kirchgessner, M. (1993) Homeostasis and homeorhesis in trace element metabolism. In: *Trace Elements in Man and Animals – TEMA 8* (eds. M. Anke, C.F. Mills & D. Meissner), pp. 4–21. Verlag Media Touristik, Gersdorf, Germany.
55. Taylor, C.M., Bacon, J.R., Aggett, P.J. & Bremner, I. (1991) The homeostatic regulation of zinc absorption and endogenous zinc losses in zinc deprived man. *American Journal of Clinical Nutrition*, **53**, 755–63.
56. King, J.C., Shames, D.M. & Woodhouse, L.R. (2000) Zinc homeostasis in humans. *Journal of Nutrition*, **130**, 1360S–6S.
57. Prasad, A.S. (1979). *Zinc in Human Nutrition*, pp. 32–34. CRC Press, Boca Raton, FL.
58. Liuzzi, J.P., Bobo, J.A., Cui, L., Mahon, R.J. & Cousins, R.J. (2003) Zinc transporters 1, 2 and 4 are differentially expressed and localized in rats during pregnancy and lactation. *Journal of Nutrition*, **133**, 342–51.
59. Harris, E.D. (2002) Cellular transport for zinc. *Nutrition Reviews*, **60**, 121–4.
60. Rolfs, A. & Hediger, M.A. (1999) Metal ion transporters in mammals: structure, function, and pathological implications. *Journal of Physiology*, **518**, 1–12.
61. Liuzzi, J.P., Blanchard, R.K. & Cousing, R.J. (2001) Differential regulation of zinc transporter 1,2 and 4 mRNA expression by dietary zinc in rats. *Journal of Nutrition*, **131**, 46–52.
62. Huang, L. & Gitschier, J. (1997) A novel gene involved in zinc transport is deficient in lethal milk mouse. *Nature Genetics*, **17**, 292–7.
63. Inoue, K., Matsuda, K., Itoh, M. *et al.* (2002) Osteopenia and male-specific sudden cardiac death in mice lacking a zinc transporter gene, ZnT5. *Human Molecular Genetics*, **11**, 1775–84.
64. Harris, E.D. (2002) Cellular transport for zinc. *Nutrition Reviews*, **60**, 121–4.
65. Gaither, L.A. & Eide, D.J. (2000) Functional expression of the human hZIP2 zinc transporter. *Journal of Biological Chemistry*, **275**, 5560–4.
66. Gaither, L.A. & Eide, D.J. (2001) The human ZIP1 transporter mediates zinc uptake in human K562 erythroleukemia cells. *Journal of Biological Chemistry*, **276**, 2258–64.
67. Grider, A. & Mouat, M.F. (1998) The acrodermatitis enteropathica mutation affects protein expression in human fibroblasts: analysis of two-dimensional gel electrophoresis. *Journal of Nutrition*, **128**, 1311–4.
68. Ituri, S. & Nunez, M.T. (1998) Effect of copper, cadmium, mercury, manganese, and lead on Fe^{2+} and Fe^{3+} absorption in perfused mouse intestine. *Digestion*, **59**, 671–5.
69. Rolfs, A. & Hediger, M.A. (1999) Metal ion transporters in mammals: structure, function and pathological implications. *Journal of Physiology*, **518.1**, 1–12.
70. Harris, E.D. (2002) Cellular transport for zinc. *Nutrition Reviews*, **60**, 121–4.

71. Johnson, P.E., Hunt, J.R. & Ralston, N.V.C. (1988) The effect of past and current dietary Zn intakes on Zn absorption and endogenous excretion in the rat. *Journal of Nutrition*, **118**, 1205–9.
72. Lee, D-Y., Prasad, A.S., Hydrick-Adair, C., Brewer, G. & Johnson, P.E. (1993) Homeostasis of zinc in marginal human zinc deficiency: the role of absorption and exogenous excretion of zinc. *Journal of Laboratory and Clinical Medicine*, **122**, 549–56.
73. Sian, L., Mingyan, X., Miller, L.V. *et al.* (1996) Zinc absorption and intestinal losses of endogenous zinc in young Chinese women with marginal zinc intakes. *American Journal of Clinical Nutrition*, **63**, 348–53.
74. King, J.C., Shames, D.M. & Woodhouse, L.R. (2000) Zinc homeostasis in humans. *Journal of Nutrition*, **130**, 1360S–6S.
75. Fung, E.B., Ritchie, L.D., Woodhouse, L.R., Roehal, R. & King, J.C. (1997) Zinc absorption of women during pregnancy and lactation: a longitudinal study. *American Journal of Clinical Nutrition*, **66**, 80–8.
76. King, J.C., Shames, D.M. & Woodhouse, L.R. (2000) Zinc homeostasis in humans. *Journal of Nutrition*, **130**, 1360S–6S.
77. Baer, M.T. & King, J.C. (1984) Tissue zinc levels and zinc excretion during experimental zinc depletion in young men. *American Journal of Clinical Nutrition*, **39**, 556–60.
78. Milne, D.B., Canfield, W.K., Mahalko, J.R. & Sandstead, H.H. (1983) Effect of dietary zinc on whole body surface loss of zinc: impact on estimation of zinc retention by balance method. *American Journal of Clinical Nutrition*, **38**, 181–6.
79. Hunt, C.D. & Johnson, P.E. (1990) The effects of dietary zinc on human sperm morphology and seminal mineral loss. In: *Trace Element Metabolism in Man and Animals – 7* (eds. L.S. Hurley, C.L. Keen, B. Lonnerdal & R.B. Rucker), pp. 35–42. Plenum, New York.
80. Jackson, M.J., Jones, D.A. & Edwards, R.H.T. (1982) Tissue zinc levels as an index of body zinc status. *Clinical Physiology*, **2**, 333–43.
81. King, J.C., Shames, D.M. & Woodhouse, L.R. (2000) Zinc homeostasis in humans. *Journal of Nutrition*, **130**, 1360S–6S.
82. Chesters, J.K. (1982) Metabolism and biochemistry of zinc. In: *Clinical, Biochemical, and Nutritional Aspects of Trace Elements* (ed. A.S. Prasad). Liss, New York.
83. Zhou, J.R., Canar, M.M. & Erdman, J.W., Jr. (1993) Bone zinc is poorly released in young, growing rats fed marginally zinc-restricted diet. *Journal of Nutrition*, **123**, 1383–8.
84. King, J.C., Shames, D.M. & Woodhouse, L.R. (2000) Zinc homeostasis in humans. *Journal of Nutrition*, **130**, 1360S–6S.
85. Cousins, R.J. (1996) Zinc. In: *Present Knowledge in Nutrition* (eds. E.F. Ziegler & I.J. Filer, Jr.), pp. 293–306. International Life Sciences Institute, Washington, DC.
86. Rink, L. & Gabriel, P. (2000) Zinc and the immune system. *Proceedings of the Nutrition Society*, **59**, 541–52.
87. Henry, R.W. & Elmes, M.E. (1975) Plasma zinc in acute starvation. *British Medical Journal*, **i**, 625–6.
88. Hambidge, K.M., Goodall, M.J., Stall, C. & Pritts, J. (1989) Postprandial and daily changes in plasma zinc. *Journal of Trace Elements and Electrolytes in Health and Disease*, **3**, 55–7.
89. Cousins, R.J. (1989) Systemic transport of zinc. In: *Zinc in Human Biology* (ed. C.F. Mills), pp. 79–93. Springer, London.
90. Brown, K.H. (1998) Effect of infections on plasma zinc concentration and implications for zinc status assessment in low-income countries. *American Journal of Clinical Nutrition*, **68**, 425S–39S.
91. Shenkin, A. (1995) Trace elements and inflammatory response: implications for nutritional support. *Nutrition*, **11**, 100–5.
92. Lukaski, H.C., Bolonchuk, W.W., Klevay, L.M. *et al.* (1984) Changes in plasma zinc content after exercise in men fed a low-zinc diet. *American Journal of Physiology*, **247**, E88–E93.

93. Prasad, A.S., Miale, A., Farid, Z., Sandstead, H.H., Schulert, A.R. & Darby, W.J. (1963) Biochemical studies on dwarfism, hypogonadism, and anemia. *Archives of Internal Medicine*, **111**, 407–28.
94. Moynahan, E.J. (1974) Acrodermatitis enteropathica: a lethal inherited human zinc-deficiency disorder. *Lancet*, **ii**, 399–400.
95. Hambidge, M. (2000) Human zinc deficiency. *Journal of Nutrition*, **130**, 1344S–9S.
96. Prasad, A.S. (1995) Zinc: an overview. *Nutrition*, **11**, 93–9.
97. Rink, L. & Gabriel, P. (2000) Zinc and the immune system. *Proceedings of the Nutrition Society*, **59**, 541–52.
98. Walravens, P.A., Van Doorninck, W.J. & Hambidge, K.M. (1978) Metals and mental function. *Journal of Pediatrics*, **93**, 535–6.
99. Hambidge, M. (2000) Human zinc deficiency. *Journal of Nutrition*, **130**, 1344S–9S.
100. Brown, K.H., Peerson, J.M. & Allen, L.H. (1998) Effect of zinc supplementation on children's growth: a meta-analysis of intervention trials. In: *Role of Trace Elements for Health Promotion and Disease Prevention* (eds B. Sandstrom & P. Walters), pp. 76–83. University of California, Davis, CA.
101. Bhutta, Z.A., Black, R.E., Brown, K.H. *et al.* (1999) Prevention of diarrhea and pneumonia by zinc supplementation in children in developing countries: pooled analysis of randomized controlled studies. *Journal of Pediatrics*, **135**, 689–97.
102. Ghishan, F.K. (1984) Transport of electrolytes, water and glucose in zinc deficiency. *Journal of Pediatric Gastroenterology and Nutrition*, **3**, 608–12.
103. Hambidge, M. (2000) Human zinc deficiency. *Journal of Nutrition*, **130**, 1344S–9S.
104. Black, R.E. (1998) Therapeutic and preventive effects of zinc on serious childhood infectious diseases in developing countries. *American Journal of Clinical Nutrition*, **68**, 476S–9S.
105. Penalnd, J.G., Sandstead, H.H., Alcock, N.W. *et al.* (1998) Zinc and micronutrients affect cognitive and psychomotor function of rural Chinese children. *Federation of American Societies of Experimental Biology Journal*, **12**, A649 (Abstract).
106. Bentley, M.E., Caulfield, L.E., Ryan, M. *et al.* (1997) Zinc supplementation affects the activity patterns of rural Guatemalan infants. *Journal of Nutrition*, **127**, 1333–8.
107. Aggett, P.J. (1989) Severe zinc deficiency. In: *Zinc in Human Biology* (ed. C.F. Mills), pp. 259–80. Springer, London.
108. Shay, N.F. & Mangan, H.F. (2000) Neurobiology of zinc-influenced eating behaviour. *Journal of Nutrition*, **130**, 1493S–9S.
109. Shankar, A.H. & Prasad, A.S. (1998) Zinc and immune function: the biological basis of altered resistance to infection. *American Journal of Clinical Nutrition*, **68**, 447S–63S.
110. Walsh, C.T., Sandstead, H.H., Prasad, A.S., Newberne, P.M. & Fraker, P.J. (1994) Zinc health effects and research priorities for the 1990s. *Environmental Health Perspectives*, **102**, 5–46.
111. Zalewski, P.D. (1996) Zinc and immunity: implications for growth, survival and function of lymphoid cells. *Journal of Nutrition and Immunology*, **4**, 39–80.
112. Shankar, A.H. & Prasad, A.S. (1998) Zinc and immune function: the biological basis of altered resistance to infection. *American Journal of Clinical Nutrition*, **68**, 447S–63S.
113. Rink, L. & Gabriel, P. (2000) Zinc and the immune system. *Proceedings of the Nutrition Society*, **59**, 541–52.
114. Shankar, A.H. & Prasad, A.S. (1998) Zinc and immune function: the biological basis of altered resistance to infection. *American Journal of Clinical Nutrition*, **68**, 447S–63S.
115. Dardenne, M. (2002) Zinc and the immune function. *European Journal of Clinical Nutrition*, **36**, S20–3.
116. Hambidge, K.M., Walravens, P.A. & Neldner, K.H. (1977) The role of zinc in the pathogenesis and treatment of acrodermatitis enteropathica. In: *Zinc Metabolism: Current Aspects in Health and Disease* (eds. G.J. Brewer & A.S. Prasad), pp. 329–40. Liss, New York.

117. Walsh, C.T., Sandstead, H.H., Prasad, A.S., Newberne, P.M. & Fraker, P.J. (1994) Zinc health effects and research priorities for the 1990s. *Environmental Health Perspectives*, **102**, 5–46.
118. Truong-Tran, A.Q., Ho, L.H., Chai, F. & Zalewski, P.D. (2000) Cellular death fluxes and regulation of apoptosis/gene-directed cell death. *Journal of Nutrition*, **130**, 1459S–66S.
119. Cohen, J.J., Duke, R.C., Fadok, V.A. & Seilins, K.S. (1992) Apoptosis and programmed cell death in immunity. *Annual Review of Immunology*, **10**, 267–93.
120. Fraker, P.J., King, L.E., Garvy, B.A. & Medina, C.A. (1993) The immunopathology of zinc deficiency in humans and rodents: a possible role for programmed cell death. In: *Human Nutrition: a Comprehensive Treatise* (ed. D.M. Kurfeld), pp. 267–83. Plenum, New York.
121. Zalewski, P.D. & Forbes, I.J. (1993) Intracellular zinc and the regulation of apoptosis. In: *Programmed Cell Death: the Cellular and Molecular Biology of Apotosis* (eds. M. Laviri & D. Watters), pp. 73–85. Harwood, Melbourne.
122. Maret, W. (1998) The glutathione redox state and zinc mobilization from metallothionein and other proteins with zinc–sulphur coordination sites. In: *Glutathione in the Nervous System* (ed. C.A. Shaw), pp. 257–73. Taylor & Francis, London.
123. Giannakis, C., Forbes, U. & Zalewski, P.D. (1991). Ca^{2+}/Mg^{2+}-dependent nuclease: tissue distribution, relationship to inter-nucleosomal DNA fragmentation and inhibition by Zn^{2+}. *Biochemical and Biophysical Research Communications*, **181**, 915–20.
124. Meflah, S. & Prasad, A.S. (1989) Nucleotides in lymphocytes from human subjects with zinc deficiency. *Journal of Laboratory and Clinical Medicine*, **114**, 114–9.
125. Zalewski, P.D., Forbes, I.J., Seamark, R.F. *et al.* (1994) Flux of intracellular labile zinc during apoptosis (gene-directed cell death) by a specific chemical probe, Zinquin. *Chemistry and Biology*, **1**, 153–61.
126. Chandra, R.K. (1984) Excessive intake of zinc impairs immune response. *Journal of the American Medical Association*, **252**, 1443–6.
127. Shankar, A.H. & Prasad, A.S. (1998) Zinc and immune function: the biological basis of altered resistance to infection. *American Journal of Clinical Nutrition*, **68**, 447S–63S.
128. Dardenne, M. (2002) Zinc and the immune function. *European Journal of Clinical Nutrition*, **36**, S20–3.
129. Lesourd, B.M. (1997) Nutrition and immunity in the elderly: modifications of immune responses with nutritional treatments. *American Journal of Clinical Nutrition*, **66**, 478S–84S.
130. Boukaiba, N., Flament, C., Acher, S. *et al.* (1993) A physiological amount of zinc supplementation: effects on nutritional, lipid, and thymic status in an elderly population. *American Journal of Clinical Nutrition*, **57**, 566–72.
131. Powell, S.R. (2000) The antioxidant properties of zinc. *Journal of Nutrition*, **130**, 1447S–54S.
132. Bray, T.M. & Bettger, W.J. (1990) The physiological role of zinc as an antioxidant. *Free Radicals in Biology and Medicine*, **8**, 281–91.
133. Powell, S.R. (2000) The antioxidant properties of zinc. *Journal of Nutrition*, **130**, 1447S–54S.
134. Alexander, I., Forre, O., Aaseth, J., Dobloug, J. & Ovrebo, S. (1982) Induction of a metallothionein-like protein in human lymphocytes. *Scandinavian Journal of Immunology*, **15**, 217–20.
135. Maret, W. (2000) The function of zinc metallothionein: a link between cellular zinc and redox state. *Journal of Nutrition*, **130**, 1455S–8S.
136. Klassen, C.D., Liu, J. & Choudhuri, S. (1999) Metallothionein: an intracellular protein to protect against cadmium toxicity. *Annual Review of Pharmacology and Toxicology*, **39**, 267–94.
137. Kang, Y.J. (2000) The antioxidant function of metallothionein in the heart. *Proceedings of the Society of Experimental Biology and Medicine*, **222**, 263–73.
138. Robbins, A.H., McRee, D.E., Williamson, M. *et al.* (1991). Refined crystal structure of Cd, Zn, metallothionein at 2.0 Å resolution. *Journal of Molecular Biology*, **221**, 1269093.

139. Maret, W. & Vallee, B.L. (1998) Thiolate ligands in metallothionein confer redox activity on zinc clusters. *Proceedings of the National Academy of Sciences*, **95**, 3478–82.
140. Maret, W. (2000) The function of zinc metallothionein: a link between cellular zinc and redox state. *Journal of Nutrition*, **130**, 1455S–8S.
141. Maret, W. (1994) Oxidative metal release from metallothionein via zinc-thiol/disulfide interchange. *Proceedings of the National Academy of Sciences*, **91**, 237–41.
142. Jacob, C., Maret, W. & Vallee, B.L. (1998a) Control of zinc transfer between thionein, metallothionein and zinc proteins. *Proceedings of the National Academy of Sciences*, **95**, 3489–94.
143. Jacob, C., Maret, W. & Vallee, B.L. (1998b) Ebselen, a selenium-containing redox drug, releases zinc from metallothionein. *Biochemical and Biophysical Research Communications*, **248**, 569–73.
144. Marletta, M.A. (2002) Trace elements and nitric oxide function. In: *Trace Elements in Man and Animals* (eds. J.C. King, B. Sutherland & L.H. Allen), Abstracts 1, p. 26. University of California, Berkley, CA.
145. Pearce, L.L., Wasserlkoos, K., StCroix, C.M. *et al.* (2000) Metallothionein, nitric oxide and zinc homeostasis in vascular endothelial cells. *Journal of Nutrition*, **130**, 1467S–70S.
146. Rink, L. & Gabriel, P. (2000) Zinc and the immune system. *Proceedings of the Nutrition Society*, **59**, 541–52.
147. Dreosti, I.E. (1990) Zinc. In: *Recommended Nutrient Intakes: Australian Papers*, (ed. A.S. Truswell), p. 264. Australian Professional Publications, Sydney.
148. World Health Organisation (1996) *Trace Elements in Human Nutrition and Health*. WHO, Geneva.
149. Brown, K.H., Wuehler, S.E. & Peerson, J.M. (2001) The importance of zinc in human nutrition and estimation of the global prevalence of zinc deficiency. *Food and Nutrition Bulletin*, **22**, 113–25.
150. Department of Health (1991) *Dietary Reference Values for Food Energy and Nutrients for the United Kingdom*, pp. 167–8. HMSO, London.
151. Fischer, P.W.F., Giroux, A. & L'Abbé, M.R. (1984) Effect of zinc supplementation on copper status in adult man. *American Journal of Clinical Nutrition*, **40**, 743–6.
152. Yadrick, M.K., Kenney, M.A. & Winterfeldt, E.A. (1989) Iron, copper and zinc status: response to supplementation with zinc or zinc and iron in adult females. *American Journal of Clinical Nutrition*, **49**, 145–50.
153. Department of Health (1991) *Dietary Reference Values for Food Energy and Nutrients for the United Kingdom*, pp. 167–8. HMSO, London
154. Sandström, B (2001) Diagnosis of zinc deficiency and excess in individuals and populations. *Food and Nutrition Bulletin*, **22**, 133–6.
155. Brown, K.H., Wuehler, S.E. & Peerson, J.M. (2001) The importance of zinc in human nutrition and estimation of the global prevalence of zinc deficiency. *Food and Nutrition Bulletin*, **22**, 113–25.
156. King, J.C. (1990) Assessment of zinc status. *Journal of Nutrition*, **120**, 1474S–9S.
157. Brown, K.H., Peerson, J.M. & Allen, L.H. (1998) Effect of zinc supplementation on children's growth: a meta-analysis of intervention trials. *Bibliotheca Nutritio Dieta*, **54**, 76–83.
158. Gibson, R.S. & Ferguson, E.L. (1999) *An Interactive 24-Hour Recall for Assessing the Adequacy of Iron and Zinc Intakes in Developing Countries*. International Life Sciences Institute Press, Washington, DC.
159. Gibson, R.S. (1994) Zinc nutrition in developing countries. *Nutrition Research Reviews*, **7**, 151–73.
160. Ruz, M., Cavan, K.R., Bettger, W.J. *et al.* (1991) Development of a dietary model for the study of mild zinc deficiency in humans and evaluation of some biochemical and functional indices of zinc status. *American Journal of Clinical Nutrition*, **53**, 1295–303.

161. Prasad, A.S., Meftah, S., Abdallah, J. *et al.* (1988) Serum thymulin in human zinc deficiency. *Journal of Clinical Investigation*, **82**, 1202–10.

162. Chesters, J.K. (1997) Zinc. In: *Handbook of Nutritionally Essential Mineral Elements* (eds. B.L. O'Dell & R.A. Sunde), pp. 185–230. Dekker, New York.

163. Grider, A., Bailey, L.B. & Cousins, R.J. (1990) Erythrocyte metallothionein as an index of zinc status in humans. *Proceedings of the National Academy of Sciences*, **87**, 1259–62.

164. Sullivan, V.K., Burnett, F.R. & Cousins, R.J. (1998) Metallothionein expression is increased in monocytes and erythrocytes of young men during zinc supplementation. *Journal of Nutrition*, **128**, 707–13.

165. Sullivan, V.K. & Cousins, R.J. (1997) Competitive reverse transcriptase-polymerase chain reaction shows that dietary zinc supplementation in humans increases monocyte metallothionein mRNA levels. *Journal of Nutrition*, **127**, 694–8.

166. McMahon, R.J. & Cousins, R.J. (1998a) Mammalian zinc transporters. *Journal of Nutrition*, **128**, 667–70.

167. Davis, S.R., McMahon, R.J. & Cousins, R.J. (1998) Metallothionein knockout and transgenic mice exhibit altered intestinal processing of zinc with uniform zinc-dependent zinc transporter-1 expression. *Journal of Nutrition*, **128**, 825–31.

168. McMahon, R.J. & Cousins, R.J. (1998b) Regulation of the zinc transporter ZnT-1 by dietary zinc. *Proceedings of the National Academy of Sciences*, **95**, 4841–6.

169. Food and Agricultural Organization (1999) Food Balance Sheets, country averages 1990–1997. In: *FAO Statistical Databases.* http://apps.fao.org/lim500/nph-wrap.pl?FoodBalanceSheet&Domain=FoodBalanceSheet

170. Brown, K.H., Wuehler, S.E. & Peerson, J.M. (2001) The importance of zinc in human nutrition and estimation of the global prevalence of zinc deficiency. *Food and Nutrition Bulletin*, **22**, 113–25.

171. World Health Organisation (1996) *Trace Elements in Human Nutrition and Health.* WHO, Geneva.

172. Brown, K.H., Wuehler, S.E. & Peerson, J.M. (2001) The importance of zinc in human nutrition and estimation of the global prevalence of zinc deficiency. *Food and Nutrition Bulletin*, **22**, 113–25.

173. Solomons, N.W. & Shrimpton, R. (1989) Zinc. In: *Tropical and Geographic Medicine* (eds. K.S. Warren & Mahoud), pp. 1059–63. McGraw-Hill, New York.

174. Solomons, N. (2001) Dietary sources of zinc and some factors affecting its bioavailability. *Food and Nutrition Bulletin*, **22**, 138–54.

175. Jorhem, L. & Sunderström, B. (1993) Levels of lead, cadmium, zinc, copper, nickel, chromium, manganese, and cobalt in foods on the Swedish market, 1983–1990. *Journal of Food Composition and Analysis*, **6**, 223–41.

176. Pennington, J.A.T. & Young, B. (1990) Iron, zinc, copper, manganese, selenium, and iodine in foods from the United States Total Diet Study. *Journal of Food Composition and Analysis*, **3**, 166–84.

177. Hunt, J.R. (2002) Moving towards a plant-based diet: are iron and zinc at risk? *Nutrition Reviews*, **60**, 127–34.

178. Lightowler, H.J. & Davies, G.J. (2000) Micronutrient intakes in a group of UK vegans and the contribution of self-selected dietary supplements. *Journal of the Royal Society for the Promotion of Health*, **120**, 117–24.

179. Hannon, E.M., Kiely, M., Flynn, A. *et al.* (2000) The North–South Ireland food consumption survey 2000: mineral intakes in 18–64 year old adults. *Proceedings of the Nutrition Society*, **60**, 41A.

180. Saini, N., Maxwell, S.M., Dugdill, L. & Miller, A.M. (2000) Micronutrient intake of free-living elderly people. *Proceedings of the Nutrition Society*, **60**, 41A.

181. Gibson, R.S. & Ferguson, E.L. (1998) Nutrition intervention strategies to combat zinc deficiency in developing countries. *Nutrition Research Reviews*, **11**, 115–31.
182. Gillespie, S., Kevany, J. & Mason, J. (1991) *Controlling Iron Deficiency: ACC/SCN State-of-the-Art Series Nutrition Policy Discussion Papers No. 9*. United Nations Administrative Committee on Coordination/Subcommittee on Nutrition, Geneva.
183. Gibson, R.S. (1994) Zinc nutrition in developing countries. *Nutrition Research Reviews*, **7**, 151–73.
184. Osendarp, S.J.M., Santosham, M., Black, R.E. *et al.* (2002) Effect of zinc supplementation between 1 and 6 months of life on growth and morbidity of Bangladeshi infants in urban slums. *American Journal of Clinical Nutrition*, **76**, 1401–8.
185. Zinc Investigators' Collaborative Group (2000) Therapeutic effects of oral zinc in acute and persistent diarrhea in children in developing countries: pooled analysis of randomised controlled trials. *American Journal of Clinical Nutrition*, **72**, 1516–22.
186. Shankar, A.H., Genton, B., Baisor, M. *et al.* (2000) The influence of zinc supplementation on morbidity due to *Plasmodium falciparum*: a randomised trial in preschool children in Papua New Guinea. *American Journal of Tropical Medicine and Hygiene*, **62**, 663–9.
187. Zinc against Plasmodium Study Group (2002) Effect of zinc on the treatment of *Plasmodium falciparum* malaria in children: a randomised controlled study. *American Journal of Clinical Nutrition*, **76**, 805–12.
188. Goldenberg, R.L., Tamura, T., Neggers, Y. *et al.* (1995) The effect of zinc supplementation on pregnancy outcome. *Journal of the American Medical Association*, **274**, 463–8.
189. Sachdev, H.P.S., Mittal, N.K. & Yadav, H.S. (1990) Oral zinc supplementation in persistent diarrhoea in infants. *Annals of Tropical Paediatrics*, **10**, 63–9.
190. Roy, S.K., Behrens, R.H., Haider, R. *et al.* (1992) Impact of zinc supplementation on intestinal permeability in Bangladeshi children with acute diarrhoea and persistent diarrhoea syndrome. *Journal of Pediatric Gastroenterology and Nutrition*, **15**, 289–96.
191. Henderson, L.M., Brewer, G.J., Dressman, J.B. *et al.* (1995) Effect of intragastric pH on the absorption of oral zinc acetate and zinc oxide in young healthy volunteers. *Journal of Parenteral and Enteral Nutrition*, **19**, 393–7.
192. Wedekind, K.J. & Baker, D.H. (1990) Zinc bioavailability in feed-grade sources of zinc. *Journal of Animal Science*, **68**, 684–9.
193. Ranum, P. (2001) Zinc enrichment of cereal staples. *Food and Nutrition Bulletin*, **22**, 169–73.
194. Golden, M.H.N., Briend, A. & Grellety, Y. (1995) Meeting report: report of the meeting on supplementary feeding programmes with particular reference to refugee populations. *European Journal of Clinical Nutrition*, **49**, 137–45.
195. International Study Group on Persistent Diarrhea – ISGPD (1996) Evaluation of an algorithm for the treatment of diarrhea: a multi-centre study. *Bulletin of the World Health Organization*, **74**, 479–88.
196. Herman, S., Griffin, I.J., Suwarti, S. *et al.* (2002) Cofortification of iron-fortified flour with zinc sulfate, but not zinc oxide, decreases iron absorption in Indonesian children. *American Journal of Clinical Nutrition*, **76**, 813–7.
197. Ruel, M.T. & Bouis, H.E. (1998) Plant breeding: a long-term strategy for the control of zinc deficiency in vulnerable populations. *American Journal of Clinical Nutrition*, **68**, 488S–94S.
198. Gibson, R.S., Yeudall, F., Drost, N., Mtitimuni, B. & Cullinan, T. (1998) Dietary intervention to prevent zinc deficiency. *American Journal of Clinical Nutrition*, **68**, 484S–7S.
199. Gibson, R.S. & Ferguson, E.L. (1998) Nutrition intervention strategies to combat zinc deficiency in developing countries. *Nutrition Research Reviews*, **11**, 115–31.

Chapter 4
Copper

4.1 Introduction

Copper was among the first of the metals to be discovered. This was most probably because it sometimes occurs in its native elemental state – a single mass of metallic copper weighing 420 tons was once found in Michigan in the US. Moreover, the metal does not require a very high level of technological skill to extract it from its ores, and these are relatively abundant and easily recognisable by their distinctive colours. Along with the other ancient metals, silver and gold, copper has long been used in coinage. There is evidence that cooking vessels and food and beverage containers made of copper, as well as of copper alloys such as brass and bronze, were in use as many as 5000 years ago[1]. Thus, as well as the copper naturally occurring in foods, humans have without doubt been ingesting the metal picked up as a contaminant from cooking utensils for many thousands of years. Yet, it is only relatively recently that serious attention has been given to the role that copper might play in human metabolism.

4.2 Copper chemistry

Copper has an atomic weight of 63.54 and is number 29 in the Periodic Table. It is a heavy metal, with a density of 8.96 and a melting point of 1083°C, is tough, though soft and ductile, and is second only to silver as a conductor of heat and electricity. It is resistant to corrosion, in the sense that, on exposure to air, a protective layer of oxide, or verdigris, builds up on its surface. Its conductivity and corrosion resistance, as well as the ease with which it can be worked by craftsmen, are properties which account for its wide commercial use, especially in the electrical industry and in the manufacture of utensils of many kinds. Its use in former times was enhanced when it was discovered that by combining copper with tin and some other metals, it could be made into tough and durable alloys suitable for making weapons and tools.

Copper belongs to Group 11/1B of the elements, along with silver and gold, two other members of the coinage group with which it shares certain chemical properties. It is also a member of the *d*-block transition elements with, in its atomic structure, valence electrons in more than one shell, and thus has several oxidation states. These are, +1 (cuprous) and +2 (cupric), both stable states. A third, unstable (+3) oxidation state occurs in some crystalline compounds. Though copper is a relatively inert element, it forms a wide range of cuprous, Cu(II), and cupric, Cu(I), compounds. Most cuprous compounds are readily oxidised to the cupric form.

Copper, in both its cuprous and cupric forms, has the ability to form chelates with O-, S- and N-containing ligands, a property which accounts for many of its biological activities. These compounds, many of which are coloured, also provide the basis for several colorimetric methods for determination of the metal, including the classical Fehling and Benedict tests. The chemistry of the many copper complexes that are to be found in biological tissues is complex. Copper proteins, structural as well as functional, contain a mixture of oxygen-, nitrogen- and sulphur-donating ligands, with predominantly tetra- and penta-coordinate Cu(II) geometry. In a few particular instances, such as in copper-metallothionein, it is present as Cu(I) and is chelated exclusively by cysteinyl sulphydryl groups with a trigonal or digonal Cu(I) coordination[2].

4.3 The biology of copper

A nutritional role of copper was first identified in animals in the early decades of the twentieth century, when a form of anaemia in cattle grazing on pastures with a low soil copper level was found to be due to deficiency of the element. In studies using rats, copper was shown to be necessary for haemoglobin formation[3]. A few years later, anaemia in humans was also found to be related to copper deficiency[4]. Subsequent elucidation of the biological role of copper has been slow. Only in recent years has its central role in human metabolism begun to be adequately recognised.

An adult human body contains about 100 mg of copper. There is still a great deal that is not known about its role in the body, but what is clear is that copper is an essential trace metal. Most of the body's copper appears to be tightly bound in several different metallo-proteins, in which it functions both structurally and as a cofactor for catalytic activity. Some two dozen copper enzymes have been characterised, with a variety of cellular and extra-cellular activities, including involvement in the body's immune reactions, neural function, bone health, blood chemistry, anti-oxidant function, energy production and others.

4.3.1 Copper proteins

Table 4.1 lists some of the copper-dependent and other copper proteins identified in humans, with an indication of their functions. Several of the enzymes utilise the ability of copper to cycle between the Cu(II) and Cu(I) states. They play roles in oxidation/reduction reactions, using molecular oxygen as a co-substrate. Others have a variety of functions, as can be seen from the selection of copper proteins discussed in the following sections.

*4.3.1.1 Cytochrome-*c *oxidase*

Cytochrome-*c* oxidase, which is embedded in the inner mitochondrial membrane, functions as the terminal link in the electron transport chain, catalysing the reduction of dioxygen to water, with the production of ATP. The enzyme contains three copper atoms per molecule in two separate active sites. At the first site, two copper atoms receive an electron from cytochrome-*c*. The electron is then transferred to the second site where the

Table 4.1 Some copper proteins in humans.

Enzyme	Functions
Blue proteins	Electron transfers
Cytochrome-*c* oxidase	Electron transport; reduction of O_2 to H_2O
Caeruloplasmin (ferroxidase I)	Iron oxidation and transport
Cu–Zn superoxide dismutase (SOD)	Antioxidant defence
Dopamine β-hydroxylase	Hydroxylation of dopa in brain
Diamine and monamine oxidase	Removal of amines and diamines
Lysyl oxidase	Collagen cross-linking
Tyrosinase	Melanin formation
Chaperone proteins	Intracellular copper transport
Chromatin scaffold proteins	Structural integrity of nuclear material
Clotting factor V, VIII	Thrombogenesis
Metallothionein	Metal sequestration
Nitrous oxide reductase	Reduction of NO_2^- to NO

Adapted from Fraústo da Silva, J.J.R. & Williams, R.J.P. (2001) *The Biological Chemistry of the Elements*, p. 419. Oxford University Press, Oxford; McAnena, L.B. & O'Connor, J.M. (2002) Measuring intakes of nutrients and their effects: the case of copper. In: *The Nutrition Handbook for Food Processors*, (eds. C.J.K. Henry & C. Chapman), p. 118. Woodhead, Cambridge, UK.

third copper atom links to molecular oxygen[5]. This terminal step is the rate-limiting step in the electron transport chain responsible for the production of the energy required by cells and tissues, and consequently, cytochrome-*c* oxidase is considered by some to be the single most important enzyme of the mammalian cell[6].

4.3.1.2 The ferroxidases

In an earlier section, the roles in iron metabolism and transport of the copper proteins ferroxidase I, and the closely related ferrodoxin II, have been discussed. They have the ability to oxidise Fe(II) to Fe(III) without forming hydrogen peroxide or oxygen radicals. Ferrodoxin I is also known as caeruloplasmin. It contains six copper atoms per molecule, three of which provide active sites for electron transfer processes. The other three form an oxygen-activating site for catalysis. Caeruloplasmin is an important cellular antioxidant, responsible for scavenging hydrogen peroxide and other active oxygen species, inhibiting lipid peroxidation and DNA degradation by free copper and iron ions[7]. It also has another important role as an acute-phase protein in the body's immune system. In response to inflammation, caeruloplasmin concentration is increased in cells and helps to sequester free circulating iron ions, and thus reduces their potential for oxidative activity.

4.3.1.3 Copper/zinc superoxide dismutase

Superoxide dismutase (SOD) occurs in several forms in human tissues, two of which have copper at their active sites. The cytosolic copper/zinc form, SOD I, occurs apparently in most cells, while an extracellular form, SOD 2, is found in plasma as well as in particular cell types in the lungs, thyroid and uterus. Both SODs are involved in oxygen metabolism.

They are active antioxidants and catalyse the dismutation of superoxide radicals to hydrogen peroxide and water[8].

4.3.1.4 *Amine oxidases*

In the amine oxidases, copper acts as a structural or allosteric component, giving the enzyme the shape it requires to function catalytically. Monoamine oxidase (MAO) inactivates a variety of amines such as serotonin and catecholamines, including adrenalin, noradrenalin and dopamine. Diamine oxidase (DAO) deaminates histamine and polyamines involved in cell proliferation. Lysyl oxidase is another amine oxidase which deaminates lysine and hydroxylysine side chains in immature collagen and elastin molecules. This is necessary for the formation of strong and elastic cross links in the maturation of the extracellular matrix.

4.3.1.5 *Tyrosinase*

Tyrosinase is also known as catechol oxidase. It catalyses the oxidation of phenols and is necessary for the synthesis of melanin from tyrosine. It brings this about by hydroxylating the tyrosine to dopa, which it then oxidises to dopaquinone. This in turn undergoes a series of non-enzymatic reactions, leading to the formation of melanin[9]. An inherited deficiency of tyrosinase results in albinism.

4.3.1.6 *Other copper proteins*

Copper plays an essential structural role as a component of chromatin scaffold proteins. There is no evidence that copper is required for DNA synthesis in mammals, though it appears to be in yeast cells.

A copper protein which is not encountered in mammals, but appears to be restricted to only a few species of molluscs and arthropods, is haemocyanin. This is a colourless extracellular protein which contains two closely associated copper atoms which have the ability to bind oxygen molecules reversibly, to give a purple $Cu(II)–O_2$ complex. Haemocyanin takes the place of the iron protein, haemoglobin, as an oxygen carrier in the organisms that contain it. Though the number of species that rely on this copper enzyme is small, compared with the many haemoglobin-dependent animal species, the actual numbers of haemocyanin users is considerable, since the arthropods are the largest group in the entire animal kingdom, with 85% of all animal species[10].

Maintenance of these diverse activities requires that the body has a dependable supply of copper for incorporation into the apocuproproteins. Food is obviously the major source of copper for humans, with additional intakes from drinking water and other beverages and, in many cases, from dietary supplements.

4.4 Dietary sources of copper

The normal intake of copper by an adult consuming a Western-style mixed diet is about 1–4 mg/d. Copper is present in all foods, with vegetables probably supplying much of

Table 4.2 Copper in UK foods.

Food group	Mean concentration (mg/kg fresh weight)
Bread	1.6
Miscellaneous cereals	1.8
Carcass meat	1.4
Offal	40
Meat products	1.5
Poultry	0.73
Fish	1.1
Oils and fats	0.05
Eggs	0.59
Sugar and preserves	1.5
Green vegetables	0.84
Potatoes	1.3
Other vegetables	0.91
Canned vegetables	1.5
Fresh fruit	0.94
Fruit products	0.73
Beverages	0.10
Milk	0.05
Dairy products	0.45
Nuts	8.5

Adapted from Ysart, G., Miller, P., Crews, H. *et al.* (1999) Dietary exposure estimates of 30 elements from the UK Total Diet Study. *Food Additives and Contaminants*, **16**, 391–403.

the copper in most diets. Overall concentrations in most foods range from about 0.5 to 2.0 mg/kg (fresh weight)[11]. There are some exceptions, such as animal offal and nuts, which can contain considerably more. Dairy products, and particularly cow's milk, are particularly poor sources of the metal. Copper concentrations in different food groups, as measured in the UK Total Diet Study, are listed in Table 4.2[12]. Similar levels in foods normally consumed are reported in other countries, such as the US[13], Italy[14] and Spain[15]. The richest food sources, apart from offal and nuts, are reported to be cereals, especially wholegrain, with about 1–4 mg/kg. Certain ready-to-eat breakfast cereals, especially those based on wheat bran, some of which are probably fortified, may contain up to 10 mg/kg of copper[16]. Foods and beverages cooked or stored in copper utensils may, on occasion, be contaminated with relatively high levels of adventitious copper[17].

4.5 Copper absorption and metabolism

Most of the copper in the human diet is probably in organic form, bound to proteins, amino acids and other large molecules. Inorganic copper may be contributed to the diet in drinking water, as contaminants from copper pipes and containers, as well as in certain types of dietary supplements. About 30–60% of ingested copper appears to be absorbed by healthy individuals, though it has been shown that the efficiency of absorption varies inversely with the levels of copper in the diet[18]. Copper deficiency can result in uptakes of up to 70%, while in copper-rich diets, it may be as low as 12%[19]. The ability to adapt to changing levels of ingestion of copper appears to develop during childhood, with absorption in infants lower than in adults[20].

4.5.1 *Effects on copper absorption of various food components*

Absorption of ingested copper mainly takes place in the duodenum, with a small amount in the stomach. A number of luminal factors, apart from copper concentration, can affect the efficiency of absorption of copper from food. Various plant components that form complexes with copper, such as lectins and glycoproteins in cereals, and are not easily solubilised by digestive enzymes, can limit the availability of the metal. In contrast, animal protein can enhance uptake. Other components that modify absorption include amino acids, other trace metals, sugars, ascorbic acid and fibre[21].

4.5.1.1 Effect of amino acids on copper absorption

While amino acids generally enhance copper absorption, by forming soluble complexes with the metal, there is evidence that, when present in quantity, they can cause malabsorption, possibly as a result of competition with binding proteins on the enterocyte membrane. Certain types of food processing, which result in the formation of Maillard compounds from amino acids and sugars, may reduce copper bioavailability by reducing the amounts of the acids available for the formation of soluble copper–amino acid complexes[22].

4.5.1.2 Competition between copper and other metals for absorption

Ingested copper competes for absorption with other divalent metals in the lumen of the gut. The competition can be due to their similarities in electronic structure and ionic size, which allows them to form similar coordination complexes with transport molecules on the brush-border membrane[23]. They may also compete for ligands necessary for uptake by these receptors. High levels of dietary zinc are known to be antagonistic to copper absorption[24]. Though it has been suggested that this is caused by zinc-induced metallothionein, which sequesters copper and prevents its absorption[25], other factors may be involved. The immediate effect of high zinc levels may be on the expression or activities of copper transport proteins in the intestinal cell membranes[26]. This antagonism between the two metals is used in the treatment of patients suffering from Wilson's disease, in which the body retains excessive amounts of copper, by giving zinc salts orally.

Copper absorption is also impaired by the presence of other metals, including iron, manganese, molybdenum and tin[27]. Infants fed iron-enriched formula have been found to absorb less copper than other infants fed a lower iron diet[28]. In animal studies, however, iron was found to interfere with copper absorption only in those with a pre-existing low copper status[29]. Antagonism between molybdenum and copper has long been known in agriculture. Teart disease, or chronic molybdenum poisoning, caused by grazing of molybdenum-rich fodder by livestock, results in reduced copper status, anaemia and bone malformations[30]. Advantage has been taken, clinically, of the antagonism between molybdenum and copper, in the use of the unabsorbable molybdenum complex, tetrathiomolybdate, which inhibits intestinal copper absorption, in the treatment of Wilson's disease[31].

4.5.1.3 Effects of dietary carbohydrates and fibre on copper absorption

There have been a number of reports of interactions between copper and various sugars and other carbohydrates which affect copper absorption from food. Very high intakes of fructose or sucrose have been found to increase dietary copper deficiency in rats[32]. In humans, a high fructose intake can increase copper requirements. This effect may be associated with alterations in energy metabolism, since a high fat intake also increases copper requirements. A recent study has found that although copper status was decreased in healthy men fed fructose in conjunction with a low-copper diet, the subjects attempted to adapt to the low intake by retaining absorbed copper longer. However, the adaptation was inadequate, and copper balance became negative[33].

An indirect effect on copper absorption has been shown to result from the presence of glucose polymers in the diet. The polymers appear to increase copper uptake from the intestinal lumen by increasing mucosal water uptake. Phytate and other dietary fibres exert an inhibitory effect on copper absorption in the gut. However, since copper is not as tightly bound to fibre as are other divalent cations, the inhibition is limited[34].

4.5.2 Copper absorption from human and cow's milk

Of some special interest is the difference between bioavailability of copper in human and cow's milk, since it can have consequences for the copper status of bottle-fed infants. Copper has a much higher bioavailability in human than in ruminant milk, apparently because of the presence in the latter of higher levels of low molecular weight ligands that can inhibit copper absorption. The difference in absorption may also be related to differences in distribution of copper in fractions of the two kinds of milk, with a higher proportion in whey and lipids in humans[35].

4.5.3 Transport of copper across the mucosal membrane

Transfer of copper from the intestinal lumen across the brush border into the enterocytes and subsequently through the basolateral membrane to the plasma involves both passive and carrier-mediated systems. It is now known that a number of distinctive and specific copper transport proteins are involved in cellular uptake and export of the metal. As with zinc, copper appears to have a family of transporters, known as Ctr. The first of these to be identified, Ctr1, was detected in yeast[36]. It has two human homologues, hCtr1 and hCtr2. These transporter proteins function primarily in the high-affinity uptake of copper across the cell membrane[37]. In contrast to what is found in the case of zinc[38], intracellular compartmentalisation, as well as efflux of copper from the cell, relies on energy-dependent P-type ATPases in the membrane and on a specialised series of smaller peptides known as *chaperones* that move copper internally[39]. Two genetic disorders, responsible for a series of defects in copper homeostasis, Menkes and Wilson diseases, are caused by mutations in genes encoding for these P-type transport ATPases. Menkes is the result of defects in the MNK protein (also known as ATP7A) responsible for the export of copper from the intestine, leading to copper deficiency and subsequent loss of copper-requiring enzyme function. Wilson disease is the result of defects in the gene encoding the WND transporter that functions in the release of copper from the liver. As a result, toxic accumulation of copper in liver and other tissues, can occur, resulting in cirrhosis and neurodegradation[40].

There is still a good deal of uncertainty about the exact distribution and function of copper transport proteins in mammals. It is unclear, for instance, how copper is delivered to the transporter for uptake into cells. Most of the copper that circulates in the blood is bound to caeruloplasmin. This multicopper oxidase is synthesised in the liver, where it binds copper and is secreted. However, there is evidence to suggest that caeruloplasmin is unlikely to mediate the distribution of copper from the liver to other tissues[41]. It is possible that this is carried out by other serum factors such as albumin and histidine. It is probable that Cu(I) is the transport substrate and that a cell surface metalloreductase is involved in uptake. It is also unclear how copper imported into the cell is loaded on to the metallochaperones[42]. A family of chaperones responsible for the intracellular transport of copper has been identified in yeast. A mammalian homologue of one of these, known as Atox1, has been identified in mice, but its mechanism of operation is unclear[43].

4.6 Distribution of copper in the body

Not a great deal is yet known about the details of copper distribution from the enterocytes to other parts of the body. It appears to occur in two phases[44]. During the first, the copper is exported from the enterocytes into the blood utilising the MNK protein transporter. Except in exceptional conditions, none of the copper in blood is in ionic form but is immediately bound to the high-affinity plasma proteins albumin and transcuprein. This protein-bound copper is then carried to the liver and kidney. Within the liver, much of the recently acquired copper is incorporated into caeruloplasmin and returned to the circulation for distribution to other tissues. Copper leaving peripheral tissues can re-enter the circulation and be taken up by the liver for re-utilisation or excretion. Excess hepatic copper is exported into bile for elimination from the body and can be stored temporarily as metallothionein[45]. Biliary excretion is the major mechanism for the control of copper homeostasis in the body, while urinary excretion plays only a minor role in this process.

Some of the protein-bound copper is also transferred directly to sites where synthesis of cytoplasmic copper-dependent and other copper-proteins occurs. A number of different copper transport proteins are involved[46], including the trans-Golgi network protein ATP7B, also known as WND. Defects in this and other copper pumps are responsible for Menkes and Wilson diseases[47].

The second phase occurs with the efflux of copper from the liver and kidney and its transfer to other tissues. It is secreted from these organs into plasma bound mainly to caeruloplasmin, which appears to be the main transporter of the metal throughout the body. Surface receptors specific for caeruloplasmin-copper are present in most tissues.

However, whether caeruloplasmin is essential for copper transport in the body is uncertain, since it can be shown that the genetic defect of acaeruloplasminaemia does not disrupt copper metabolism severely. It may be that tissues absorb copper preferentially from caeruloplasmin but can also utilise other pathways for cellular acquisition of the metal if caeruloplasmin is not available[48].

4.7 Assessment of copper status

There is, as yet, no widely accepted and totally reliable, sensitive method for assessing copper status. Determination of marginal status is particularly difficult, and it has not been possible to define optimal intakes of the trace nutrient with certainty[49]. Consequently, dietary recommendations for the metal are either unavailable or, at best, doubtful estimates.

As has been seen in the case of both zinc and iron, while no single method is entirely satisfactory on its own, a combination of several different procedures can be used to assess copper status with reasonable reliability in practice. In a recent review, Hambidge has summarised the categories of biomarkers of trace element intake and status that are normally used for this purpose[50]. These are measurement of tissue concentration, homeostasis and metabolism, body stores, functional indices and response to increase of intake. Not all of these biomarkers are of equal importance for the determination of status of each of the trace metal nutrients. The most significant of these in the case of copper are discussed below.

4.7.1 Assessment of copper status using plasma copper and caeruloplasmin

The most frequently used biomarkers for copper are plasma copper and caeruloplasmin levels. Both are depressed in deficiency states and rise with increased intake. However, levels plateau when intake reaches adequacy and do not reflect higher intakes.

Changes in caeruloplasmin levels are brought about by a number of factors, in addition to copper intake. The protein is an acute phase reactant and is elevated during infections, inflammatory response and other stress conditions. Production of caeruloplasmin may be depressed by protein deficiency and increased by oestrogens, rather than by changes in copper intake. Its levels are also age-dependent. Thus, the value of caeruloplasmin, and of plasma copper, as biomarkers of copper status, is diminished by their lack of specificity and the effects of various confounding factors that complicate interpretation of data[51]. Nevertheless, both are widely used to assess copper status, mainly because of the simplicity of assays involved.

4.7.2 Copper enzyme activity

The activities of several copper-dependent enzymes are reduced by dietary copper restriction and have potential as biomarkers of copper status. These include erythrocyte and extracellular superoxide dismutase and cytochrome-*c* oxidase, in platelets and leukocytes. However, measurement of their activities requires procedures which are not suitable for routine and especially epidemiological studies, and results appear to lack adequate sensitivity and specificity[52].

A number of other copper enzymes have also been examined and appear to offer better prospects as biomarkers of copper status. A simple assay on a finger-stick plasma sample that measures the activity of the neuroendocrine peptide peptidylglycine α-amidating monooxygenase (PAM) and indicates a relatively sensitive response to changes in copper levels has been developed, though so far only *in vitro*[53]. Another enzyme that is sensitive to changes in copper levels and also may be suitable as a sensitive biomarker of copper status is plasma diamine oxidase. It has been shown to respond to copper supplementation in normal subjects[54].

4.7.3 Relation of immunity to copper status

Maturation and signal-mediated activity of immune cells depend on the availability of adequate copper. This relationship has been proposed as a novel biomarker of copper status, though its use is likely to be confined to research and specialist studies[55].

4.7.4 Responses to copper supplementation

As with some of the other trace metal nutrients, response to supplementation in well controlled trials may provide clues to inadequate copper intake in the absence of detectable abnormalities of any of the biomarkers discussed above. As has been observed in the case of zinc, a positive feature of this approach is that it links inadequate intakes with otherwise non-specific disturbances of normal physiology and with otherwise non-specific morbidity[56].

4.8 Copper requirements

The determination of dietary requirements for copper has proved far from easy for those advisory bodies with responsibility for determining dietary requirements. The lack of uniformity in official recommendations published in different countries points to the lack of consensus between experts.

4.8.1 Copper deficiency

Though there is no doubt that copper is an essential nutrient, severe copper deficiency has only rarely been reported in humans[57]. Because of the element's wide distribution in foodstuffs, diet-related copper deficiency is unlikely to occur, except in extreme circumstances. Clinical copper deficiency is far more often seen in premature infants and in malnourished children. Copper stores are laid down late in fetal development. Full-term infants, but not those that are premature, can be expected to start life with adequate stores of the element[58]. The situation in premature infants may also be made more serious if their diet is highly refined carbohydrate- or cow's milk-based, from which copper does not appear to be easily absorbed[59].

Copper deficiency has been known to occur in patients maintained on total parenteral nutrition (TPN). Copper is now usually added to the infusion fluid to prevent this occurring, though there are still occasional reports of TPN-induced copper deficiency[60].

Increased intestinal copper loss in patients suffering from a number of clinical conditions, such as coeliac disease and cystic fibrosis, as well as chronic diarrhoea in children, can also result in copper deficiency[61]. Probably, the best known and most widely studied cause of copper deficiency is Menkes syndrome, the inherited condition in which the body's ability to transport absorbed copper to its tissues is impaired.

The consequences of copper deficiency can be severe. In Menkes disease, for instance, symptoms appear within the first few months of life, and death may follow in early childhood[62]. The symptoms include a variety of cardiovascular and haematological disorders such as iron-resistant anaemia, neutropenia and thrombocytopenia. There may also be bone abnormalities, including osteoporosis and fractures, as well as alterations to skin and hair texture and colour[63], and immunological problems[64].

4.8.1.1 Copper deficiency and heart disease

There is growing evidence that copper deficiency is a risk factor for ischaemic heart disease. A positive correlation between the zinc-to-copper ratio in the diet and the incidence of cardiovascular disease has been postulated[65]. Copper deficiency has been shown to lead to elevated plasma cholesterol levels, impaired glucose tolerance and heart-related abnormalities including blood pressure changes, electrocardiograph irregularities, cardiac enlargement, myocardial degeneration and infarction[66].

4.8.2 Recommended and safe intakes of copper

In 1989, in its 10th edition of recommended dietary allowances, the Food and Nutrition Board of the US National Research Council noted that, because of uncertainties about the quantitative human requirement for copper, it was unable to establish an RDA and could only propose an ESADDI for adults of 1.5–3 mg/d[67]. More than a decade later, in the 2001 review of dietary recommendations, the US experts again noted that the absence of adequate data made it difficult to derive even an Estimated Adequate Requirement (EAR) for the metal[68]. No single indicator of copper requirements was, they believed, sufficiently sensitive, specific and consistent, to be used on its own, and a combination of biochemical indicators had to be used to derive the EAR of 0.7 mg/d, for adults. By extrapolating the EAR to take account of inter-individual variations in requirements, it was possible to derive an RDA for adults of 0.9 mg/d for copper, they proposed. The RDAs for other age groups are listed in Table 4.3.

The UK's expert panel on dietary intakes also noted the inadequacy of data available on copper requirements. They concluded that it was impossible to establish either an EAR or an LNRI for the metal, but that there were sufficient data for infants and biochemical changes in adults on which to base RNIs. These were 1.2 mg/d for adults, with an additional 0.3 mg for women who were lactating. Recommendations for other age groups, including children, are listed in Table 4.4. These UK recommendations are similar to the European Community Population Reference Intake (PRI)[69], as well as to the WHO Acceptable Range of Oral Intake (AROI) of 1.2 to 2 or 3 mg/d[70].

Table 4.3 US Dietary Reference Values for copper.

Life-stage group	RDA (mg/d)	UL (mg/d)
Infants		
0–6 months	0.20 (AI)	ND
7–12 months	0.22 (AI)	ND
Children		
1–3 years	0.34	1.00
4–8 years	0.44	3.00
Males		
9–13 years	0.70	5.00
14–18 years	0.89	8.00
19–30 years	0.90	10.00
31–50 years	0.90	10.00
50–70 years	0.90	10.00
> 70 years	0.90	10.00
Females		
9–13 years	0.70	5.00
14–18 years	0.89	8.00
19–30 years	0.90	10.00
31–50 years	0.90	10.00
50–70 years	0.90	10.00
> 70 years	0.90	10.00
Pregnancy		
≤18 years	1.00	8.00
19–30 years	1.00	10.00
31–50 years	1.00	10.00
Lactation		
≤18 years	1.3	8.00
19–30 years	1.3	10.00
31–50 years	1.3	10.00

Adapted from: Food and Nutrition Board National Academy of Sciences (2003) http://www4.nationalacademies.org/10M/10Mhome.nst/pages/Food+and+Nutrition+Board

AI: Adequate Intake.

RDA: Recommended Dietary Allowance.

UL: Tolerable Upper Intake Level.

4.8.2.1 Upper limits of intake

Copper, as well as being an essential nutrient, is also toxic. Acute toxicity occurs normally at high levels of intake, but chronic poisoning can also be caused by regular intakes of relatively small amounts of the metal. Symptoms of acute toxicity include abdominal pain, nausea, vomiting and diarrhoea, and in extreme cases, death may result. Chronic copper poisoning is often caused by contaminated water supplies or food, as a result of contact with copper pipes and cooking utensils. The long-term effects can be serious, resulting in

Table 4.4 UK Dietary Reference Values for copper.

Age	RNI (mg/d)
0–3 months	0.3
4–6 months	0.3
7–9 months	0.3
10–12 months	0.3
1–3 years	0.4
4–6 years	0.6
7–10 years	0.7
11–14 years	0.8
15–16 years	1.0
18–50 years	1.2
50+ years	1.2
Pregnancy	No increment
Lactation	+0.3

No Estimated Average Requirement (EAR) or Lower Reference Nutrient Intakes (LRNI).
From Department of Health (1991) *Dietary Reference Values for Food Energy and Nutrients in the United Kingdom*, p. 172. HMSO, London.

copper-induced liver cirrhosis, especially in children[71]. Official data, in the UK and the US, indicate that overt toxicity from dietary sources of copper is extremely rare. However, because of the possibility of copper contamination of food and beverage supplies from a number of sources, international and national health authorities have established recommended water and dietary limits for copper. In the UK, a limit of 3.0 mg/l has been set for drinking water. This is higher than the WHO and the EU standard of 2.0 mg/l, while the US EPA has set 1.3 mg/l as the maximum contaminant level. In the US, as can be seen in Table 4.4, a UL of 10 mg has been set for adults, with lesser quantities for younger people[72].

4.8.3 Dietary intakes of copper

In the UK, total dietary exposure of adults to copper, according to estimates based on the 1994 Total Diet Study, is 1.2 mg/d (mean intake), with an upper range of 3.0 mg/d[73]. Similar levels have been reported in the US[74] and in several other countries[75]. These are in keeping with dietary recommendations and are unlikely to result in either deficiency or excess. Indeed, since sources of copper in most diets are numerous, and excessively high levels of the metal are found only where serious contamination of food or beverages has occurred, overt copper deficiency or toxicity is unlikely to occur in those consuming a mixed diet. However, it is believed by some nutritionists that many Western diets provide a level of copper only barely adequate to meet the body's requirements and that it is possible that marginal deficiency may be quite common but difficult to diagnose[76].

References

1. Tylecote, R.F. (1976) *A History of Metallurgy*, pp. 148–9. The Metals Society, London.
2. Stillman, M.J. & Presta, A. (2000) Characterizing metal ion interactions with biological molecules – the spectroscopy of metallothionein. In: *Molecular Biology and Toxicology of Metals* (eds. R.K. Zalups & J. Koropatnick), pp. 5–6. Taylor & Francis, London.
3. Harte, E.B., Steenbock, H., Waddell, J. & Elvenhjem, C.A. (1928) Iron nutrition VII. Copper is a supplement to iron for hemoglobin building in the rat. *Journal of Biological Chemistry*, **77**, 797–812.
4. Mills, E.S. (1930) The treatment of idiopathic (hypochromic) anaemia with iron and copper. *Canadian Medical Association Journal*, **22**, 175–8.
5. Uauy, R., Olivares, M. & Gonzalez, M. (1998) Essentiality of copper in humans. *American Journal of Clinical Nutrition*, **67**, 952S–9S.
6. McAnena, L.B. & O'Connor, J.M. (2001) Measuring intake of nutrients and their effects: the case of copper. In: *The Nutrition Handbook for Food Processors* (eds. C.J.K. Henry & C. Chapman), pp. 117–41. Woodhead, Cambridge, UK.
7. Johnson, M.A., Fischer, J.G. & Kays, S.E. (1992) Is copper an anti-oxidant nutrient? *Critical Reviews in Food Science and Nutrition*, **32**, 1–31.
8. Malmström, B.G. & Leckner, R. (1998) The chemical biology of copper. *Current Opinion in Chemical Biology*, **2**, 286–92.
9. Weser, U. (1997) Biological chemistry of copper. In: *Biological Chemistry* (ed. A.X. Trautwein), Wiley-VCH, Weinheim, Germany.
10. Fraústo da Silva, J.J.R. & Williams, R.J.P. (2001) *The Biological Chemistry of the Elements*, pp. 421–2. Oxford University Press, Oxford.
11. Reilly, C. (2002) *Metal Contamination of Food*, 3rd ed., pp. 161–3.
12. Ysart, G., Miller, P., Crews, H. *et al.* (1999) Dietary exposure estimates of 30 elements from the UK Total Diet Study. *Food Additives and Contaminants*, **16**, 391–403.
13. Pennington, J.A.T. & Young, B. (1990) Iron, zinc, copper, manganese, selenium and iodine in foods from the United States Total Diet Study. *Journal of Food Composition and Analysis*, **3**, 166–84.
14. Lombardo-Boccia, G., Aguzzi, A., Cappelloni, M. & DiLullo, G. (2000) Content of some trace elements and minerals in the Italian total-diet. *Journal of Food Composition and Analysis*, **13**, 525–7.
15. Cuadrado, C., Kumpulainen, J., Carbajal, A. & Moreiras, O. (2000) Cereals contribution to the total dietary intake of heavy metals in Madrid, Spain. *Journal of Food Composition and Analysis*, **13**, 495–503.
16. Booth, C.K., Reilly, C. & Farmakalidis, E. (1996) Mineral composition of Australian ready-to-eat breakfast cereals. *Journal of Food Composition and Analysis*, **9**, 135–47.
17. Reilly, C. (1985) The dietary significance of adventitious iron, zinc, copper and lead in domestically-prepared food. *Food Additives and Contaminants*, **2**, 209–15.
18. Turnland, J.R., Keyes, W.R., Anderson, H.L. & Acord, L.L. (1989) Copper absorption and retention in young men at three levels of dietary copper by use of the stable isotope ^{65}Cu. *American Journal of Clinical Nutrition*, **49**, 870–8.
19. Turnland, J.R. (1998) Human whole body copper metabolism. *American Journal of Clinical Nutrition*, **67**, 960S–4S.
20. Bremner, I. (1998) Manifestations of copper excess. *American Journal of Clinical Nutrition*, **67**, 1069S–73S.
21. Cousins, R.J. (1985) Absorption, transport and hepatic metabolism of copper and zinc: special reference to metallothionein and caeruloplasmin. *Physiological Reviews*, **65**, 238–309.

22. Langhendries, J.P., Hurrell, R.F., Furniss, D.E. *et al.* (1992) Maillard reaction products and lysoalanine: urinary excretion and the effects on kidney function of preterm infants fed heat-processed milk formula. *Journal of Pediatric Gastroenterology and Nutrition*, **14**, 62–70.
23. Vulpe, C.D. & Packman, S. (1995) Cellular copper transport. *Annual Review of Nutrition*, **15**, 768–73.
24. Fischer, P.W., Giroux, A. & L'Abbé, M.R. (1981) The effect of dietary zinc on intestinal copper absorption. *American Journal of Clinical Nutrition*, **34**, 1670–5.
25. Cousins, R.J. (1985) Absorption, transport and hepatic metabolism of copper and zinc: special reference to metallothionein and caeruloplasmin. *Physiological Reviews*, **65**, 238–309.
26. Reeves, P.G., Briske-Anderson, M. & Johnson, L. (1998) Physiologic concentrations of zinc affect the kinetics of copper uptake and transport in the human intestinal cell model, Caco-2. *Journal of Nutrition*, **128**, 1794–1801.
27. Yu, S. & Beynen, A.C. (1995) High tin intake reduces copper status in rats through inhibition of copper absorption. *British Journal of Nutrition*, **73**, 863–9.
28. Haschke, F., Ziegler, E.E., Edwards, B.B. & Foman, S.J. (1986) Effect of iron fortification of infant formula on trace mineral absorption. *Journal of Pediatric Gastroenterology and Nutrition*, **5**, 768–73.
29. Boobis, S. (1999) *Review of Copper*. Expert Group on Vitamins and Minerals. Ministry of Agriculture, Fisheries and Food, London.
30. Poole, D.B.R. (1982) Bovine copper deficiency in Ireland – the clinical disease. *Irish Veterinary Journal*, **36**, 169–73.
31. Brewer, G.J., Dick, R.D., Yuzbasiyan-Gurkan, V. *et al.* (1991) Initial therapy of patients with Wilson's Disease with tetrathiomolybdate. *Archives of Neurology*, **48**, 42–7.
32. Fields, M., Ferretti, R.J., Smith, J.R. & Reiser, S. (1984) The interaction of type of dietary carbohydrate with copper deficiency. *American Journal of Clinical Nutrition*, **39**, 289–95.
33. Milne, D.B. & Nielsen, F.H. (2003) High dietary corn starch compared with fructose does not heighten changes in copper absorption, or status indicators in dietary copper status. *Journal of Trace Elements in Experimental Medicine*, **16**, 27–38.
34. Wapnir, R.A. (1998) Copper absorption and bioavailability. *American Journal of Clinical Nutrition*, **67**, 1054S–60S.
35. Wapnier, R.A. (1998) Copper absorption and bioavailability. *American Journal of Clinical Nutrition*, **67**, 1054S–60S.
36. Dancis, A., Yuan, D.S., Haile, D. *et al.* (1994) Molecular characteristic of a copper transport protein in *S. cerevisae*: an unexpected role for copper in iron transport. *Cell*, **76**, 393–402.
37. Zhou, B. & Gitschier, J. (1997) hCTRI: a human gene for copper uptake identified by complementation in yeast. *Proceedings of the National Academy for Sciences*, **94**, 7481–6.
38. Harris, E.D. (2002) Cellular transporters of zinc. *Nutrition Reviews*, **60**, 121–4.
39. Harris, E.D. (2001) Copper homeostasis: the role of cellular transporters. *Nutrition Reviews*, **59**, 281–5.
40. Failla, M.L. (1999) Considerations for determining 'optimal nutrition' for copper, zinc, manganese and molybdenum. *Proceedings of the Nutrition Society*, **58**, 497–505.
41. Meyer, L.A., Durley, A.P., Prohaska, J.R. & Harris, Z.L. (2001) Copper transport and metabolism are normal in aceruloplasminemic mice. *Journal of Biological Chemistry*, **276**, 36857–61.
42. Wessling-Resnick, M. (2002) Understanding copper uptake at the molecular level. *Nutrition Reviews*, **60**, 177–86.
43. Hamsa, I., Faisst, A., Prohaska, J. *et al.* (2001) The metallochaperone Atox1 plays a critical role in perinatal copper homeostasis. *Proceedings of the National Academy of Sciences*, **98**, 6848–52.
44. Linder, M.C., Wooten, L., Cerveza, P. *et al.* (1998) Copper transport. *American Journal of Clinical Nutrition*, **67**, 965S–71S.

45. Dameron, C.T. & Harrison, M.D. (1998) Mechanisms for protection against copper toxicity. *American Journal of Clinical Nutrition*, **67**, 1091S–7S.
46. Harris, E.D. (2000) Cellular copper transport and metabolism. *Annual Review of Nutrition*, **20**, 291–310.
47. Harris, Z.L. & Gitlin, J.D. (1996) Genetic and molecular basis for copper toxicity. *American Journal of Clinical Nutrition*, **63**, 836S–41S.
48. Linder, M.C., Wooten, L., Cerveza, P. *et al.* (1998) Copper transport. *American Journal of Clinical Nutrition*, **67**, 965S–71S.
49. Failla, M.L. (1999) Considerations for determining 'optimal nutrition' for copper, zinc, manganese and molybdenum. *Proceedings of the Nutrition Society*, **58**, 497–505.
50. Hambidge, M. (2003) Biomarkers of trace mineral intake and status. *Journal of Nutrition*, **133**, 948S–55S.
51. Milne, D.B. & Nielsen, F.H. (1996) Effects of a diet low in copper on copper-status indicators in postmenopausal women. *American Journal of Clinical Nutrition*, **63**, 358–64.
52. Milne, D.B. (1994) Assessment of copper nutritional status. *Clinical Chemistry*, **40**, 1479–84.
53. Prohaska, J.R., Tamura, T., Perecy, A.K. & Tumlund, J.R. (1997) *In vitro* copper stimulation of plasma peptidylglycine alpha-amidating monooxygenase in Menkes disease variant with occipital horns. *Pediatric Research*, **42**, 862–5.
54. Kehoe, C.A., Faughman, M.S., Gilmore, W.S. *et al.* (2000) Plasma diamine oxidase activity is greater in copper-adequate than copper-marginal or copper-deficient rats. *Journal of Nutrition*, **130**, 30–3.
55. Failla, M.L. & Hopkins, R.G. (1998) Is low copper status immunosuppressive? *Nutrition Reviews*, **56**, S59–S64.
56. Hambidge, M. (2003) Biomarkers of trace mineral intake and status. *Journal of Nutrition*, **133**, 948S–55S.
57. Danks, D.M. (1988) Copper deficiency in humans. *Annual Review of Nutrition*, **8**, 235–7.
58. Olivares, M. & Uauy, R. (1996) Copper as an essential nutrient. *American Journal of Clinical Nutrition*, **63**, 791S–6S.
59. Beshgetoor, D. & Hambidge, M. (1998) Clinical conditions altering copper metabolism in humans. *American Journal of Clinical Nutrition*, **67**, 107S–21S.
60. Spiegel, J.E. & Willenbucher, R.F. (1999) Rapid development of severe copper deficiency in a patient with Crohn's disease receiving parenteral nutrition. *Journal of Parenteral and Enteral Nutrition*, **24**, 169–72.
61. Beshgetoor, D. & Hambidge, M. (1998) Clinical conditions altering copper metabolism in humans. *American Journal of Clinical Nutrition*, **67**, 107S–21S.
62. Mercer, J.B. (2001) The molecular basis of copper-transport diseases. *Trends in Molecular Medicine*, **7**, 64–9.
63. Olivares, M. & Uauy, R. (1996) Copper as an essential nutrient. *American Journal of Clinical Nutrition*, **63**, 791S–6S.
64. Hopkins, R.G. & Failla, M.K. (1997) Copper deficiency reduces interleukin-2 (IL-2) production and IL-2 mRNA in human T-lymphocytes. *Journal of Nutrition*, **127**, 257–62.
65. Klevay, L.M. (1984) The role of copper, zinc, and other chemical elements in ischemic heart disease. In: *Metabolism of Trace Metals in Man* (eds. O.M. Rennert & W.Y. Chan), Vol. 1, pp. 129–57. CRC Press, Boca Raton, FL.
66. Klevay, L.M. (2000) Cardiovascular disease from copper deficiency – a history. *Journal of Nutrition*, **130**, 489S–92S.
67. National Research Council, Food and Nutrition Board, Commission on Life Sciences (1989) *Recommended Dietary Allowances*, 10th ed. National Academy Press, Washington, DC.

68. Institute of Medicine (2001) *Dietary Reference Intakes for vitamin A, vitamin K, Arsenic, Boron, Chromium, Copper, Iodine, Iron, Molybdenum, Nickel, Silicon, Vanadium and Zinc.* Food and Nutrition Board, National Academy Press, Washington, DC.
69. European Community Scientific Committee for Food (1992) *Reference Nutrient Intakes for the European Community.* European Community, Brussels.
70. World Health Organisation (2003) *International Programme on Chemical Safety.* http://www.inchem.org
71. Tanner, M.S. (1998) Role of copper in Indian childhood cirrhosis. *American Journal of Clinical Nutrition*, **67**, 1074S–81S.
72. McAnena, L.B. & O'Connor, J.M. (2001) Measuring intake of nutrients and their effects: the case of copper. In: *The Nutrition Handbook for Food Processors* (eds. C.J.K. Henry & C. Chapman), pp. 117–41. Woodhead, Cambridge, UK.
73. Ysart, G., Miller, P., Crews, H. *et al.* (1999) Dietary exposure estimates of 30 elements from the UK Total Diet Study. *Food Additives and Contaminants*, **16**, 391–403.
74. National Research Council, Food and Nutrition Board, Commission on Life Sciences (1989) *Recommended Dietary Allowances*, 10th ed. National Academy Press, Washington, DC.
75. Van Dokkum, W. (1995) The intake of selected minerals and trace elements in European countries. *Nutrition Research Reviews*, **8**, 271–302.
76. Failla, M.L. (1999) Considerations for determining 'optimal nutrition' for copper, zinc, manganese and molybdenum. *Proceedings of the Nutrition Society*, **58**, 497–505.

Chapter 5
Selenium

5.1 Introduction

Some 50 years ago, Schwarz and Foltz presented evidence that selenium was essential for animal life, when they reported that the element was an integral part of what was known as 'Factor 3', a component of brewer's yeast able to prevent liver necrosis in rats and chicks[1]. Their discovery was a milestone in our understanding of the biological significance of selenium, an element which, until that time, had been known only for its toxic properties but was now shown to play a positive role in animal health.

Though selenium was first isolated, and named, by the Swedish chemist Jöns Jakob Berzelius in 1817, the element had already been known, at least for its toxic properties, for several hundred years. In the early thirteenth century, the Venetian traveller Marco Polo, journeying through western China, observed that in one region, merchants prevented their pack animals from eating certain local plants[2]. If they did not, the animals went lame and showed symptoms that today would be recognised as those of selenosis, or selenium poisoning. The plants were most probably selenium accumulators, growing in an area where there was a high level of selenium in the soil from which they took it up and concentrated it in their leaves[3]. A similar type of toxicity has been reported since Polo's time in many other countries besides China. In the mid-US it was known as 'alkali disease' and 'blind staggers' by the stockmen whose cattle succumbed to it; in Queensland, Australia it was called 'hoof drop disease' after the effect it had on horses. Its cause has been shown to be selenium, accumulated to toxic levels from selenium-rich soil, by certain plants, such as *Astragalus racemosus* or milk vetch – 'locoweed' to the cowboys of the 'bad lands' of Nebraska and other mid-west states of the US[4]. Today, selenosis in farm animals is still occasionally reported – as recently as 1993 in India, where buffaloes were poisoned when fed selenium-rich rice straw[5].

Even after selenium was identified and isolated in the early nineteenth century and subjected to investigation by chemists, there was no inkling that the element was anything other than an unpleasant substance, with toxic properties. Some of its compounds had appalling smells – a story is told of an early twentieth-century Cambridge chemist, whose work on organic selenium compounds produced such a terrible stench that he was banned from his laboratory and had to carry on his investigations in the distant fens[6]. Selenium was also believed to have far worse properties than simply a bad smell. As late as the 1960s, it was listed by the US National Cancer Institute as a carcinogen, and a warning was given that any unnecessary exposure of the general population to its compounds was to be avoided[7].

It was a considerable surprise, therefore, when this obnoxious substance turned out to be an essential trace nutrient, for farm animals as well as for humans. Even more surprising was the discovery that in the country where Marco Polo first came across its toxic trail are regions where selenium is in such short supply that endemic deficiency occurs, while in others there is such a high level in the diet that inhabitants suffer from selenosis. Indeed, China is in the unhappy situation of having within its borders three endemic maladies, all selenium-related, one of excess (human selenosis) and the others of deficiency (Keshan and Kashin–Beck diseases)[8].

5.2 Selenium chemistry

Selenium occurs in Group 16/VIA of the periodic table, along with sulphur (S). These two elements, together with tellurium (Te) and polonium (Po), make up what is known as the sulphur family. Selenium is one of the metalloids, or half metals. It has an atomic weight of 78.96 and is number 34 in the table. It has six stable isotopes, ^{74}Se, ^{76}Se, ^{77}Se, ^{78}Se, ^{80}Se and ^{82}Se. Its density is 4.9. It boils at 685°C and volatilises easily on heating. Selenium exists in a number of allotropic forms, one of which is metallic or grey selenium, a crystalline form that is stable at room temperature. Another form is monoclinic or red selenium, an amorphous powder, analogous to yellow 'flowers of sulphur'.

Selenium has unique properties that make it of exceptional value industrially. Its electrical conductivity, which is low in the dark, is increased several hundredfold in light, which also generates a small electrical current in the element. It is, in addition, a semiconductor, possessing asymmetrical conductivity, which allows it to transmit a current more easily in one direction than in another.

5.2.1 Selenium compounds

Chemically, selenium is close to sulphur and forms similar types of compounds[9]. It has four oxidation states, 0, -2, $+4$ and $+6$. The oxidation state Se^0 is the elemental form. In its -2 oxidation state, it combines with metallic and non-metallic elements to form selenides, such as FeSe, Al_3Se_2 and Na_2Se. Most of these are readily decomposed by water or dilute acid, producing hydrogen selenide, H_2Se, a colourless, highly toxic and inflammable gas with a foul odour. It is also a strong reducing agent and a relatively strong acid with a pK_a of 3.73.

The oxides and oxy-acids of selenium correspond to those of sulphur. In its $+4$ oxidation state, it forms the dioxide, SeO_2. This is a white crystalline substance and is a strong oxidising agent. It is readily soluble in water with which it forms selenious acid, H_2SeO_3, which gives rise to the selenite series of compounds, such as sodium selenite, Na_2SeO_3. The selenites tend to oxidise slowly to the $+6$ state when exposed to air, under alkaline or neutral conditions. They are readily reduced to elemental selenium, Se^0, by reducing agents, such as ascorbate.

The $+6$ trioxide of selenium, SeO_3, dissolves in water to form selenic acid, H_2SeO_4, corresponding to sulphuric acid, H_2SO_4. Selenic acid is a strong oxidant and reacts with many organic and inorganic substances. It parallels the S-acid by forming a series of compounds, the selenates, for example, sodium selenate, Na_2SeO_4.

5.2.1.1 Organo-selenium products

Organic compounds of selenium are of considerable interest, and several of them play important roles in cell biochemistry and nutrition. These include selenoamino-carboxylic acids, selenium-containing peptides and selenium derivatives of nucleic acids. Particularly important are selenomethionine, the Se analogue of the S-amino acid methionine, and selenocysteine. The latter is of crucial importance in human metabolism and is known as the '21st amino acid', the only non-S amino acid to have its own specific codon to direct its incorporation into a protein in ribosome-mediated synthesis. Some of the naturally occurring inorganic and organic selenium compounds are shown in Table 5.1.

While organoselenium compounds are similar in chemical and biochemical properties to organosulphur compounds, they are not identical. For instance, because an increase in atomic number results in a decrease in bond stability, selenium compounds are less stable on exposure to light or heat and are more easily oxidised than are their sulphur analogues. Selenols and selenide anions are also more potent nucleophiles, with a greater facility for making carbon–Se bonds, than their S-analogues[10]. Selenols are much stronger acids than are thiols (the pK_a for the selenohydryl group of selenocysteine is 5.2 compared with 8.3 for the sulphydryl group of cysteine). Furthermore, selenols are readily dissociated at physiological pH, whereas the corresponding thiols are mostly undissociated, with implications for catalytic function[11].

5.3 Production of selenium

There are no commercially exploitable ores of selenium, and it is obtained as a by-product of the refining of copper. It is recovered from the electrolytic sludges, along with a variety of other rare and precious metals. A minor source is the dust and sludge remaining when sulphuric acid is made from copper and other sulphide ores. It was from this source that selenium was first extracted and identified by Berzelius. Annual world production today is about 2500 tonnes and is growing[12].

Table 5.1 Naturally occurring inorganic and organic compounds of selenium.

Compound	Formula
Selenite	SeO_3^{2-}
Selenate	SeO_4^{2-}
Selenomethionine	$CH_3\text{-Se-}CH_2CH_2CH(NH_2)COOH$
Selenocysteine	$HSe\text{-}CH_2CH(NH_2)COOH$
Selenocystathionine	$HOOC(NH_2)CHCH_2\text{-Se-}CH_2CH_2CH(NH_2)COOH$
Selenocystine	$HOOC(NH_2)CHCH_2\text{-Se-Se-}CH_2CH(NH_2)COOH$
Se–Me-selenocysteine	$CH_3\text{-Se-}CH_2CH(NH_2)COOH$
γ-Glutamyl-Se-methyl-selenocysteine	$CH_3\text{-Se-}CH_2(COOH)CH\text{-NH-CO-}CH_2CH_2CH(NH_2)COOH$
Dimethylselenide	$CH_3\text{-Se-}CH_3$
Trimethylselenonium ion	$(CH_3)_3\text{-Se}^+$

5.3.1 *Uses of selenium*

Selenium has a considerable number of industrial as well as agricultural and pharmaceutical applications. The electrical and electronic industries take about one-third of total production. It is used on photoreceptive drums of plain paper copiers, though this use has been decreasing as selenium is replaced by other more environmentally friendly photo-sensitive materials. Other uses are in laser printers, rectifiers, photovoltaic cells and X-ray machines. It is also used both to decolourise and to colour glass. The addition of cadmium sulphoselenide to the glass mix gives it a brilliant ruby colour, one of the most brilliant reds known to glass makers, which is widely used in airfield and other warning lights and in stained glass. Selenium compounds are used to produce a variety of other colours, as well as the bronze and smoky glass found in the curtain walls of many modern buildings.

In metallurgy, the addition of small amounts of selenium to alloys improves the machinability of wrought iron products and castings. It enhances corrosion resistance in chromium and other steel alloys. Its other industrial uses include pigments in plastics, a hardener in grids of lead-acid batteries and a catalyst. Selenium dithiocarbamate is used in the processing of natural and synthetic rubber.

There are many agricultural applications of selenium. These include use as an additive and dietary supplement in animal feeds. Soil deficiencies are corrected by the addition of selenium compounds to fertilisers and top dressings. Potassium ammonium sulphoselenide, which is a strong insecticide, was the first systemic insecticide to be marketed. Its use is now restricted to non-food plants because of its toxicity.

Considerable amounts of selenium are used in the pharmaceutical industry, as prescribed and over-the-counter dietary supplements. This use has increased considerably in recent years following reports of the possible protective role of selenium against cancer. A surprisingly large amount of selenium is used as a treatment of seborrhoeic dermatitis and tinea versicolor. A buffered solution of selenium sulphide is marketed as an anti-dandruff shampoo[13].

As a result of these and other applications, selenium, which was once just a rare and low level constituent of our diet, has become one of the normal adventitious environmental contaminants of the modern technological world. This development, which has occurred with increasing rapidity in recent years, has undeniable consequences for human health. Though now well established as an essential nutrient, selenium remains a highly toxic element and selenosis can still occur.

5.4 Sources and distribution of selenium in the environment

Selenium is widely, though unevenly, distributed over the surface of the earth, at overall concentrations of about 50–200 $\mu g/kg$ in rocks and soils. In some places, depending on geological, climatological and other factors, it can be present in greater or lesser amounts. It occurs in igneous rocks as selenides and in volcanic deposits where it is isomorphous with sulphur. In certain sedimentary rocks, such as limestones, shales and coal deposits, its concentration can be relatively high.

Selenium is particularly concentrated in soils of some dry regions, such as the mid-west states of Wyoming, Nebraska and South Dakota in the US, as well as some inland regions of Central China. It occurs in alkaline soils as selenates, which are readily dissolved in water and are available for uptake by plants. In acid soils, it is present mainly as selenide, which is less available to plants.

5.4.1 Selenium in soil and water

Selenium is probably ubiquitous, occurring in all soils, at concentrations, from as little as 0.1 $\mu g/g$ in some areas to more than 1 mg/g in others. Generally, however, most agricultural soils will contain between 0.1 and 1.5 $\mu g/g$[14]. The level of selenium in a soil is determined mainly by geochemical factors, especially the nature of the parent rock. Whereas highly siliceous rocks, such as granite, give rise to soils low in selenium, those originating in coals and shales can contain high levels[15]. Soils that are rich in organic matter, including plant debris and peat, may also have high levels of selenium[16]. Soil concentrations can be affected by rainfall, and by percolating ground and surface water, as well as by other natural and human activities. Climate, especially with regard to rainfall, can result in low levels as a result of leaching out when the element is present as soluble selenate. Selenium-enriched fertilisers are used in many countries to increase levels in deficient soils. Accidental increases in levels have occurred through mining and industrial activities and the spreading of selenium-containing sewage sludge and fly ash on farmland.

5.4.2 Availability of selenium in different soils

Even more important than total concentration, from the point of view of uptake by plants, is the form in which selenium occurs in the soil. This can be as elemental selenium, selenite, selenate, in association with other elements, or in organic form[17]. Elemental selenium is moderately stable in soil and is thus not readily available to plants. In lateritic soils, with a high iron content, Se^0 binds tightly to the iron. Selenides are also largely insoluble, though weathering can increase their solubility.

Selenites are the most important source of selenium in many soils. Under acid conditions, selenite tends to bind tightly to clay particles and iron complexes, and thus its availability is reduced. Alkaline conditions favour conversion of selenite into selenate, which is readily soluble. In dry areas, such as South Dakota in the US, selenate can build up to toxic levels in soil. In wetter regions, the soluble selenate is leached out, leaving selenium-depleted soil.

5.4.3 Selenium in surface waters

Selenium concentrations in natural and domestic waters are generally very low, usually only a few micrograms per litre. A maximum standard of 0.01 mg/l has been set by the WHO for selenium in drinking water[18]. This has been adopted by several countries, including the US[19]. Typical concentrations in domestic water supplies in many other countries are between about 0.05 and 5 $\mu g/l$[20]. A range of 1.6 to 5.3 $\mu g/l$ has been reported in both tap and well water in Germany. A mean concentration of 0.06 μg/l has been reported in an Australian urban water supply[21].

There have been reports of higher concentrations in domestic water supplies in certain regions. In an area of China in which human selenosis occurs, levels of up to 12.27 μg/l occur[22]. Well water in a small municipality in northern Italy was found to have a mean concentration of 7 μg/l of selenium, leading to a ban by health authorities on its use[23]. Levels of 1.6 mg/l have been found in well water used for human consumption in South Dakota[24]. An extreme case, though not in domestic water, was the finding of levels of 260 mg/l in run-off from irrigated crops into the Kesterton reservoir in the San Joaquin Valley, California, where environmental contamination by selenium is a serious problem[25]. However, apart from such isolated situations, water is unlikely to be a significant source of selenium from either a nutritional or toxicity point of view[26].

5.5 Selenium in foods and beverages

Levels of selenium in plant foods, and in the animals that feed on them, reflect levels in the soil on which they grow. Because of the wide regional and other variations in soil selenium concentrations, levels in different foods can show a wide range. For example, in parts of China, where soil levels are very low, locally produced cereals can have as little as 0.02 μg/g selenium. In contrast, in the US, where soil selenium levels are mainly high in cereal-growing regions, levels in grain are approximately 0.30 μg/g[27]. Such variations in concentrations in cereals, as in other foods, can have significant implications for dietary intakes. Thus, in the US, the average daily intakes of selenium range from 62 to 216 μg, while in some regions of China, they are 3–22 μg. In the UK, where, as in most other European countries, soil levels are relatively low, average intake is about 40 μg/d[28].

5.5.1 Variations in selenium levels in foods

Normally, data reported in published documents on levels of selenium, as well as on other nutritional trace metals, represent average concentrations in foods, not levels in individual samples. These can show a wide range. The US TDS reported coefficients of variation (CVs) for selenium of 19–47%, with an average of 32%, higher than the CVs for other trace metals, in the 234 different foods surveyed. The high CV in animal tissues was attributed to variable amounts of selenium consumed, and this in turn was related to variable levels in plant materials attributed to variations in soil selenium[29]. The wide range of CVs found in foods in other countries, in some cases up to a hundredfold, has been attributed to similar causes[30].

An example of the level of variability in selenium levels in a particular, widely consumed foodstuff is seen in the case of cow's milk, which ranges from 10 to 260 μg/kg in different parts of the US[31]. There can even be significant differences between levels in milk produced on different farms, even in a single farming area. An Australian study found that raw milk from one farm contained 38.5 μg/l, while that from a neighbouring farm, collected on the same day, had only 21.0 μg/l. Overall, concentrations in processed (pasteurised and homogenised) milk collected over two years across Australia ranged from 38.34 ± 6.01 to 15.87 ± 4.49 μg/l[32]. The range of selenium in UK milk has been reported as 7–43 μg/l[33], and in a high soil selenium region of the US (South Dakota) 32–138 μg/l[34]. In contrast, milk products in a region of low soil selenium in China contained 2–10 μg/l[35]. It is of interest to note that though wheat grown in North America is generally believed to be a good source of dietary selenium, in fact its selenium concentrations range overall from 6 to 66 μg/kg[36]. This may be compared with the reported range of 2–53 μg/kg in the UK, where dietary selenium intake is moderate to low[37].

A conclusion that can be drawn from consideration of the wide variations to be found in selenium levels in foodstuffs is that, in general, food composition tables cannot be used to provide an accurate estimate of dietary intakes of selenium by particular population groups. This has implications for official investigations that annually determine the range of selenium, and other trace nutrients, in a variety of foodstuffs.

5.5.2 *Sources of dietary selenium*

Levels of selenium in different foods consumed in the UK are summarised in Table 5.2. As this table indicates, the richest sources of selenium are organ meat, such as liver (0.05–1.33 mg/kg), muscle meat (0.06–0.42 mg/kg) and fish (0.05–0.54 mg/kg). Though cereals contain only 0.01–0.31 mg/kg, cereal products make a major contribution to intake of selenium because of the relatively large amounts of cereal products consumed in many diets. Another good source is nuts, but because they are not usually consumed in quantity, they do not normally make a significant contribution to intake. Vegetables, fruit and dairy products are poor sources of selenium.

5.5.2.1 Brazil nuts

Brazil nuts have been reported to be the richest natural source of dietary selenium. Levels of up to 53 μg/g have been found in some sold in the UK[38]. In the US, nuts purchased in supermarkets averaged 36 ± 50 μg selenium/g, with the extraordinarily high level of 512 μg in an individual nut. However, not all Brazil nuts contain such high levels. The selenium concentration in batches of the nuts, even from the same source, can be highly variable. These depend on how effectively the Amazonian rain forest tree *Bertholletia excelsa,* from which the nuts are harvested, takes up the element from the soil. This is determined by the maturity of the root system and the variety of the tree, as well as by the concentration and the chemical form of the selenium in the soil, soil pH and other factors[39].

Brazil nuts are harvested over an enormous area of the Amazon basin, in Brazil, Bolivia and neighbouring countries in tropical South America. Not all soil types and conditions across the growing areas are the same. In some, such as the Manaus to Belem region, stretching for nearly a thousand miles across the lower reaches of the Amazon basin, soil levels of available selenium are high. Nuts from the region contain between 1.25 and 512.0 μg selenium/g, with an average of 36.0 ± 50.0 μg/g. In contrast, nuts from the Acre-Rondonia region, on the upper Amazon where soil levels of selenium are low, contain on average 3.06 ± 4.01 μg/g, with a range of 0.03–3.17 μg/g[40]. Such differences can account for the range of 0.085–6.86 μg/g found in Brazil nuts sold in the UK[41].

Table 5.2 Selenium in UK foods.

Food group	Mean concentration (μg/kg fresh weight)
Bread	44
Miscellaneous cereals	39
Carcass meat	115
Offal	492
Meat products	130
Poultry	185
Fish	360
Oil and fats	30
Eggs	194
Sugar and preserves	9
Green vegetables	8
Potatoes	3
Other vegetables	22
Canned vegetables	14
Fresh fruit	1
Fruit products	0.7
Beverages	0.4
Milk	14
Dairy products	32
Nuts	251

Adapted from British Nutrition Foundation (2001) *Briefing Papers: Selenium and Health*. BNF, London.

While Brazil nuts can be considered a good, if somewhat variable, source of selenium, it is well to recognise that they could also be a health hazard. Brazil nut kernels average about three grams in weight. If these were to contain 50 μg/g of selenium, a level not infrequently found in some selenium-rich samples[42], consumption of three nuts would result in ingestion of about 450 μg of the element. This is the amount of selenium that the UK Department of Health considers the safe maximum intake for an adult. Half a nut could exceed the safe maximum for a 10 kg infant[43].

5.5.3 *Dietary intakes of selenium*

Since selenium concentrations in the diet generally depend on levels of the element in soils in the area in which foods are produced, and since soil selenium levels can show considerable differences across the globe, estimates of per capita intakes vary widely between countries. This can be seen in Table 5.3, in which daily intakes range from as low as 3 μg in parts of China, where human disease has been correlated with selenium deficiency, to a high of nearly 7 mg in another part of the same country where human selenosis has been reported. In a country like New Zealand that has a history of selenium-deficiency diseases in farm animals, human intakes are almost two to 10 times higher than in selenium-deficient parts of China. In contrast, residents of the US normally have an intake twice as high, or more, than that of New Zealanders[44].

Table 5.3 Estimated selenium intakes of adults in different countries.

Country	Intake (mean and/or range, μg/d)
Australia	57–87
Bangladesh	63–122
Belgium	30
Canada	98–224
China	
Enshi Province	3200–6690
Keshan area	3–11
Finland	
Pre-1984	25–60
Post-1984	67–110
France	47
Germany	47
Greece	110–220
Italy	49
Japan	133
Mexico	9.8–223.0
New Zealand	5–102
Spain	60
Sweden	38
Turkey	32
UK	
1974	60
1997	39
USA	98 (60–220)
Venezuela	80–500

Adapted from Reilly, C. (1996) *Selenium in Food and Health.* Blackie/Chapman & Hall, London.

In the diets of most countries, the main sources of selenium are cereals, meat and fish, with only a small contribution from dairy products and vegetables. A US survey found that five foods, beef, white bread, pork, chicken and eggs, contributed about 50% of the total selenium in a typical diet[45]. In the UK diet, bread, cereals, fish, poultry and meat are the main contributors. Percentage intakes from different foods are: bread and cereals 22, meat and meat products 32, fish 13, dairy products and eggs 22, vegetables 6, other foods 5. Of these, nuts provide 1.2%[46].

The dominance of cereal-based foods as core sources of dietary selenium means that intakes can be affected by a variety of unexpected circumstances. These include the success or failure of domestic harvests, fluctuations in international grain prices, and national agricultural and trade policies that affect importation of grain from the world market[47].

The consequences for human nutrition of changes in the international grain market can be significant. Europe, for example, which relied in the past on imported North American wheat to provide high-quality flour for bread-making, has, with the development of new baking technology, been able to rely increasingly on home-grown wheat. But since European wheat is mostly grown on soils which have lower selenium levels than do those of the Canadian and US wheat producing areas, this means that the dietary selenium intake of Europeans has been falling in recent years. Selenium levels in the bread and other bakery products they consume are lower now than they were in immediate post-World War II years. As a result, in the UK, for instance, there has been a substantial drop in daily selenium intake, from an average of 60 μg in 1978, to 43 μg in 1994 and 39 μg in 1997[48], with a corresponding decline in blood selenium levels. Similar changes have been reported elsewhere in Europe[49].

5.5.3.1 Changes in dietary intakes of selenium: Finland and New Zealand

In Finland where, in the 1980s, health authorities became concerned that selenium intakes of the general population were sub-optimal and that consequently there was the possibility of a serious public health problem, a dramatic dietary intervention was undertaken to improve the situation[50]. A law was passed which required that sodium selenate was to be added to all multi-element fertilisers used in agriculture. The intention was that, by increasing the amount of available selenium in soil, the levels in crops and animal feeds, and consequently in human foods, would also be increased.

The decision was based on the knowledge that Finnish soils were selenium deficient and that locally produced plant and animal foodstuffs had lower levels of the element than imported foodstuffs, especially those produced in North America[51]. Surveys had shown that dietary intakes of selenium of the population were possibly among the lowest in the world, at about 25–60 μg/d[52].

The enrichment law required that, from spring 1985, sodium selenate was to be added to NPK (nitrogen–phosphorus–potassium) fertilisers used on cereal crops and grasslands, at a rate of 16 and 6 mg/kg, respectively. The effects were immediate and remarkable. Within the first growing season, increased levels of selenium were observed in feeds and a variety of human foods, initially in cow's milk, rising from 0.02 to 0.19 μg/g (dry weight), followed by meat (pork up from 0.02 to 0.70 μg/g, dry weight). Notable increases were also observed in vegetables and cereals. A particularly impressive increase was in broccoli, over a somewhat longer period, with a rise from <0.01–0.01 to 0.27–1.70 μg/g, dry weight[53]. The effects were also seen in humans, with an increased selenium intake by adults of two- to threefold compared with the pre-supplementation levels during the first year. By the third year, following introduction of the supplemented fertiliser, intakes had reached 110–120 μg/10 MJ, or approximately 100 μg/d[54]. So successful was the outcome of the fertiliser-enrichment programme that concerns were raised about possible adverse health effects of high selenium intakes. As a result, in 1990 a decision was made to decrease levels of selenate in all NPK fertilisers to 6 mg/kg. By 1993, dietary intakes had fallen back to a mean of 85 μg/10 MJ, with a mean serum level of 100 μg/l in both urban and rural populations. The requirement for addition of selenate to fertilisers remains in force in Finland to this day. Blood selenium levels of Finnish residents continue to be among the highest in Europe and on a par with those observed in North America[55].

In contrast to the Finnish strategy, authorities in New Zealand, where soil selenium levels and dietary intakes were, in the 1980s, similar to those in Finland, decided that compulsory nationwide supplementation through the addition of selenium to all fertilisers was not appropriate. Voluntary use of selenium-enriched fertilisers and animal feed, was, however, approved. The practice was adopted on a wide scale by farmers whose animals were suffering from white muscle disease and other selenium deficiency-related conditions[56]. Although selenium intakes by farm animals were increased by such measures, with resulting decreases in selenium-deficiency disease, levels in human foods did not rise significantly. Dietary intakes remained low, at about 28 μg/d in adults, and blood levels continued at a mean level of 68 μg/l, similar to those in pre-supplementation Finland[57]. In spite of this, it was reported that there was no convincing evidence of selenium-responsive clinical conditions in the general population, and the authorities maintained their policy of non-intervention[58].

Surprisingly, in spite of this, selenium intakes have, in fact, increased in New Zealand in recent years. This has been attributed largely to a change in trade laws affecting cereal importation into the country, along with changes in some dietary practices, especially increased use of imported foods. Since the wheat market was deregulated in 1987 and sale of Australian grain allowed in New Zealand, blood selenium levels of New Zealanders have increased significantly, reflecting to a large extent the replacement of low-selenium local flour with a relatively selenium-rich replacement from across the Tasman Sea. Today, the selenium intake of New Zealanders, which was formerly among the lowest in the world, outside the Keshan-disease endemic areas of China, is now considered to be close to that required for saturation of the selenium-dependent enzyme glutathione peroxidase[59].

5.6 Absorption of selenium from ingested foods

Selenium is present in foods mainly as the seleno-amino acids, selenomethionine (mainly in cereals) and selenocysteine (in animal products). In some plants, it also occurs as selenate, for example in cabbage, beets and garlic in which up to 50% may be in the inorganic form[60].

Various other selenium compounds are found, generally in small amounts, in certain plants; for example, methyl derivatives responsible for the distinctive odour of garlic[61], and selenocystathione, which is a toxic factor in the South American nut, Coco de Mono[62]. A number of metabolic intermediates of selenium also occur in plants and animals. Selenium is also consumed in nutritional supplements in the form of selenite, selenate, selenomethionine and other selenium compounds, as well as in enriched yeast preparations.

Absorption of selenium in the GI tract is efficient, with uptake of around 80%. Selenomethionine appears to be actively absorbed, sharing a transport mechanism with the amino acid methionine. Selenocysteine may also share a common active transport mechanism with basic amino acids. Selenate is absorbed by a sodium-mediated carrier transport mechanism shared with sulphur, while selenite uses passive diffusion. A number of dietary factors, in addition to the chemical form, can affect absorption from food. Bioavailability is enhanced by the simultaneous presence in food of protein, vitamin E and vitamin A, while it is decreased by sulphur, arsenic, mercury, guar gum and vitamin C[63].

5.6.1 Retention of absorbed selenium

How much selenium is absorbed from the GI tract appears to depend mainly on its chemical form and subsequent use in the body. Thus, selenomethionine is absorbed and retained more efficiently than are selenate or selenite. However, it is not as efficient at maintaining selenium status. The reason for this appears to be that though selenomethionine is retained in muscle and other tissue proteins to a greater extent than are selenocysteine or the inorganic forms, this retention is non-specific, and the seleno-amino acid is used immediately as a substitute for methionine in protein structure, not as a component of glutathione peroxidase or other functional selenoproteins[64].

5.6.1.1 *The nutritional significance of selenomethionine*

Though selenomethionine is the main selenoprotein of cereals and other plant foods, as well as of 'high-selenium yeast', which is widely used as a nutritional supplement, it was once believed to be a toxic component of seleniferous plants[65]. In more recent years, concern has been expressed that consumption of selenomethionine-containing supplements might, under some circumstances, result in its accumulation in body tissues and its subsequent release with toxic effects. However, it has been claimed that selenomethionine could have beneficial physiological effects not shared by other selenium compounds and that further research may uncover specific therapeutic roles for the seleno-amino acid, especially in tissues such as skeletal muscles, brain and cells of the immune system which have a high affinity for it[66].

5.6.2 Excretion of selenium

Selenium is excreted from the body primarily in urine[67], with about 50% in the form of the trimethylselenonium ion, $(CH_3)_3Se^+$. A small amount is exhaled through the skin and lungs as dimethyl selenide, CH_3-Se-CH_3, and dimethyl diselenide, CH_3-Se-Se-CH_3. These are the compounds that account for the strong 'garlic' smell on the breath of people who consume high amounts of selenium.

A small amount of the body's selenium is lost in hair, nails and breast milk[68]. The relation of maternal intake to the selenium status of the breast-fed infant is of considerable importance and is the subject of extensive investigation[69]. Levels in the milk appear to reflect intakes, though there is evidence from animal studies that females who had previously consumed a high selenium diet may be able to retain a store of the element for use by their sucklings in subsequent times of deficiency[70].

5.6.3 Selenium distribution in the human body

Selenium is transported in a protein-bound form to various organs and tissues of the body. The total selenium content of a US adult has been calculated to be approximately 15 mg (range 13.0–20.3 mg)[71]. Values of less than half these have been reported for New Zealand adult women, with a range of 2.3–10.0 mg[72], and with intermediate levels of about 6.6 mg for adult male Germans[73].

Concentrations in selenium in different organs appear to be related to the total amount and the chemical form of the element ingested[74]. There is, in addition, evidence of a clear order of priority between organs for available selenium, under different conditions of supply. When intakes are adequate, selenium levels are higher in liver and kidney than in other organs; at lower intakes, levels in muscle can be markedly reduced while still remaining high in the kidneys[75]. It has been suggested that the liver has a 'saturation level' for selenium and a minimum requirement at the expense of other organs, suggesting that it plays a special role in selenium balance[76]. Though concentrations of selenium are generally lower in muscle than in other tissues, because of its relative bulk compared with other tissues, muscle appears to be a major storage compartment for the element[77]. Table 5.4, in which concentrations of selenium in tissues of residents of several countries are shown, suggests that these are related to the country of residence, and thus to dietary levels, except in the kidney which is to some extent independent of intake.[78]

5.6.4 Selenium levels in blood

Selenium levels are commonly measured in whole blood in clinical practice. A correlation between whole blood levels and dietary intakes has been shown in farm animals[79]. In humans, whole blood selenium can vary significantly between different populations, depending on dietary intakes[80].

5.6.4.1 Selenium in whole blood

Table 5.5 presents a selection from the literature of data on selenium levels in whole blood of subjects in different countries. They range from extremes such as those in parts of China where human selenosis occurs, to lows as in pre-supplementation Finland. Selenium levels in blood can be affected by changes in place of residence. Thus, blood selenium levels in visitors to New Zealand from the US were found to drop during their first year of residence, from more than 0.15, to less than 0.10 μg/ml whole blood, levels found in native New Zealanders[81].

Table 5.4 Selenium concentrations in organs: international comparison (μg/g, wet weight).

Country	Liver	Kidney	Muscle	Heart
Canada	0.390	0.840	0.370	–
USA	0.540	1.090	0.240	0.280
Japan	2.300	1.500	1.700	1.900
New Zealand	0.209	0.750	0.061	0.190
Germany	0.291	0.771	0.111	0.170

Adapted from Oster, O., Schmiedel, G. & Prellwitz, W. (1988) The organ distribution of selenium in German adults. *Biological Trace Elements Research,* **15**, 23–45.

Table 5.5 Whole blood selenium concentrations of residents of different countries.

Country	Reported concentrations (μg/ml, range or mean ± SD)
Australia	0.210–0.110
China	0.440–0.027
Finland (pre-1984)	0.081–0.056
New Zealand	0.072 ± 0.005
Sweden	> 0.070
UK	0.120–0.091
USA	0.300–0.150

Adapted from Reilly, C. (1996) *Selenium in Food and Health*, p. 39. Blackie/Chapman & Hall, London.

5.6.4.2 *Selenium in serum and plasma*

Plasma and serum contain about 75% of the selenium found in whole blood. Levels in these blood fractions represent recent dietary intakes. They appear to be age-related and can be altered in various diseases and health conditions, as shown in Table 5.6[82]. A world reference range for serum selenium levels in healthy human adults, based on extensive surveys of the scientific literature, of 0.046–0.143 μg/ml has been proposed[83]. Actual levels observed in residents of several different countries are shown in Table 5.7. The figures have been taken from the extensive data, based on findings in more than 70 countries, from Austria to Zambia, published by Combs in his recent review of selenium in global food systems[84].

Table 5.6 Plasma and serum selenium levels in different disease states.

Disease	Selenium level, μg/ml (control)
Cancer (gastrointestinal)	0.486 ± 0.015
	(0.0543 ± 0.016)
Diabetes (children)	0.074 ± 0.008
	(0.065 ± 0.008)
Myocardial infarction	0.055 ± 0.015
	(0.078 ± 0.011)
Crohn's disease	0.110 ± 0.036
	(0.096 ± 0.035)
Liver cirrhosis, alcoholic	0.058 ± 0.011
	(0.080 ± 0.011)
Renal disease	0.078 ± 0.016
	(0.103 ± 0.018)

Adapted from Reilly, C. (1996) *Selenium in Food and Health*, p. 42. Blackie/Chapman & Hall, London.

Table 5.7 Plasma and serum selenium levels in different countries.

Country	Selenium level, μg/ml (control)
Austria	0.067 ± 0.025
Australia	0.092 ± 0.015
Canada	0.135 ± 0.013
England	0.088 ± 0.021
France	0.083 ± 0.004
Italy	0.082 ± 0.023
New Zealand	0.065 ± 0.012
South Africa	0.177 ± 0.011
USA	0.140 ± 0.041
Zambia	0.040 ± 0.010

Adapted from Combs, G.F., Jr. (2001) Selenium in global food systems. *British Journal of Nutrition*, **85**, 517–547.

5.6.4.3 Selenium levels in other blood fractions

Levels of selenium in serum and/or plasma are very widely used in the assessment of trace element status in clinical practice, though there is good evidence that these parameters do not necessarily reflect body stores or dietary intakes. In order to overcome this problem, various other blood fractions are also used by a number of investigators[85]. Erythrocytes are considered to provide a measure of long-term status, unlike serum or plasma levels[86]. Platelets, which have a relatively high concentration of selenium, are believed to reflect recent changes in dietary intake and body stores[87]. They can be separated from whole blood by gradient-density centrifugation, a technique available in many clinical laboratories, and are thus increasingly used in the assessment of selenium status[88].

5.7 Biological roles of selenium

The primary fate of most of the selenium absorbed in the gastrointestinal tract is to be incorporated into selenoproteins that perform a number of essential functions in the body. None of the element remains in inorganic and non-complexed form. Selenium metabolism and the mechanisms by which it is incorporated into selenoproteins are complex and, as has been noted by one of the experts in the field, have probably evolved to deal with the potential for selenium compounds to participate in spontaneous chemical reaction. Because of its chemical reactivity, it is essential that the element be handled mainly in a relatively unreactive organic form before its incorporation into catalytically reactive selenoproteins[89].

5.7.1 Selenium-responsive conditions in farm animals

Selenium has been recognised as an essential micronutrient for farm animals for more than half a century. A number of selenium-responsive illnesses, such as white muscle disease

(WMD), or nutritional myopathy, were found to occur in areas with low soil selenium and, consequently, inadequate selenium in animal feed. These diseases generally occurred in conjunction with vitamin E deficiency[90]. An adequate explanation of the biochemical role of the element and its relationship to vitamin E seemed to have been provided when it was shown that the peroxide-metabolising enzyme glutathione peroxidase contained an integral, stoichiometric quantity of selenium[91]. It was believed that these selenium-deficiency diseases were the result of uncontrolled oxidation in the tissues of animals[92]. However, this hypothesis proved to be only part of the truth, and subsequent investigation made it clear that selenium had other roles. It was found that, even in the presence of adequate vitamin E, deficiency of selenium was linked with enzymic and functional effects that were not oxidation-linked. We now know that selenium acts through the expression of a wide range of selenoproteins that have diverse functions. These functions include, in addition to acting as a powerful antioxidant, roles as a growth factor, an inhibitor of cancer, involvement in thyroid metabolism, immune function and fertility[93].

5.7.2 Functional selenoproteins in humans

In recent years our understanding of the key role that selenium plays in human metabolism and health has expanded dramatically with the availability of the techniques of molecular biology. As noted in a recent review[94], evidence obtained from molecular and bioinformatic studies indicates that between 20 and 30 selenoproteins are expressed in mammals. These proteins may arise from 25 genes identified by computer-searching of the human genome.

With the use of ^{75}Se labelling in mammals *in vivo* or in cells in culture, it has been possible to show the presence of upwards of 40 selenoproteins in mammals. Some 20 of these have so far been characterised by purification and cloning[95]. These include four glutathione peroxidases (GPXs), three iodothyronine deiodinases (IDIs) and three thioredoxin reductases (Trxs). These functional selenoproteins are involved in at least three key areas of cell biochemistry, namely antioxidant function, thyroid hormone metabolism and redox balance[96]. In addition to these three 'families' of enzymes, a number of other selenoproteins have been identified, but their functional roles are still uncertain.

5.7.2.1 Glutathione peroxidases (GPXs)

Each of the four GPXs is located in different cellular compartments and is impaired to a different degree by selenium deficiency. Thus, depending on the sensitivity of each GPX to selenium deficiency, loss of activity from a particular tissue or cellular compartment could cause a specific organ-related condition. This may account for the involvement of selenium deficiency in the pathogenesis of apparently unrelated clinical conditions[97].

'Classical' intracellular GPX (GPXI or cGPX) was the first functional selenoprotein to be clearly characterised. It was originally recognised in 1957, but its selenium dependence was not shown until 1971[98]. It was found in erythrocytes where it protected haemoglobin against oxidative damage by hydrogen peroxide[99]. The enzyme consists of four identical 22-kDa subunits, each of which contains one selenocysteine residue, with the ionised selenol moiety acting as the redox centre in the peroxidase[100]. It can metabolise a wide range of free hydroperoxides as well as hydrogen peroxide, but not hydroperoxides of fatty acids esterified in phospholipids, such as those in cell membranes[101]. In addition, GPXI may function as a selenium store, a role that could account for its usefulness, at least under certain conditions, as an indicator of selenium status[102].

GPXII and GPXIII have similar tetrameric structures to GPXI. They are also antioxidants, though they operate in different compartments, with GPXII in the gastrointestinal tract and GPXIII in plasma[103].

GPXIV, or phospholipid hydroperoxide GPX, is a protein monomer of 20–30 kDa, similar in structure to a single subunit of the other GPXs. It is found in the same organs as GPXI, but not in the same relative amounts. In rat liver, for example, there is relatively little, but it is abundant in the testis, where it may be regulated by gonadotrophins[104]. It is more resistant to the effects of selenium deficiency than are other GPXs, which may indicate that GPXIV has a more important antioxidant role than the other enzymes[105]. It has also been suggested that the major nutritional interaction between selenium and vitamin E may be protection of cell membranes by GPXIV and the vitamin against oxidative damage[106]. Besides acting as an antioxidant, GPXIV is believed to have a number of other roles, for example in eicosanoid metabolism[107], and in maintaining the structure of spermatozoa[108].

5.7.2.2 Iodothyronine deiodinase (ID)

The discovery that selenium was involved in iodine metabolism was a clear indication that the element had roles other than as those of a peroxidase. Type I deiodinase (IDI) was tentatively identified as a selenoprotein when it was shown that selenium deficiency increased levels of thyroxine (T4), while reducing those of 3,3′,5-triiodothyronine (T3) in rat plasma, and that these changes were due to decreased hepatic deiodinase activity[109]. The enzyme was subsequently isolated and its identity as a selenoprotein substantiated by cloning. Its mRNA has been shown to contain a single in-frame UGA codon specifying selenocysteine at the active site in each substrate-binding subunit[110]. IDI is a homodimer with two 27-kDa subunits, each of which contains one selenocysteine residue[111]. The other two deiodinases have also been shown to be selenoproteins. IDI cooperates with IDII in the catalysis of T4 to the active triiodo-form, while, in collaboration with IDIII, it catalyses the conversion of T4 to the inactive 3,3′,5′ reverse triiodothyronine

5.7.2.3 Thioredoxin reductase (TR)

TR is a member of the pyridine nucleotide-disulphide family of proteins. It is a flavine adenine dinucleotide (FAD)-containing homodimeric selenoenzyme that, in conjunction with thioredoxin (Trx) and NADPH, forms a powerful dithiol-disulphide oxidoreductase with multiple roles, known as the TR/Trx system[112].

Each TR subunit has a single selenocysteine as the penultimate C-terminal residue[113]. A number of isoforms of TR have been identified, including cytosolic (TR1), mitochondrial (TR2), which is believed to provide a mitochondrial-specific defence against reactive oxygen species produced by the respiratory chain[114], and TR-β found in high levels in the prostate, testis, liver, uterus and small intestine[115]. TRs affect many different cellular processes. Mammalian TR can catalyse a number of different substrates in addition to Trx, including low molecular weight disulphides and non-sulphides, including selenite, selenodiglutathione, vitamin K, alloxan and lipid hydroperoxides, as well as dehydroascorbic acid[116].

The TR/Trx system is a key player in DNA synthesis, with Trx as a hydrogen donor for ribonucleotide reductase in the initial and rate-limiting step. TR also regulates gene expression through the activation of DNA-binding activity of transcription factors[117]. The TR/Trx system is involved in a variety of other key functions in the cell, including regulation of cell growth, inhibition of apoptosis, regeneration of proteins inactivated by oxidative stress and regulation of the cellular redox state[118]. In a cell-free environment, the system can directly reduce hydrogen peroxide, as well as organic and lipid hydroperoxides, and serve as an electron donor to plasma GPX[119] and IDI[120].

5.7.2.4 Other selenoproteins

Selenoprotein P (Se-P) is a glycoprotein with a single polypeptide chain of 41-kDa and contains 10–12 selenocysteine residues per molecule. Four isoforms of Se-P that share the same amino acid sequence have been characterised[121]. It is the major selenoprotein of blood, providing between 60–70% of the element in plasma[122]. Its role has not yet been clearly determined. It possibly functions as an antioxidant, especially in extracellular fluids. It may protect endothelial cells against peroxidative damage during inflammation, particularly from peroxynitrite, a reactive nitrogen species formed by the reaction between nitric oxide and superoxide under inflammatory conditions[123]. It may also have a role as a transporter of selenium from the liver to sites where it is required for incorporation into other Se-proteins. Se-P is highly sensitive to the selenium nutritional status, making it a useful biomarker of selenium status[124].

Selenoprotein W (Se-W) is located in muscle and other tissues, including brain, testis and spleen. It is a low molecular weight protein of approximately 10 kDa, with a single selenium atom in each molecule as selenocysteine[125]. Its function is unknown, but it appears to be involved in the metabolism of heart muscle. In lambs and other farm animals, it may be necessary for prevention, in conjunction with vitamin E, of white muscle disease. Levels of Se-W respond rapidly to changes in selenium intake[126], and it has been suggested that the enzyme might be a useful biomarker of selenium status[127].

The other selenoproteins that have been either purified or identified by bioinformatic methods remain only partially characterised and their full roles undetermined. Nevertheless, as has been noted by McKenzie and colleagues, their existence as specific proteins emphasises the wide range of metabolic processes that can potentially be influenced by changes in selenium intakes[128]. This has important consequences in relation to selenium status and, in particular, the use of supplements to increase intake of the nutrient.

5.7.3 Selenoprotein synthesis

As has been noted, in all the functional selenoproteins discovered so far, selenium occurs in the form of the selenoamino acid, selenocysteine, which is synthesised by the body in a complex series of operations, from selenium ingested in the diet. Elucidation of the steps involved in this synthesis is one of the remarkable achievements of modern nutrition. It was achieved by the collaboration of investigators from a number of different fields, especially that of molecular biology[129]. Details of these investigations, briefly summarised here, can be consulted elsewhere[130].

The synthesis of selenocysteine and its incorporation into mammalian selenoproteins involve a number of complicated steps, some of which are not yet fully understood. The processes have been characterised in some detail in bacterial and other prokaryotes, but less is known about it in eukaryotes. It is a cotranslational event directed, surprisingly, by an inframe UGA codon which was originally known as a stop or termination or 'nonsense' codon[131]. In selenoprotein synthesis, the UGA is recognised as a code to insert a selenocysteine residue rather than terminate synthesis.

5.7.3.1 Selenocysteine, the 21st amino acid

The finding that a UGA codon specified the insertion of an amino acid other than one of the 20 S-amino acids so far recognised as components of protein was a momentous discovery. For the first time, a non-standard amino acid was shown to be incorporated into a protein during translation. Selenocysteine was, as has been remarked by one of the pioneers in the study of the selenoproteins, the 21st amino acid in terms of ribosome-mediated protein synthesis[132].

5.7.3.2 Selenocysteine synthesis

It has been shown in *E. coli* that selenoprotein synthesis involves the products of four genes (*selA, selB, selC, selD*)[133]. These products are: a selenocysteine-specific tRNA species ($tRNA^{Sec}$), which carries the anticodon for UGA (*selC*); selenocysteine synthase (*selA*) and selenophosphate synthetase (*selD*); two enzymes essential for the formation of selenocysteine-tRNA from seryl-$tRNA^{Sec}$; and an elongation factor that specifically recognises the selenocysteine-tRNA (*selB*)[134].

The process of selenoprotein synthesis in eukaryotes is similar in many respects to that in prokaryotes. There are, however, significant differences, for example, in the nature of what is known as SECIS, the mRNA selenocysteine insertion sequence. In eukaryotes, but not in prokaryotes, this sequence, which is responsible for the recognition of the UGA as a selenocysteine insertion codon, is located in the 3′-untranslated region of the mRNA[135]. Eukaryotes also differ from prokaryotes in having two selenophosphate synthetases, *Sps1* and *Sps2*, rather than a single enzyme. *Sps2* has itself been shown to be a selenoprotein, and this may provide a sensitive autoregulation of selenoprotein synthesis, if its activity decreases when selenium supplies are reduced[136].

Because of their similarities in structure, it might be expected that selenocysteine would be synthesised by the body directly from either serine or cysteine, by replacing an oxygen atom in the former or a sulphur atom in the latter with selenium. However, this is not the pathway followed by Nature[137]. Serine is used to make selenocysteine, but not in a simple substitution reaction. The first step in the synthesis is the charging of $tRNA^{sec}$ with L-serine by the enzyme seryl-tRNA synthetase to form seryl-$tRNA^{Sec}$ and requires ATP[138]. Seryl-$tRNA^{Sec}$ is then converted into an intermediate compound, aminoacrylyl-$tRNA^{Sec}$, by the enzyme selenocysteine synthase.

In the next step of the synthesis, selenium, in its selenide form, is joined to the aminoacrylyl intermediate, under the influence of selenophosphate synthetase, and involves hydrolysis of ATP in the presence of magnesium ions. The highly reactive selenophosphate produced then combines with aminoacrylyl-tRNA^{Sec} to produce selenocysteyl-tRNA^{Sec}[139].

In the final stage of the synthesis, the selenocysteyl-tRNA^{Sec} is incorporated into a growing polypeptide chain to produce selenoprotein. This is an equivalent function to that carried out in prokaryotes by Sel B and involves two proteins. One of these binds to the SECIS sequence. The second is a selenocysteyl-tRNA$^{[Ser]Sec}$-specific elongation factor. Together, they allow the translation of UGA as selenocysteine instead of a termination codon[140].

5.8 Selenium in human health and disease

It was inevitable that once the importance of selenium to farm animals had been recognised, the question was asked whether it also had significance for human health and disease. This has, indeed, been shown to be the case, with numerous reports of adverse effects of both selenium excess and deficiency and a growing recognition that an adequate intake was of importance in the maintenance of health.

5.8.1 Selenium toxicity

The possibility that humans, as well as animals, could be adversely affected by a high intake of selenium in food began to be investigated by the US Public Health Services in the early 1930s, following the identification of selenosis in farm animals in seleniferous areas of the Rocky Mountain states. The health status of rural families in parts of South Dakota with a history of selenium toxicity in farm animals was investigated, along with their intakes of locally grown foods and levels of selenium in their urine. No clear indication of selenium poisoning was found, though there were vague symptoms of ill health and a higher than normal incidence of bad teeth, damaged nails and other less clearly defined symptoms, none of which were specific to selenium poisoning[141]. Subsequently, on the basis of these findings and results from animal experiments, the FDA restricted levels of selenium permitted in animal rations and, later, in human diets, on the grounds that the element was carcinogenic[142].

In the 1970s, there were a number of reports of apparent selenium poisoning, especially of children, in seleniferous regions of South America[143]. One of these described cases of acute intoxication among residents of an area of Venezuela where nuts of *Lecythis ollaria*, a close relation of the Brazil nut, were commonly consumed. The condition was attributed to high levels of selenium in the nuts[144]. About the same time, cases of selenium intoxication due to excessive consumption of selenium supplements intended for agricultural use were reported. One of these from New Zealand described an incident of acute poisoning in a girl who consumed selenium-containing sheep drench[145].

The first large-scale incidence of endemic selenium intoxication due to consumption of selenium-contaminated food was reported in 1983. It occurred in a seleniferous region in China, a remote mountainous area in the mid-west of the country, about 1100 km west of

Shanghai[146]. It has been suggested that this was the area where, many hundreds of years earlier, Marco Polo had observed what is believed to have been selenosis among pack animals[147].

At its peak, the illness affected nearly half the inhabitants of villages in the area. Symptoms included loss of colour and breaking of hair, brittle nails, skin rash, mottled and eroded teeth, and disturbance of the nervous system. Many of those affected suffered from peripheral anaesthesia, 'pins and needles', and pain in the extremities. There was, however, only one report of death. The poisoning was traced to very high levels of selenium in locally grown food, with total daily intakes ranging from 3.20 to 6.99 mg, more than 40 times those encountered in neighbouring, non-seleniferous areas of the country. Changes in the diet, with increased consumption of foods produced in non-seleniferous regions and consequently a significant reduction in selenium intake, have largely eliminated endemic selenosis in the region in more recent years[148].

High intakes of selenium, whether from food or other sources, such as dietary supplements, have been responsible for a number of less dramatic illnesses than the endemic selenosis of Enshi County in China. These include dental caries[149], amyotrophic lateral sclerosis[150], infertility and spontaneous abortion in women[151], and teratogenic effects[152].

5.8.2 *Effects of selenium deficiency*

As was the case with selenium toxicity, so it was with the discovery of selenium deficiency-related diseases in humans. The finding of such conditions in farm animals directed the attention of investigators to the possibility that humans could, under certain circumstances, also be at risk from an inadequate intake of the element. However, in spite of some earlier indications that such conditions did occur, it was not until the 1970s that the possibility was widely acknowledged. This was when selenium deficiency-related illness on an endemic scale was first reported in the international scientific literature.

5.8.2.1 Keshan disease

In the 1930s, an outbreak of an unknown disease with a sudden onset of pericardial oppression and pain, nausea and vomiting, in some cases ending in death, was reported to have occurred in Keshan County, a remote region of Heilongiang Province in north-eastern China. Since the aetiology of the disease was unknown, it was given the name Keshan disease (KD) after the place where it was first observed[153]. Though KD has been found to occur elsewhere in China and neighbouring countries, the name has not been changed.

Because of wartime and other difficulties, the early findings of KD and subsequent research into its distribution and cause were not reported in the international scientific literature for nearly 50 years, though there had been reports in local scientific journals. However, that changed with the publication in English of information presented in Beijing in 1973 at the *First National Symposium of the Etiology of Keshan Disease*[154]. This was followed by a stream of publications in overseas journals, by Chinese investigators and their collaborators from the larger scientific community. KD is now well recognised as a selenium deficiency-related disease of considerable significance, not only in China but also worldwide.

KD occurs in a belt-like zone more than 4000 km in length, which forms an arc through Central China, from the Amur River in the north-east to Lasa in Tibet, touching Myanamar, Vietnam and Laos in the south-west. The disease is encountered mainly in hilly regions, with heavily eroded soils. Epidemics are seasonal and irregular from year to year, with a sharp decline in recent years. Women of childbearing age and children of age 2–10 years, mainly from peasant and non-industrial worker families, are mostly affected. Features include acute or chronic cardiac insufficiency and enlargement, congestive heart failure and arrhythmias. Multiple necrosis and fibrous replacement are seen in the myocardium. The disease may be acute, chronic or latent, with symptoms varying from dizziness, malaise, nausea and loss of appetite, to restlessness and slight dilation of the heart[155].

The aetiology of KD is still uncertain, though there is little doubt that it is related to selenium deficiency[156]. However, other factors appear to be involved. It has been suggested that an infectious myocarditis, possibly caused by enteroviruses, including Coxsachie virus, may play a part in its development[157]. Nutrient deficiencies, especially of vitamins B_1 and E, and of minerals, including magnesium and molybdenum, as well as selenium, may also be involved[158].

The connection with selenium deficiency was established when residents of KD areas were shown to have very low blood and hair levels, as well as urinary excretion rates of selenium compared with people living elsewhere. The low status was attributed to a low dietary intake as a result of consumption of a simple and monotonous diet largely composed of cereals produced on selenium-depleted soil. For example, the two main cereals consumed, rice and maize contained, respectively 0.007 ± 0.003 and $0.005 \pm 0.002\,\mu g/g$, compared with 0.024 ± 0.038 and $0.036 \pm 0.056\,\mu g/g$ in non-KD areas[159]. Several successful intervention trials, in which sodium selenite was provided as a dietary supplement, were carried out. These trials and subsequent interventions in other low selenium areas of China have confirmed that oral administration of a sodium selenite supplement is effective in reducing the incidence, morbidity and fatality of KD. Control of the disease is continued today by the use of selenised salt in affected areas of China[160].

The occurrence of KD has also been reported in other countries. An outbreak of an illness, with symptoms similar to those of KD, occurred in the late 1980s in southern Siberia, in the Lake Baikal region neighbouring Mongolia. Soil selenium levels and dietary intakes in the region were found to be very low, and local farm animals suffered from selenium deficiency conditions, such as white muscle disease. Similar incidents have been reported elsewhere in Russia. Oral supplementation with sodium selenite has been used to treat the condition[161].

5.8.2.2 Kashin–Beck disease (KBD)

This endemic condition is sometimes known as Urov disease, after the River Urov, in eastern Siberia, where it was first reported to occur in 1854. It is more usually named after two Russian scientists, H.I. Kashin and E.V. Beck, who were the first to investigate the condition in the nineteenth and early twentieth centuries[162]. It is an osteopathy believed to be related to selenium deficiency, though that is unlikely to be its sole cause. It is characterised by chronic disabling degeneration and necrosis of the joints and the epiphyseal-plate cartilages of the arms and legs. It is most commonly observed in growing children[163].

Kashin–Beck disease (KBD) has been reported to occur in isolated, usually mountainous areas of China, as well as in the Transbaikalia district of Siberia. Incidents have also been reported in Japan, Korea and other districts of Russia. Most of the areas where it occurs have low levels of selenium in the soil, and dietary intakes of its victims are generally low. Though it occurs in areas in China where KD is also found, the two diseases are not identical. Its aetiology is far from clear. In addition to selenium deficiency, other nutritional imbalances, including a low intake of iodine, may be involved[164]. In addition, there is some evidence that mycotoxin contamination of cereals by certain strains of *Fusarium* mould[165] may contribute to KBD by interfering with collagen formation[166]. An additional factor may be stress of a poor diet and harsh living conditions experienced in the prolonged winter in many KBD areas. Oral supplementation with selenium has been found to be effective. It is believed that general improvements in food supply and overall standards of nutrition have led to a decrease in incidence of KBD in China in recent years[167].

5.8.3 Non-endemic selenium deficiency-related conditions

There are no other reports of endemic selenium deficiency-related conditions similar to KD and KBD. However, illnesses which show some of the features of these two diseases, and which are not confined to any particular geographical region, have been reported. These are normally associated with an inadequate dietary intake of selenium and may be iatrogenic in origin.

5.8.3.1 TPN-induced selenium deficiency

Patients sustained for long periods on infusion fluids have, on occasion, been found to have a low selenium status. Some of these have suffered from muscular pain and tenderness, particularly in the lower limbs. Addition of selenium to the infusion fluid led to a rapid improvement in the patients' condition[168]. Cardiopathy associated with selenium deficiency in parenteral nutrition has also been reported, sometimes resulting in death. Symptoms similar to, though not normally as severe as, those found in Chinese KD patients have been observed in some of these cases[169]. A patient with Crohn's disease receiving long-term TPN exhibited lassitude of the legs, changes in nail colour and macrocytosis. The symptoms cleared up after intravenous administration of sodium selenite[170]. Selenium deficiency associated with cardiomyopathy has been observed in a patient receiving a ketogenic diet as treatment for intractable epilepsy[171].

5.8.3.2 Other iatrogenic selenium deficiencies

Restricted diets followed for therapeutic purposes may result in unexpected deficiencies of micronutrients, including selenium. This is a particular risk where there is an absence of natural proteins in the diet. Patients suffering from the inherited disorder phenylketonuria (PKU), who have a defect in their metabolic pathway for the conversion of the essential amino acid phenylalanine into tyrosine and are maintained on a semi-synthetic diet in which a mixture of amino acids replaces natural, phenylalanine-rich protein foods, have been found in several studies to have a low selenium status. In an Australian study, daily selenium intakes of about 8 μg have been recorded for young PKU children, comparable with intakes reported in Chinese KD sufferers. Yet, no overt signs of selenium deficiency such as growth retardation, nail damage or cardiac myopathy were observed. It would appear that the otherwise well balanced diet consumed by the PKU children, unlike those in KD areas of China, was able to compensate for the low selenium intake[172]. Similar findings have been reported in a number of other countries, including Germany[173] and the US[174].

More recent studies have, however, found some evidence of certain differences between PKU and other children that may be related to their selenium status. Blood T4 levels in the low selenium children were found to be significantly higher than in healthy children from a reference group[175]. A negative correlation was found between plasma selenium levels and whole blood and plasma activity of the transaminase enzyme aspartate amino-transferase (ASAT), which may indicate a subclinical stage of heart or skeletal muscle myopathy. Nevertheless, no evidence was found that these differences between the two groups of children were of clinical importance[176].

5.8.3.3 Selenium deficiency and iodine deficiency disorders

There is a close connection between selenium and iodine metabolism. There are two principal ways in which this connection occurs. First, the three deiodinases, IDI, IDII and IDIII, that regulate the synthesis and degradation of T3 are selenium-containing enzymes. Second, glutathione peroxidases and, possibly, thioredoxin reductase protect the thyroid gland from oxidative damage that could be caused by hydrogen peroxide produced during synthesis of thyroid hormones. Thus, selenium deficiency can exacerbate hypothyroidism due to iodine deficiency[177]. However, in contrast to this adverse effect, concurrent selenium deficiency may also cause changes in deiodinase activity that can protect the brain from low T3 concentrations in iodine deficiency, thus affording protection against neurological cretinism[178].

Studies in some regions of central Africa where iodine deficiency is endemic, and soils are also depleted of selenium, have found that the prevalence of the iodine-deficiency diseases, goitre and myxoedematous cretinism, is greater among populations of relatively low selenium status than among those that are selenium-replete[179]. This suggests that the efficacy of iodine supplementation programmes may be limited in selenium-deficient populations and that treatment with both trace elements may be indicated[180]. In addition to the combined deficiencies of iodine and selenium, it is likely that other factors, such as goitrogens, are also implicated in the development of cretinism[181].

5.8.3.4 Selenium deficiency and other diseases

Selenium deficiency may also be related to several other health conditions. A low selenium status has been linked with an increased risk of pre-eclampsia and spontaneous abortions[182]. A number of studies have found evidence that an adequate supply of selenium is essential for male fertility[183]. Selenium deficiency has also been linked to the occurrence and severity of viral infections. It has been shown, under experimental conditions, that severe selenium deficiency in vitamin E-deficient hosts can change the mutation rates of RNA viruses, such as influenza, measles, hepatitis and HIV[184], and thus increase their virulence[185]. It has been shown, for example, that a mild strain of influenza virus exhibits increased virulence when given to selenium-deficient mice and that this is accompanied by multiple changes in the viral genome in a segment previously thought to be relatively stable[186].

A number of studies have indicated that selenium deficiency may be a risk factor in CVD[187]. A protective effect against the disease could be accounted for by the antioxidant role of GPX in protecting membrane lipids and reducing platelet aggregation. Several epidemiological studies have found evidence of an inverse relationship between dietary selenium levels and incidence of coronary diseases. It has been suggested that the high level of incidence of CVD in Scotland and Northern Ireland, for example, is related to a low level of selenium, and other antioxidants, in the diet[188]. Other epidemiological studies, for example in Sweden[189] and in Finland[190], have also indicated a link between selenium deficiency and cardiovascular disease (CVD)[191].

5.8.4 Selenium and cancer

Though selenium was once considered by the US FDA to be carcinogenic, its positive role as a protectant against cancer has also been postulated for more than 50 years[192]. Epidemiological data collected in 27 countries in the 1970s were believed to indicate that there was an inverse relationship between selenium intake and cancer[193]. Other reports of a similar nature have been published since then[194], though several have been criticised on the grounds of a lack of strength and consistency in the evidence on which they are based[195].

There is little doubt that selenium has anti-carcinogenic properties, as has been shown in studies using animal models. It has long been known that addition of sodium selenite to their diet can reduce the incidence of azo dye-induced tumours in rats[196]. Several other studies have also demonstrated that selenium can inhibit tumourigenesis in experimental animals[197].

There is growing evidence, from human studies, that selenium supplementation of non-deficient subjects may be effective in reducing cancer risk. One of the largest of these investigations involved 34 000 men from the Harvard-based Health Professionals' Cohort. This prospective study looked at the association between selenium intake and prostate cancer, and found that those in the lowest quintile of selenium status were three times more likely to develop advanced prostate cancer than those in the highest quintile[198].

Several large intervention trials involving selenium, and other micronutrients, have been carried out in China. Two of these were conducted in Linxian, a remote rural county in the north of the country where some of the highest rates of oesophageal cancer in the world have been recorded. More than 30 000 subjects were involved, in four separate groups, each of which was given a different combination of nutritional supplements daily over a period of more than six years. In those receiving a mixture of β-carotene, vitamin E and selenium, all at doses two to three times the US RDAs, a significant reduction in cancer mortality was observed[199]. Whether this was due to selenium alone or to the other antioxidants was impossible to say[200].

Another large scale Chinese intervention trial was carried out in Qidong, Jiansu Province, a region noted for its high level of incidence of primary liver cancer (PLC). More than 130 000 people were involved in the trial. Salt fortified with sodium selenite was provided to one group of subjects, while unfortified salt was provided to control groups. After six years, the incidence of PLC had fallen significantly in the fortified area, while there was no change in those receiving the unfortified salt[201].

The Nutritional Prevention of Cancer (NPC) Trial carried out in the US in the late 1990s was the first randomised double-blind, placebo-controlled intervention trial in a Western population, designed to test the hypothesis that supplementation with selenium could reduce the risk of cancer[202]. Though the results did not show that selenium supplementation could reduce the risk of basal or squamous cell carcinomas, they did indicate that it was associated with significantly fewer incidents of total non-skin cancers (37%), total carcinomas (45%) and cancer of the prostate (63%), colon–rectum (58%) and lung (46%), as well as mortality due to lung (53%) and total cancers (50%). The 1312 subjects who took part in the trial received a daily intake of 200 μg of selenium in the form of selenium-enriched yeast, a dose nearly four times the current US RDA. The results have been widely accepted by many health professionals, as well as the general public, as supporting the view that high-level exposure to at least some selenium compounds can be anti-tumorigenic[203] and have led to widescale self-medication with high doses of selenium as a preventive against cancer[204].

A further randomised, prospective, double-blind trial has been planned to investigate whether selenium and vitamin E alone and in combination can reduce the risk of prostate cancer among healthy men. This is the Selenium and Vitamin E Cancer Prevention Trial (SELECT) that will study some 32 400 men with a low serum prostate specific antigen (PSA) level. The trial was started in 2001, with results expected in 2013[205].

Some investigators believe that not enough is yet known about the effects of using selenium, especially in high doses, as a health supplement, or about cancer risks, and that such large scale intervention trials are premature. Criticism has been made especially of an earlier proposal, since modified, for a very large international study, known as the Prevention of Cancer with Selenium in Europe and America Trial (PRECISE), with more than 50 000 subjects from six countries taking either a placebo or a dose of 100, 200 or 300 μg of selenium per day for five years[206]. One of the major concerns is that the anticarcinogenic activity of selenium compounds most probably depends not on their nutritional role but on their toxicity, both oxidative and genotoxic. Before large numbers of people are exposed to long-term and high doses, some argue, it must be clear that doing so carries no risk[207].

As has been pointed out by Combs[208], the anti-tumorigenic effects seen in experimental carcinogenic models have been consistently associated with very high levels of intake of selenium. These 'supranutritional' intakes are at least 10-fold those required to prevent clinical signs of selenium deficiency and are considerably higher than the level of intake at which GPX and other selenoproteins are maximally expressed[209]. Thus, the effects are believed to be due not to selenium acting simply as a nutrient, but to the production of selenium metabolites with anticarcinogenic properties[210]. These most probably include methylselenol (CH_3SeH) and related compounds that enhance carcinogen metabolism.

5.8.5 Selenium and the immune response

Since selenium is involved in most aspects of cell biochemistry and function, it can be expected that it also is able to influence the immune system of the body[211]. How it performs this function is not clearly understood, in spite of the considerable amount of investigation carried out in recent years. These investigations are discussed in a number of reviews, such as those by Arthur and colleagues[212], on which much of the following brief account is based.

Immunity and the immune system involve a very complex collection of processes that act together to protect the organism against attacks by pathogens and malignancy. The system operates at several levels. A first line of defence is innate or natural immunity, which provides formidable physical and chemical protection against infection. This is the function of skin and other epithelial and mucous-membrane barriers and surface secretions of the respiratory and other tracts. The process includes phagocytosis and killing of invading organisms as well as secretions of enzymes and other compounds that provide a chemical barrier, a non-specific and not always effective form of defence. The most important of these defensive secretions are the lysozymes, with, as the next line of defence, acute-phase proteins and interferons. Phagocytosis, the ingestion and destruction of foreign material entering the cell, is the work of polymorphonuclear neutrophil leucocytes, white blood cells, followed by the monocyte–macrophage system[213].

Selenium supplementation can substantially decrease the level of skin damage, tumour formation and overall mortality in mice exposed to ultraviolet B (UVB) radiation[214]. Langerhans cells (LCs) are the most abundant dendritic antigen-presenting cells in the skin and are the prime initiators of cutaneous immune response[215]. Recent research has shown that selenium deficiency reduces epidermal LC numbers and thus may contribute to reduced cutaneous immunity[216].

Adaptive or acquired immunity is the body's second line of defence and comes into play when invading organisms manage to pass the non-specific defences. Both T- and B-lymphocytes form the major effector cells of the acquired system that respond to immune challenges. Selenium-deficient lymphocytes are less able to proliferate in response to mitogen than they are when selenium is in adequate supply. The deficiency also impairs leucotriene B4 synthesis, which is essential for neutrophil chemotaxis. In addition, production of immunoglobulins is impaired with, in humans, decreases in IgG and IgM titres[217].

It has been shown that selenium deficiency in experimental animals impairs the ability of neutrophils and macrophages to kill ingested pathogens. In selenium-replete animals, the invaders are killed by free radicals produced by neutrophils in a respiratory burst. Any surplus reactive species which could damage the cell's microbicidal and metabolic functions are immediately mopped up by cytosolic GPX. However, when there is inadequate selenium, GPX activity is reduced, with the result that neutrophils themselves are damaged by the free radicals[218].

There is some evidence, though so far inconclusive, that GPXIV which is able to metabolise fatty acid hydroperoxides esterified to phospholipids in membranes undergoing oxidative stress, plays an important role in protecting cells against free-radical damage[219]. The ability of selenium at normal levels of intake to modulate GPX activities is believed to indicate that this role constitutes a plausible explanation for its effects on inflammation[220]. This view is supported by the finding that selenium supplementation of normal subjects in the UK leads to changes that stimulate the immune system by, for example, improving lymphocyte response to a challenge with poliovirus[221]. There are several other reports of the effectiveness of selenium in boosting immune responses. Supplementation of institutionalised elderly subjects has been found to increase their production of T-cells[222]. Similarly, supplementation of selenium-replete subjects resulted in a significant increase in cytoxic lymphocytes and natural killer cell activity, even though there was no significant change in blood selenium levels[223].

5.8.6 Selenium and brain function

There are good grounds for believing that selenium plays a role in brain function. The supply of the element to the brain is maintained at the expense of other organs during deficiency[224]. This preferential retention suggests that the element has a special role in psychological functioning of the brain[225]. Evidence exists of a connection between low selenium status and mental depression[226], and selenium supplementation has been found to decrease anxiety significantly in some cases[227]. It has been suggested that the beneficial effect of selenium in such cases is associated with thyroid-hormone metabolism

Use of a trace element and vitamin supplement, which included selenium, has been found to be beneficial in the treatment of mood lability and explosive rage in certain children. Whether selenium alone would have a similar effect was not investigated[228]. Supplementation with selenium has been found to improve depression and behavioural problems in patients undergoing dialysis, suggesting that selenium deficiency may play a role in the mechanisms of psychiatric disorders.[229]. Changes in selenium concentrations in brain tissue have been reported in Alzheimer's disease and in brain tumours. Glutathione peroxidase has been localised in glial cells, and its expression is increased in the damaged area in Parkinson's disease and occlusive cerebrovascular disease. There are suggestions that selenium supplementation may be beneficial in the treatment of Alzheimer's patients and schizophrenics[230].

5.8.7 Selenium and other health conditions.

It has been claimed that there are at least 50 specific diseases against which selenium may have a protective role[231]. While this may be an exaggeration, it is true that oxidative damage has been implicated in a range of degenerative disorders, and selenium undoubtedly plays an antioxidant role in the body. Burk was probably too harsh, when he observed that our vacuum of knowledge about the pathological conditions in human beings related to selenium deficiency was being filled by speculation[232]. That may have been true to a certain extent when he wrote in 1988, but today there is little doubt that selenium does play a very wide role in the maintenance of human health.

There are many degenerative disorders, in addition to cancer and heart disease, in which oxidative damage is known to have a role, and in these it is not unlikely that antioxidant selenoproteins play a protective role. These disorders include stroke, macular degeneration and age-related cataract[233], rheumatoid arthritis and various conditions that are part of the ageing process. Selenium deficiency may also be involved in asthma. A New

Zealand study has provided evidence pointing to a connection between a low intake of dietary selenium and the high prevalence of asthma in the country[234]. Certain conditions such as cystic fibrosis and coeliac disease, in which nutrient absorption from the diet is compromised, may also have a selenium deficiency connection[235].

Many of the human health conditions for which claims have been made of a connection with selenium deficiency appear to be of similar origin to diseases to which farm animals have been shown to be predisposed by an inadequate intake of the element. Considerable interest worldwide was generated by the report in the late 1960s that sudden death in selenium-deficient pigs had close similarities to human cot death or Sudden Infant Death Syndrome (SIDS)[236]. Subsequent investigations have produced contradictory findings and, in general, have failed to support any connection between selenium deficiency and SIDS[237]. Though the debate continues sporadically in the medical literature, it seems likely that SIDS is multifactorial in origin and that physical conditions as well as nutritional factors are involved.

5.9 Recommended allowances, intakes and dietary reference values for selenium

Dietary recommendations have been the subject of considerable debate since they were first published in a number of countries in the late 1980s. The main reason for this has been the difficulties encountered by expert committees in attempting to arrive at a definition of requirements based on the interpretation of biochemical markers of selenium status[238]. In recent years, the controversy has been further stimulated by changing attitudes in nutrition and the development of new concepts of 'optimal' nutrition, which are complementary to 'adequate' nutrition[239]. As a consequence, there are uncertainties and a lack of uniformity between intake recommendations in different countries, and expert committees are currently undertaking a review of the recommendations or have already done so and have issued new guidelines. Their recommendations have been controversial in some cases, not least in the US where, in spite of strong pressure from several leading nutritionists for an increase in the RDA, it has been lowered[240].

The first country to establish an official recommended intake for selenium was Australia when, in 1987, the NHMRC proposed an RDI of 80 and 70 μg/d for adult men and women, respectively[241]. Two years later, the US National Research Council followed the Australians with a selenium RDA of 70 and 55 μg/d for men and women, respectively[242]. In 1991, the UK's COMA established an RNI of 75 μg/d for men and 60 μg/d for women, with an LRNI of 40 μg/d for both male and female adults, as shown in Table 5.8. Several other national and international bodies have also established dietary recommendations for selenium. The WHO's recommendation is 40 and 30 μg/d[243], and that of the Nordic countries 60 and 30 μg/d for adult men and women, respectively. The current US RDA for both males and females is 55 μg/d. Details of the full US recommendations are given in Table 5.9.

The differences between intake recommendations for different countries reflect differences in approaches and in interpretations of data by the experts charged with responsibility for making recommendations. Nève has discussed the problems caused by such differences in a review which provides a useful comment on the problem, especially as it impinges on the reasoning behind the decision of the US experts to reduce the adult

Table 5.8 UK recommendations for selenium intake (μg/d).

Age	Lower reference nutrient intake (LRNI)	Reference nutrient intake (RNI)
0–3 months	4	10
4–6 months	5	13
7–9 months	5	10
10–12 months	6	10
1–3 years	7	15
4–6 years	10	20
7–10 years	16	30
Men		
11–14 years	25	45
15–18 years	40	70
19–50 years	40	75
50+ years	40	75
Women		
11–14 years	25	45
15–18 years	40	60
19–50 years	40	60
50+ years	40	60
Lactation	+15	+15

Department of Health (1991) *Dietary Reference Values for Food Energy and Nutrients for the UK*. COMA, HMSO, London.

RDA to 55 μg/d[244]. Interestingly, in spite of the view expressed by some experts that dietary recommendations for selenium should be increased to reflect possible beneficial effects for chronic diseases such as cancer and heart disease[245], the outcome of at least some of the current reviews is likely to be a reduction in dietary reference values for selenium. The proposed joint Australian and New Zealand nutrient reference values, which will replace the current Australian standards[246], are for an RNI of 60 and 55 μg/d, for adult males and females, respectively. In addition, however, there is a proposal for an additional reference value, known as the Provisional Functional Range (PFR) of 50–125 μg/d, to allow for possible health benefits of higher selenium doses[247]. This innovation is an approach that may well be followed in other countries.

5.10 Perspectives for the future

There are still many unanswered questions about selenium's metabolic roles and its place in human health. The importance of the element, once known only for its toxic effects on farm animals and humans, is now universally accepted, as is its essentiality for several key metabolic functions. Some populations, however, have a dietary intake that is insufficient for maximum expression of many of the selenoproteins that play key roles in the body. Selenium supplementation has been shown to be able to increase selenium

Table 5.9 US recommendations for selenium intake (μg/d)

Life-stage group	RDA/AI*	UL
Infants		
0–6 months	15*	45
7–12 months	20*	60
Children		
1–3 years	**20**	90
4–8 years	**30**	150
Males		
9–13 years	**40**	280
14–18 years	**55**	400
19–30 years	**55**	400
31–50 years	**55**	400
50–70 years	**55**	400
>70 years	**55**	400
Females		
9–13 years	**40**	280
14–18 years	**55**	400
19–30 years	**55**	400
31–50 years	**55**	400
50–70 years	**55**	400
>70 years	**55**	400
Pregnancy		
≤ 18 years	**60**	400
19–30 years	**60**	400
31–50 years	**60**	400
Lactation		
≤ 18 years	**70**	400
19–30 years	**70**	400
31–50 years	**70**	400

RDA: Recommended Dietary Allowances are shown in bold. Adequate Intakes (AIs) are shown in ordinary type followed by an asterisk; RDAs are set to meet the needs of almost all (97–98%) individuals in a group. For healthy breastfed infants, the AI is the mean intake. The AI for other life-stage and gender groups is believed to cover the needs of all individuals in a group, but because of the lack of data, the percentage of individuals covered by this intake cannot be specified with confidence. UL: the maximum level of daily intake (from all sources) that is likely to pose no risk of adverse effects.

Adapted from: Food and Nutrition Board National Academy of Sciences (2002) *US Dietary Reference Intakes: Elements.* http://www4.nationalacademies.org/10M/10MHome.nst/pages/Food+and+Nutrition+Board

status and to restore levels of expression of glutathione peroxidases and other functional selenoproteins. Such an improvement could have potential benefits, including prevention of cancer, improved thyroid metabolism and a number of other effects such as prevention of male infertility. This was the sort of reasoning that lay behind the Finnish authorities' decision to legislate for the addition of selenium to fertilisers. A similar policy has been advocated in the UK[248]. However, COMA has concluded that such measures should not be encouraged without evidence of adverse effects from the UK's current relatively low selenium intakes[249]. Moreover, even though selenium supplementation trials that have already been carried out indicate that such increases in dietary intake can change the activity of selenium-dependent metabolic pathways, the actual benefits can only be predicted after extensive trials in which the effects of the micronutrient can be separated from other dietary or medical interventions that may be taking place[250].

Two further points need to be taken into account when the question of selenium supplementation, whether on an individual or a community scale, is being considered. The first is that there are variations in the way in which people respond to selenium supplementation. The second is that many of the reported beneficial effects of selenium supplementation, for example in cancer prevention, have been achieved with the use of 'supranutritional' intakes of the element. To take the second point first, it has been noted by Combs that the anti-tumorigenic effects in experimental carcinogenesis models have been consistently associated with intakes of selenium that are at least 10-fold those required to prevent signs of selenium deficiency[251]. They are also much greater than the dietary intakes of most people worldwide and greater than the recommended dietary intakes in the US, UK and other countries. Dietary supplement preparations containing up to 200 μg of selenium are available in the UK and elsewhere without medical certificate and are consumed by many people. The intervention study of Clark and colleagues in the US provided doses of up to 200 μg/d to participants over a period of 4.5 years[252]. Doses of 300 μg/d were considered for a follow-up intervention study[253].

Though intakes of 200–300 μg/d are below the upper safe limit of 400 μg/d of selenium set by WHO[254], and also the UK's recommended maximum safe intake of 450 μg/d[255], concern has been expressed by some experts about the long-term use of high doses on the basis of findings in a study of the effects of high intakes of naturally occurring selenium in drinking water[256]. However, a review by the US EPA has concluded that the NOAEL for an adult is 853 μg of selenium per day[257]. The agency's current Reference Dose (RfD) for a 70-kg human is 350 μg/d, which is what on average an American adult, consuming a normal diet, with an additional supplement intake of 200 μg might be expected to consume in a day[258]. A similar intake level in the UK would require consumption of a supplement of at least 300 μg/d.

To return to the first point, as has been pointed out by Arthur, differences in responses to selenium supplementation, in part, may be explained by single nucleotide polymorphisms[259]. Searches of the human genome have revealed the potential for many single nucleotide polymorphisms in selenium-containing proteins, and investigation of these polymorphisms may shed further light on individual variations in response to selenium deficiency or supplementation. However, until these investigations are carried out, the actual health effects of selenium supplementation, especially if carried out, as in Finland, on a nationwide basis, cannot be predicted with reliability.

References

1. Schwarz, K. & Foltz, C.M. (1957) Selenium as an integral part of Factor 3 against dietary necrotic liver degeneration. *Journal of the American Chemical Society*, **79**, 3292–3.
2. Polo, M. (1967) *The Travels of Marco Polo*, translated by E.W. Marsden, revised by T. Wright, Chapter XL, pp. 110–11. Everyman's Library, Dent, London.
3. Yang, G., Wang, S., Zhou, R. & Sun, S. (1983) Endemic selenium intoxication of humans in China. *American Journal of Clinical Nutrition*, **37**, 872–31.
4. Jukes, T.H. (1983) Nuggets on the surface: selenium an 'essential poison'. *Journal of Applied Biochemistry*, **5**, 233–4.
5. Subramanian R. & Muhuntha, A. (1993) Soil–fodder–animal relationship of selenium toxicity in buffalos. In: *Trace Elements in Man and Animals – TEMA 8* (eds. M. Anke, D. Meissner & C.F. Mills), pp. 498–501. Verlag Media Touristik, Gersdorf, Germany.
6. Frost, D.V. (1972) The two faces of selenium – can selenophobia be cured? In: *Critical Reviews in Toxicology* (ed. D. Hemphill), pp. 467–514. CRC Press, Boca Raton, FL.
7. Hueper, W.C. (1961) Carcinogens in the human environment. *Archives of Pathology*, **71**, 237–44.
8. Reilly, C. (1991) *Selenium in Food and Health*, pp. 4–21. Chapman & Hall/Blackie, London.
9. Tinggi, U. & Reilly, C. (2002) Selenium: its molecular chemistry and role in health and disease. In: *Proceedings of the Malaysian Chemistry Congress*, 12–14 December, Kuching, Malaysia.
10. Monahan, R., Brown, D., Waykole, L. & Liotta, D. (1987) Nucleophilic selenium. In: *Organoselenium Chemistry* (ed. D. Liotta), pp. 207–41. Wiley-Interscience, New York.
11. Ursini, R. & Bindoli, A. (1987) The role of selenium peroxidases in the protection against oxidative damage of membranes. *Chemistry and Physics of Lipids*, **44**, 255–76.
12. Hoyne, E. (1992) The selenium and tellurium markets. *Selenium–Tellurium Development Association Bulletin*, September, 1–3. Selenium–Tellurium Development Association, Grimbergen, Belgium.
13. Selenium-Tellurium Development Association (1993) *Information on the Uses, Handling and Storage of Selenium*. Selenium–Tellurium Development Association, Grimbergen, Belgium.
14. Berrow, M.L. & Ure, A.M. (1989) Geological materials and soils. In: *Occurrence and Distribution of Selenium* (ed. M. Ihnat), pp. 226–8. CRC Press, Boca Raton, FL.
15. Thornton, I., Kinniburgh, D.G., Pullen, G. & Smith, C.A. (1983) Geochemical aspects of selenium in British soils and implications for animal health. In: *Trace Substances in Environmental Health* (ed. D.D. Hemphill), pp. 391–405. University of Missouri Press, Columbia, MO
16. Fleming, G.A. (1962) Selenium in Irish soils and plants. *Soil Science*, **94**, 28–35.
17. Olson, O.E. (1967) Soil, plant, animal cycling of excessive levels of selenium. In: *Selenium in Biomedicine* (ed. O.H. Muth, J.E. Oldfield & P.H. Wesig), pp. 251–73. AVI, Westport, CT.
18. World Health Organisation (1971) *International Standards for Drinking Water*. World Health Organisation, Geneva.
19. US Public Health Service (1967) *Code of Regulations. Drinking Water*. Title 42.
20. Oelschlager, W. & Menke, K.H. (1969) Concerning the selenium content of plant, animal and other materials. II. The selenium and sulfur content of foods (in German, English Abstract). *Zeitschrift für Ernahrungswissenschaft*, **9**, 216–22.
21. Tinggi, U., Reilly, C. & Patterson, C.M. (1992) Determination of selenium in foodstuffs using spectrofluorometry and hydride generation atomic absorption spectrometry. *Journal of Food Composition and Analysis*, **5**, 269–80.
22. Yang, G., Zhou, R., Gu, L., Liu, Y. & Li, X. (1989) Studies of safe maximal daily dietary selenium intake in the seleniferous area of China. I. Selenium intake and tissue selenium levels of the inhabitants. *Trace Elements and Electrolytes in Health and Disease*, **3**, 77–87.

23. Vivoli, G., Vinceti, M., Rovesti, M. & Bergomi, M. (1993) Selenium in drinking water and mortality for chronic diseases. In: *Trace Elements in Man and Animals – TEMA 8* (eds. M. Anke, D. Meissner & C.F. Mills), pp. 951–4. Verlag Media Touristik, Gersdorf, Germany.
24. Byers, H.G. (1936) Selenium occurrence in certain soils in the United States with a discussion of certain topics. *US Department of Agriculture Technical Bulletin*, No. 530, pp. 1–78. USDA, Washington, DC.
25. University of California Agricultural Issues Center (1998) Selenium, human health and irrigated agriculture. In: *Resources at Risk in the San Joaquin Valley*. University of California, Davis, CA.
26. National Academy of Sciences/National Research Council (1989) *Recommended Dietary Allowances*, 10th ed., pp. 217–24. Food and Nutrition Board, National Academy of Sciences/ National Research Council, Washington, DC.
27. Reilly, C. (1996) *Selenium in Food and Health*, p. 29. Blackie, London.
28. British Nutrition Foundation (2001) *Selenium and Health*, 5. British Nutrition Foundation, London.
29. Pennington, J.A.T. & Young, B. (1990) Iron, zinc, copper, manganese, selenium and iodine in foods from the United States Total Diet Study. *Journal of Food Composition and Analysis*, **3**, 166–84.
30. Molnar, J., MacPherson, A., Barclay, I. & Molnar, P. (1995) Selenium content of convenience and fast foods in Ayrshire, Scotland. *International Journal of Food Science and Nutrition*, **46**, 343–52.
31. Combs, G.F. (2001) Selenium in global food systems. *British Journal of Nutrition*, **85**, 517–47.
32. Tinggi, U., Patterson, C. & Reilly, C. (2001) Selenium levels in cow's milk from different regions of Australia. *International Journal of Food Science and Nutrition*, **52**, 43–51.
33. Barclay, M.N.I., MacPherson, A. & Dixon, J. (1995) Selenium content of a range of UK foods. *Journal of Food Composition and Analysis*, **8**, 307–18.
34. Olsen, O.E. & Palmer, I.S. (1984) Selenium in foods purchased or produced in South Dakota. *Journal of Food Science*, **49**, 446–52.
35. Combs, G.F., Jr. & Combs, S.B. (1986) The biological variability of selenium in foods and feeds. In: *The Role of Selenium in Nutrition* (eds. G.F. Combs & S.B. Combs), pp. 127–77. Academic Press, New York.
36. United States Department of Agriculture (1999) *Nutrient Database for Standard Reference*. http://www.nal.usda.gov/fnic/foodcomp/Data/SR13/sr13.html
37. Barclay, M.N.I., MacPherson, A. & Dixon, J. (1995) Selenium content of a range of UK foods. *Journal of Food Composition and Analysis*, **8**, 307–18.
38. Thorn, J., Robertson, J. & Buss, D.H. (1978) Trace nutrients. Selenium in British foods. *British Journal of Nutrition*, **39**, 391–6.
39. Reilly, C. (1999) Brazil nuts – a selenium supplement? *BNF Nutrition Bulletin*, **24**, 177–84.
40. Sector, C.L. & Lisk, D.J. (1989) Variation in the selenium content of individual Brazil nuts. *Journal of Food Safety*, **9**, 279–81.
41. Molnar, J., MacPherson, A., Barclay, I. & Molnar, P. (1995) Selenium content of convenience and fast foods in Ayrshire, Scotland. *International Journal of Food Science and Nutrition*, **46**, 343–52.
42. United States Department of Agriculture (1999) *Nutrient Database for Standard Reference*. http://www.nal.usda.gov/fnic/foodcomp/Data/SR13/sr13.html
43. Department of Health (1991) *Dietary Reference Values for Food Energy and Nutrients for the United Kingdom. Report on Health and Social Subjects 41*. HMSO, London.
44. Combs, G.F. (2001) Selenium in global food systems. *British Journal of Nutrition*, **85**, 517–47.
45. Schubert, A., Holden, J.M. & Wolf, W.R. (1987) Selenium content of a core group of foods based on a critical evaluation of published analytical data. *Journal of the American Dietetic Association*, **87**, 285–92.

46. Ministry of Agriculture, Fisheries and Food (1999) 1997 Total Diet Study – aluminium, arsenic, cadmium, chromium, copper, lead, mercury, nickel, selenium, tin and zinc. In: *Food Surveillance Sheet, No. 191*. Ministry of Agriculture, Fisheries and Food, London.
47. Combs, G.F. (2001) Selenium in global food systems. *British Journal of Nutrition*, **85**, 517–47.
48. Rayman, M.P. (2000) The importance of selenium to human health. *Lancet*, **356**, 233–41.
49. Rayman, M.P. (1997) Dietary selenium: time to act. *British Medical Journal*, **314**, 387–8.
50. Ministry of Agriculture and Forestry (1984) *Proposal for Addition of Selenium to Fertilizers. Working Group Report No. 7*. Helsinki (in Finnish); cited in Eurola, M., Ekholm, P., Koivistoinen, P. *et al.* (1989) Effects of selenium fertilization on the selenium content of selected Finnish fruits and vegetables. *Acta Agriculturae Scandinavica*, **39**, 345–50.
51. Koljonen, T. (1975) The behaviour of selenium in Finnish soils. *Annales Agriculturae Fenniae*, **41**, 240–7.
52. Mutanen, M. & Koivistoinen, P. (1983) The role of imported grain in the selenium intake of the Finnish population in 1941–1948. *International Journal of Vitamin Nutrition Research*, **53**, 102–8.
53. Eurola, M., Ekholm, P., Ylinen, M. *et al.* (1989) Effects of selenium fertilization on the selenium content of selected Finnish fruits and vegetables. *Acta Agriculturae Scandinavica*, **39**, 345–50.
54. Varo, P., Alfthan, G., Huttunen, J.K. & Aro, A. (1994) Nationwide selenium supplementation in Finland – effects on diet, blood and tissue levels, and health. In: *Selenium in Biology and Medicine* (ed. R.F. Burk), pp. 198–218. Springer, New York.
55. Reilly, C (1996) Selenium supplementation – the Finnish experiment. *BNF Nutrition Bulletin*, **21**, 167–73.
56. Thomson, C.D. & Robinson, M.F. (1980) Selenium in human health and disease with emphasis on those aspects peculiar to New Zealand. *American Journal of Clinical Nutrition*, **33**, 303–23.
57. Griffiths, N.M. & Thomson, C.D. (1974) Selenium in whole blood in New Zealand residents. *New Zealand Medical Journal*, **80**, 199–201.
58. Thomson, C.D. (1992) Is there a case for selenium supplementation in New Zealand? In: *Fifth International Symposium on Selenium in Biology and Medicine, Abstracts*, 20–23 July, p. 152. Vanderbilt University, Nashville, TN.
59. Thomson, C.D. & Robinson, M.F. (1996) The changing selenium status of New Zealand residents. *European Journal of Clinical Nutrition*, **50**, 107–14.
60. Agency for Toxic Substances and Disease Registry (1996) *Toxicology Profile for Selenium (Update)*. US Department of Health and Human Services, Washington, DC.
61. Block, E. (1998) The organosulfur and organoselenium components of garlic and onion. In: *Phytochemicals – a New Paradigm* (eds. W.R. Bidlack, S.T. Omaye, M.S. Meskin & D. Jahner), pp. 129–41. Technomic, Lancaster, PA.
62. Kerdel-Vergas, F. (1996) The depilatory and cytotoxic action of 'Coco de Mono' (*Lecythis ollaria*) and its relation to chronic selenosis. *Economic Botany*, **20**, 187–95.
63. Fairweather-Tait, S.J. (1997) Bioavailability of selenium. *European Journal of Clinical Nutrition*, **51**, S20–3.
64. Thomson, C. (1998) Selenium speciation in the human body. *Analyst*, **123**, 827–31.
65. Franke, K.W. & Painter, E.P. (1938) A study of the toxicity and selenium content of seleniferous diets: with statistical consideration. *Cereal Chemistry*, **15**, 1–24, cited in: Schrauzer, G.N. (2000) Selenomethionine: a review of its nutritional significance, metabolism and toxicity. *Journal of Nutrition*, **130**, 1653–6.
66. Schrauzer, G.N. (2000) Selenomethionine: a review of its nutritional significance, metabolism and toxicity. *Journal of Nutrition*, **130**, 1653–6.
67. Levander, O.A. (1972) Metabolic interrelationships and adaptations in selenium toxicity. *Annals of the New York Academy of Sciences*, **192**, 181–92.

68. Diplock, A.T. (1993) Indexes of selenium status in human populations. *American Journal of Clinical Nutrition*, **57**, 256S–8S.
69. Dorea, J.G. (2002) Selenium and breast-feeding. *British Journal of Nutrition*, **88**, 443–61.
70. Allaway, W.H., Moore, D.P., Oldfield, J.E. & Muth, O.H. (1966) Movement of physiological levels of selenium from soils through plants to animals. *Journal of Nutrition*, **88**, 414–8.
71. Schroeder, H.A., Frost, D.V. & Balassa, J.J. (1970) Essential trace elements in man: selenium. *Journal of Chronic Diseases*, **23**, 227–43.
72. Griffith, N.M., Stewart, R.D.H. & Robinson, M.F. (1976) The metabolism of ^{75}Se-selenomethionine in four women. *British Journal of Nutrition*, **35**, 373–82.
73. Oster, O., Schmiedel, G. & Prellwitz, W. (1988) The organ distribution of selenium in German adults. *Biological Trace Element Research*, **15**, 23–45.
74. Committee on Animal Nutrition Subcommittee on Selenium (1983) *Selenium in Nutrition*. National Research Council/National Academy of Sciences, Washington, DC.
75. Oldfield, J.E. (1992) *Selenium in Fertilizers*, pp. 281–6. Selenium–Tellurium Development Association, Grimbergen, Belgium.
76. Oster, O., Schmiedel, G. & Prellwitz, W. (1988) The organ distribution of selenium in German adults. *Biological Trace Element Research*, **15**, 23–45.
77. Whanger, P., Xia, V. & Thomson, C. (1993) Metabolism of different forms of selenium in humans. *Journal of Trace Elements and Electrolytes in Health and Disease*, **7**, 121–9.
78. Oster, O., Schmiedel, G. & Prellwitz, W. (1988) The organ distribution of selenium in German adults. *Biological Trace Element Research*, **15**, 23–45.
79. Lindberg, P. & Jacobsson, S.O. (1970) Relationship between selenium content of forage, blood, and organs of sheep, and lamb mortality rates. *Acta Veterinaria Scandinavica*, **11**, 49–58.
80. Ihnat, M. & Aaseth, J. (1989) Human tissues. In: *Occurrence and Distribution of Selenium* (ed. M. Ihnat), pp. 169–212. CRC Press, Boca Raton, FL.
81. Rea, H.M., Thomson, C.D., Campbell, D.R. & Robinson, M.F. (1979) Relation betweeen erythrocyte selenium concentrations and gluthatione peroxidase (EC 1.11.19) activities of New Zealand residents and visitors to New Zealand. *British Journal of Nutrition*, **42**, 201–8.
82. Lombeck, I., Kasparek, K., Harbisch, H.D. *et al.* (1977) The selenium status of healthy children. 1. Serum selenium concentrations at different ages, activity of glutathione peroxidase of erythrocytes at different ages; selenium content of food of infants. *European Journal of Pediatrics*, **125**, 81–89.
83. Iyengar. V. & Woittiez, J. (1988) Trace elements in human clinical specimens: evaluation of literature data to identify reference values. *Clinical Chemistry*, **34**, 474–81.
84. Combs, G.F., Jr. (2001) Selenium in global food systems. *British Journal of Nutrition*, **85**, 517–47.
85. Bibow, K., Meltzer, H.M., Mundal, H.H. *et al.* (1993) Platelet selenium as indicator of wheat selenium intake. *Journal of Trace Elements and Electrolytes in Health and Disease*, **7**, 171–6.
86. Thomson, C.D., Robinson, M.F., Butler, J.A. & Whanger, P.D. (1993) Long-term supplementation with selenate and selenomethionine: selenium and glutathione peroxidase (EC 1.11.1.9) in blood components of New Zealand women. *British Journal of Nutrition*, **69**, 577–88.
87. Levander, O.A., Alfthan, G., Arvilommi, H. *et al.* (1983) Bioavailability of selenium to Finnish men as assessed by platelet glutathione peroxidase and other blood parameters. *American Journal of Clinical Nutrition*, **37**, 887–97.
88. Kaspareck, K., Iyengar, G.V., Keiem, J. *et al.* (1979) Elemental composition of platelets. Part iii. Determination of Ag, Cd, Co, Cr, Cs, Mo, Rb, Sb, and Se in normal human platelets by neutron activation analysis. *Clinical Chemistry*, **25**, 711–5.
89. Arthur, J.R. (2003) Selenium supplementation: does soil supplementation help and why? *Proceedings of the Nutrition Society*, **62**, 393–7.

90. Schwartz, K. (1965) Role of vitamin E, selenium and related factors in experimental nutritional liver disease. *Federation Proceedings*, **24**, 58–67.
91. Rotruck, J.T., Pope, A.L., Ganther, H.E. *et al.* (1973) Selenium: biochemical role as a component of glutathione peroxidase. *Science*, **179**, 588–90.
92. Combs, G.F. & Combs, S.B. (1986) *The Role of Selenium in Nutrition.* Academic Press, New York.
93. McKenzie, R.C., Arthur, J.R. & Beckett, G.J. (2002) Selenium and the regulation of cell signalling, growth, and survival: molecular and mechanistic aspects. *Antioxidants and Redox Signalling*, **4**, 339–51.
94. Arthur, J.R. (2003) Selenium supplementation: does soil supplementation help and why? *Proceedings of the Nutrition Society*, **62**, 393–7.
95. Arthur, J.R. & Beckett, G.J. (1994) Newer aspects of micronutrients in at risk groups. New metabolic roles for selenium. *Proceedings of the Nutrition Society*, **53**, 615–24.
96. McKenzie, R.C., Arthur, J.R. & Beckett, G.J. (2002) Selenium and the regulation of cell signalling, growth, and survival: molecular and mechanistic aspects. *Antioxidants and Redox Signalling*, **4**, 339–51.
97. Arthur, J.R., Morrice, P.C., Nicol, F. *et al.* (1987) The effects of selenium and copper deficiencies on glutathione *S*-transferase and glutathione peroxidase in rat liver. *Biochemical Journal*, **248**, 539–44.
98. Rotruck, J.T., Pope, A.L., Ganther, H.E. *et al.* (1973) Selenium: biochemical role as a component of glutathione peroxidase. *Science*, **179**, 588–90.
99. Mills, G.C. (1957) Hemoglobin catabolism. 1. Glutathione peroxidase, an erythrocyte enzyme which protects hemoglobin from oxidative breakdown. *Journal of Biological Chemistry*, **229**, 189–97.
100. Forstrom, J.W., Zakowski, J.J. & Tappel, A.L. (1978) Identification of the catalytic site of rat liver glutathione peroxidase as selenocysteine. *Biochemistry*, **17**, 2639–44.
101. Grossman, A. & Wendel, A. (1983) Non-reactivity of the selenoenzyme glutathione peroxidase with enzymatically hydroperoxidized phospholipids. *European Journal of Biochemistry*, **135**, 549–52.
102. Burk, R.F. & Gregory, P.E. (1982) Characteristics of ^{75}Se–P, a selenoprotein found in rat liver and plasma and comparisons of it with selenoglutathione peroxidase. *Archives of Biochemistry and Biophysics*, **213**, 73–80.
103. Takahashi, K. & Cohen, H.J. (1986) Selenium-dependent glutathione peroxidase protein and activity: immunological investigations of cellular and plasma enzymes. *Blood*, **68**, 640–5.
104. Roveri, A., Casasco, A., Mairoini, M. *et al.* (1992) Phospholipid hydroperoxide glutathione peroxidase of rat testis. *Journal of Biological Chemistry*, **267**, 6142–6.
105. Arthur, J.R. (1992) Selenium metabolism and function. *Proceedings of the Nutrition Society of Australia*, **17**, 91–8.
106. Ursini, F. & Bindoli, A. (1987) The role of selenium peroxidase in the protection against oxidative damage of membranes. *Chemistry and Physics of Lipids*, **44**, 225–76.
107. Ursini, F., Pelosi, G., Tomassi, G. *et al.* (1987) Effects of dietary fats on hydroperoxide-induced chemiluminescence emission and eicosanoid release in the rat heart. *Biochimia et Biophysica Acta*, **919**, 93–6.
108. McKenzie, R.C., Arthur, J.R. & Beckett, G.J. (2002) Selenium and the regulation of cell signalling, growth, and survival: molecular and mechanistic aspects. *Antioxidants and Redox Signalling*, **4**, 339–51.
109. Beckett, G.J., Beddoes, S.E., Morrice, P.C. *et al.* (1987) Inhibition of hepatic deiodination of thyroxine is caused by selenium deficiency in rats. *Biochemical Journal*, **248**, 443–7.

110. Berry, M.J., Banu, L., Chen, Y. *et al.* (1991) Recognition of UGA as a selenocysteine codon in Type 1 deiodinase requires sequences in the 3′ untranslated region. *Nature (London)*, **353**, 273–6.
111. Berry, M.J., Banu, L. & Larsen, P.R. (1991) Type I deiodinase is a selenocysteine-containing enzyme. *Nature (London)*, **349**, 438–40.
112. McKenzie, R.C., Arthur, J.R. & Beckett, G.J. (2002) Selenium and the regulation of cell signalling, growth, and survival: molecular and mechanistic aspects. *Antioxidants and Redox Signalling*, **4**, 339–51.
113. Gladyshev, V.N., Jeang, K. & Stadman, T.C. (1996) Selenocysteine, identified as the penultimate C-terminal residue in human T-cell thioredoxin reductase, corresponds to TGA in the human placental gene. *Proceedings of the National Academy of Sciences USA*, **93**, 6146–51.
114. Lee, R., Kim, J., Kwon, K. *et al.* (1999) Molecular cloning and characterization of a mitochondrial selenocysteine-containing thioredoxin reductase from rat liver. *Journal of Biological Chemistry*, **274**, 4722–34.
115. Arner, E.S.J. & Holmgren, A. (2000) Physiological functions of thioredoxin and thioredoxin reductase. *European Journal of Biochemistry*, **267**, 6102–9.
116. Holmgren, A. (2001) Selenoproteins of the thioredoxin system. In: *Selenium, its Molecular Biology and Role in Human Health* (ed. D.L. Hatfield), pp. 178–88. Kluwer, Boston, MA.
117. Berggren, M., Gallegos, A., Gasdaska, J.R. *et al.* (1996) Thioredoxin and thioredoxin reductase gene expression in human tumors and cell lines, and the effects of serum stimulation and hypoxia. *Anticancer Research*, **16**, 3459–66.
118. Holmgren, A. (2001) Selenoproteins of the thioredoxin system. In: *Selenium, its Molecular Biology and Role in Human Health* (ed. D.L. Hatfield), pp. 178–88. Kluwer, Boston, MA
119. Björnstedt, M., Xue, J., Huang, W. *et al.* (1994) The thioredoxin and glutathione systems are efficient electron donors to human plasma glutathione peroxidase. *Journal of Biological Chemistry*, **269**, 29382–4.
120. McKenzie, R.C., Arthur, J.R. & Beckett, G.J. (2002) Selenium and the regulation of cell signalling, growth, and survival: molecular and mechanistic aspects. *Antioxidants and Redox Signalling*, **4**, 339–51.
121. Ma, S., Hill, K.E., Caprioloi, R.M. & Burk, R.F. (2002) Mass spectrometric characterization of full-length rat selenoprotein P and three isoforms shortened at the C terminus. Evidence that three UGA codons in the mRNA open reading frame have alternative functions of specifying selenocysteine insertion or translation termination. *Journal of Biological Chemistry*, **277**, 12749–54.
122. Read, R., Bellew, T., Yang, J.G. *et al.* (1990) Selenium and amino acid composition of selenoprotein P, the major selenoprotein in rat serum. *Journal of Biological Chemistry*, **265**, 17899–905.
123. Arteel, G.E., Briviba, K. & Sies, H. (1999) Protection against peroxynitrite. *Federation of European Biological Societies Letters*, **445**, 226–30.
124. Burk, R.F., Hill, K.E. & Motley, A.K. (2003) Selenoprotein metabolism and function: evidence for more than one function for selenoprotein P. *Journal of Nutrition*, **133**, 1517S–20S.
125. Vendeland, S.C., Beilstein, M.A., Chen, C.L. *et al.* (1993) Purification and properties of selenoprotein-W from rat muscle. *Journal of Biological Chemistry*, **268**, 17103–7.
126. Sun, Y., Ha, P., Butler, J. *et al.* (1998) Effect of dietary selenium on selenoprotein W and glutathione peroxidase in 28 tissues of the rat. *Nutritional Biochemistry*, **9**, 23–7.
127. Whanger, P.D., Vendeland, S.C. & Beilstein, M.A. (1993) Some biochemical properties of selenoprotein W. In: *Trace Elements in Man and Animals – TEMA* 8 (ed. M. Anke, D. Meissner & C.F. Mills), pp. 119–26. Verlag Media Touristik, Gersdorf, Germany.

128. McKenzie, R.C., Arthur, J.R. & Beckett, G.J. (2002) Selenium and the regulation of cell signalling, growth, and survival: molecular and mechanistic aspects. *Antioxidants and Redox Signalling*, **4**, 339–51.
129. Stadman, T.C. (1990) Selenium biochemistry. *Annual Review of Biochemistry*, **59**, 111–27.
130. Reilly, C. (1996) *Selenium in Food and Health*, pp. 53–67. Blackie/Chapman & Hall, London.
131. Heider, J., Baron, C. & Böck, A. (1992) Codeing from a distance: dissection of the mRNA determinants required for the incorporation of selenocysteine into protein. *EMBO Journal*, **11**, 3759–66.
132. Stadman, T.C. (1990) Selenium biochemistry. *Annual Review of Biochemistry*, **59**, 111–27.
133. McKenzie, R.C., Arthur, J.R. & Beckett, G.J. (2002) Selenium and the regulation of cell signalling, growth, and survival: molecular and mechanistic aspects. *Antioxidants and Redox Signalling*, **4**, 339–51.
134. Heider, J., Baron, C. & Böck, A. (1992) Coding from a distance: dissection of the mRNA determinants required for the incorporation of selenocysteine into protein. *EMBO Journal*, **11**, 3759–66.
135. Grunder-Culemann, G.W., Martin, R., Tujebajeva, J.W. Harney, J. & Berry, M.J. (2001) Interplay between termination and translation machinery in eukaryotic selenoprotein synthesis. *Journal of Molecular Biology*, **310**, 699–701.
136. McKenzie, R.C., Arthur, J.R. & Beckett, G.J. (2002) Selenium and the regulation of cell signalling, growth, and survival: molecular and mechanistic aspects. *Antioxidants and Redox Signalling*, **4**, 339–51.
137. Burk, R.F. & Hill, K.E. (1993) Regulation of selenoproteins. *Annual Review of Nutrition*, **13**, 65–81.
138. Leinfelder, W., Zehelein, E., Mandrad-Bertholet, M.A. & Böck, A. (1986) Gene for a novel transfer-RNA species that accepts L-serine and cotranslationally inserts selenocysteine. *Nature (London)*, **331**, 723–5.
139. Forchammer, K. & Böck, A. (1991) Selenocysteine synthetase from *Escherichia coli*. Analysis of the reaction sequence. *Journal of Biological Chemistry*, **266**, 6324–8.
140. Mansell, J.B. & Berry, M.J. (2001) Towards a mechanism for selenoprotein incorporation into eukaryotes. In: *Selenium, its Molecular Biology and Role in Human Health* (eds. D.L. Hatfield & M.A. Boston), pp. 69–80. Kluwer, New York.
141. Smith, M.I., Franke, K.W. & Westfall, B.B. (1936) The selenium problem in relation to public health. A preliminary survey to determine the possibility of selenium intoxication in the rural population living on seleniferous soil. *US Public Health Reports,* **51**, 1496–1505.
142. Frost, D.V. (1972) The two faces of selenium – can selenophobia be cured? In: *Critical Reviews in Toxicology* (ed. D. Hemphill), pp. 467–514. CRC Press, Boca Raton, FL.
143. Jaffe, W.G., Raphael, M.D., Mondragon, M.C. & Cuevas, M.A. (1972) Clinical and biochemical studies on school children from a seleniferous zone. *Archivos Latioamericanos de Nutricion,* **22**, 595–611.
144. Kerdel-Vegas, F. (1966) The depilatory and cytotoxic action of 'Coco de Mono' (*Lecythis ollaria)* and its relationship to chronic selenosis. *Economic Botany,* **20**, 187–95.
145. Civil, I.D.S. & McDonald, M.J.A. (1978) Acute selenium poisoning: case report. *New Zealand Medical Journal,* **87**, 345–6.
146. Yang, G., Wang, S., Zhou, R. & Sun, S. (1983) Endemic selenium intoxication of humans in China. *American Journal of Clinical Nutrition,* **37**, 872–81.
147. Polo, M. (1967) *The Travels of Marco Polo,* translated by E.W. Marsden, revised by T. Wright, Chapter XL, pp. 110–11. Everyman's Library, Dent, London.
148. Yang, G., Wang, S., Zhou, R. & Sun, S. (1983) Endemic selenium intoxication of humans in China. *American Journal of Clinical Nutrition,* **37**, 872–81.

149. Hadjimarkos, D.M., Storvick, C.A. & Remmert, L.F. (1952) Selenium and dental caries. An investigation among school children of Oregon. *Journal of Pediatrics,* **40**, 451–5.
150. Kilness, A.W. & Hochberg, F.H. (1977) Amyotrophic lateral sclerosis in a high selenium environment. *Journal of the American Medical Association,* **238**, 2365.
151. Jaffe, W.G. & Velez, B.F. (1973) Selenium intake and congenital malformations in humans. *Archivos Latinoamericanos de Nutricion,* **23**, 514–6.
152. Robertson, D.S.F. (1970) Selenium, a possible teratogen? *Lancet,* **i**, 518–9.
153. Yang, G., Chen, J., Wen, Z. *et al.* (1984) The role of selenium in Keshan disease. In: *Advances in Nutritional Research* (ed. H.H. Draper), Vol. 6, pp. 203–31. Plenum, New York.
154. Keshan Disease Research Group of the Chinese Academy of Medical Sciences (1979) Epidemiological studies in the etiologic relationship of selenium and Keshan disease. *Chinese Medical Journal,* **92**, 477–82.
155. Gu, B. (1993) Pathology of Keshan disease: a comprehensive review. *Chinese Medical Journal,* **96**, 251–61.
156. Ge, K. & Yang, G. (1993) The epidemiology of selenium deficiency in the etiology of endemic diseases in China. *American Journal of Clinical Nutrition,* **57**, 259S–63S.
157. Ge, K.Y., Wang, S.Q., Bai, J. *et al.* (1987) The protective effect of selenium against viral myocarditis in mice. In: *Selenium in Biology and Medicine* (ed. G.F. Combs, J.E. Spallholz, O.A. Levander & J.E. Oldfield), pp. 761–8. Van Nostrand Reinhold, New York.
158. Yang, G., Chen, J., Wen, Z. *et al.* (1984) The role of selenium in Keshan Disease. In: *Advances in Nutritional Research* (ed. H.H. Draper), Vol. 6, pp. 203–31. Plenum, New York.
159. Yang, G., Ying, T., Sun, S. *et al.* (1980) Selenium status of susceptible populations in Keshan disease area. *Chinese Journal of Preventive Medicine,* **14**, 14–6.
160. Xia, Y., Hill, K.E. & Burk, R.E. (1990) Biochemical characterisation of selenium deficiency in China. In: *Trace Elements in Clinical Medicine, Proceedings of the 2nd Meeting of the International Society for Trace Element Research in Humans (ISTERH),* 28 August 1 September 1980, pp. 349–52. Springer, Tokyo.
161. Voschenko, A.V., Anikina, L.V. & Dimova, S.N. (1992) Towards the mechanism of selenium-deficient cardiomyopathy in sporadic cases. In: *Fifth International Symposium on Selenium in Biology and Medicine, Abstracts,* 20–23 July, p. 153. Vanderbilt University, Nashville TN.
162. Allander, E. (1994) Kashin–Beck disease: an analysis of research and public health activities based on a bibliography 1849–1992. *Scandinavian Journal of Rheumatology,* **S99**, 1–36.
163. Research Group of Environment and Endemic Diseases, Institute of Geography, Beijing (1990) Kashin–Beck disease in China: geographical epidemiology and its environmental pathogenicity. *Journal of Chinese Geography,* **1**, 71–83.
164. Moreno-Reyes, R., Suetens, C., Mathieu, F. *et al.* (1998) Kashin–Beck osteoarthropathy in rural Tibet in relation to selenium and iodine status. *New England Journal of Medicine,* **339**, 1112–20.
165. Chasseur, C., Suetens, C., Nolard, N. *et al.* (1997) Fungal contamination of barley and Kashin–Beck disease in Tibet. *Lancet*, **350**, 1074.
166. Yang, C., Niu, C.R., Bodo, M. *et al.* (1992) Selenium deficiency and fulvic acid supplementation disturb the post translational modification of collagen in the skeletal system of mice. In: *Fifth International Symposium on Selenium in Biology and Medicine. Abstracts*, 20–23 July, p. 117. Vanderbilt University, Nashville, TN.
167. Wang, Z.W., Li, I.Q., Liu, J.X. *et al.* (1987) The analysis of the development of Kaschin–Beck disease in Hulin County, Heilongiang Province. *Chinese Journal of Epidemiology,* **6**, 299–331 (in Chinese); cited in Ge, K. & Yang, G. (1993) The epidemiology of selenium deficiency in the etiology of endemic diseases in China. *American Journal of Clinical Nutrition,* **57**, 259S–63S.

168. Van Rij, A.M., Thomson, C.D., McKenzie, J.M. *et al.* (1979) Selenium deficiency in total parenteral nutrition. *American Journal of Clinical Nutrition,* **32**, 2076–85.
169. Lockitch, G., Taylor, G.P., Wong, L.T.K. *et al.* (1990) Cardiomyopathy associated with nonendemic selenium deficiency in a Caucasian adolescent. *American Journal of Clinical Nutrition,* **52**, 572–7.
170. Inoue, M., Wakisaka,O., Tabuki, T. *et al.* (2003) Selenium deficiency in a patient with Crohn's disease receiving long-term total parenteral nutrition. *Internal Medicine,* **42**, 154–7.
171. Berggvist, A.G.C., Chee, C.M., Lutchka, L., Rychik, J. & Stallings, V.A. (2003) Selenium deficiency associated with cardiomyopathy: a complication of the ketogenic diet. *Epilepsia,* **44**, 618–20.
172. Reilly, C., Barrett, J.E., Patterson, C.M. *et al.* (1990) Trace element nutritional status and dietary intake of children with phenylketonuria. *American Journal of Clinical Nutrition,* **52**, 159–62.
173. Lombeck, I., Ebert, K.H., Kasparek, K. *et al.* (1984) Selenium intake of infants and young children, healthy children and dietetically treated patients with phenylketonuria. *European Journal of Pediatrics,* **143**, 99–102.
174. Acosta, P.B., Gropper, S.S., Clarke-Sheehan, N. *et al.* (1978) Trace element intake of PKU children ingesting an elemental diet. *Journal of Parenteral and Enteral Nutrition,* **11**, 287–92.
175. Terwolbeck, K., Behne, D., Meinhold, H. *et al.* (1993) Low selenium status, thyroid hormones, and other parameters in children with phenylketonuria. In: *Trace Elements in Man and Animals – TEMA 8* (eds. M. Anke, D. Meissner & C.F. Mills), pp. 535–8. Verlag Media Touristik, Gersdorf, Germany.
176. Jocum, F., Terwolbeck, K., Meinhold, H. *et al.* (1999) Is there any health risk of low dietary selenium supply in PKU-children? *Nutrition Research,* **19**, 349–60.
177. Arthur, J.R., Beckett, G.J. & Mitchell, J.H. (1999) the interaction between selenium and iodine deficiencies in man and animals. *Nutrition Research Reviews,* **12**, 55–73.
178. Contempre, B., Dumont, J.E., Ngo, B. *et al.* (1991) Effect of selenium supplementation in hypothyroid subjects of an iodine and selenium deficient area – the possible danger of indiscriminate supplementation of I-deficient subjects with selenium. *Journal of Clinical Endocrinology and Metabolism,* **73**, 213–5.
179. Vanderpas, J.B., Contrempré, B., Duale, N. *et al.* (1990) Iodine and selenium deficiency associated with cretenism in Northern Zaire. *American Journal of Clinical Nutrition,* **52**, 1087–93.
180. Combs, G.F. (2001) Selenium in global food systems. *British Journal of Nutrition,* **85**, 517–47.
181. Morenoreyes, R., Suetens, C., Mathieu, F. *et al.* (1998) Iodine and selenium deficiency in Kashin–Beck disease (Tibet). *New England Journal of Medicine,* **339**, 1112–20.
182. Rayman, M.P. (2000) The importance of selenium to human health. *The Lancet,* **356**, 233–41.
183. Scott, R. & MacPherson, A. (1998) Selenium supplementation in sub-fertile human males. *British Journal of Urology,* **82**, 76–80.
184. Baum, M.K., Shor-Posner, G., Lai, S. *et al.* (1997) High risk of HIV-related mortality is associated with selenium deficiency. *Journal of Acquired Immune Deficiency Syndrome,* **15**, 370–4.
185. Beck, M.A. (1997) Rapid genomic evolution of a non-virulent Coxsackievirus B3 in selenium-deficient mice. *Biomedical and Environmental Science,* **10**, 307–15.
186. Beck, M.A., Levander, O.A. & Handy, J. (2003) Selenium deficiency and viral infection. *Journal of Nutrition,* **133**, 1463S–7S.
187. Néve, J. (1996) Selenium deficiency as a risk factor for cardiovascular disease. *Journal of Cardiovascular Risk,* **3**, 42–7.
188. Brown, A.J. (1993) Regional differences in coronary heart disease in Britain: do antioxidant nutrients provide the key? *Asia Pacific Journal of Clinical Nutrition,* **2**, Supplement 1, 33–6.

189. Bostrom, H.J. & Wester, P.O. (1967) Trace elements in drinking water and death rates of cardiovascular disease. *Acta Medica Scandinavica,* **181**, 465–70.
190. Salonen, J.T., Alfthan, G., Huttenen, J.K. *et al.* (1982) Association between cardiovascular death and myocardial infarction and serum selenium in a matched pair longitudinal study. *Lancet,* **ii**, 175–9.
191. Korpela, H. (1993) Selenium in cardiovascular diseases. *Journal of Trace Elements and Electrolytes in Health and Disease,* **7**, 115–20.
192. Schrauzer, C.N. (1979) Trace elements in carcinogenesis. In: *Advances in Nutritional Research* (ed. H.H. Draper), Vol. 2, pp. 219–44. Plenum, New York.
193. Schrauzer, G.N. (1976) Cancer mortality correlation studies. II. Regional associations of mortalities with the consumption of foods and other commodities. *Medical Hypotheses,* **2**, 39–49.
194. Clark, L.C. (1985) The epidemiology of selenium and cancer. *Federation Proceedings,* **44**, 2584–9.
195. Diplock, A.T. (1987) Trace elements in human health with special reference to selenium. *American Journal of Clinical Nutrition,* **45**, 1313–22.
196. Clayton, C.C. & Baumann, C.A. (1949) Diet and azo dye tumors: dimethylaminobenzene. *Cancer Research,* **9**, 1313–22.
197. El-Bayoumy, K. (1991) The role of selenium in cancer prevention. In: *Practice of Oncology* (eds. V.T. DeVita, S. Hellman & S.S. Rosenberg), 4th ed., pp. 1–15. Lippincott, Philadelphia, PA.
198. Yoshizawa, K., Willet, W.C., Morris, S.J. *et al.* (1998) Study of prediagnostic selenium levels in toenails and the risk of advanced prostate cancer. *Journal of the National Cancer Institute,* **90**, 1219–24.
199. Zou, X.N., Taylor, P.R., Mark, S.D. *et al.* (2003) Seasonal variation of food consumption and selected nutrient intake, in Linxian, a high risk area for oesophageal cancer in China. *International Journal for Vitamin and Nutrition Research,* **72**, 375–82.
200. Blot, W.J., Li, B., Taylor, W. *et al.* (1993) Nutrition trials in Linxian, China: supplementation with specific vitamin/mineral combinations, cancer incidence and disease specific mortality in the general population. *Journal of the National Cancer Institute,* **85**, 1483–92.
201. Li, W.G., Yu, S.Y., Zhu, Y.J. *et al.* (1992) Six years prospective observation of ingesting selenium-salt to prevent primary liver cancer. In: *Fifth International Symposium on Selenium in Biology and Medicine, Abstracts,* 20–23 July 1992, p. 140. Vanderbilt University, Nashville, TN.
202. Clark, L.C., Combs, G.F., Jr., Turnbill, B.W. *et al.* (1996) Effects of selenium supplementation for cancer prevention in patients with carcinoma of the skin: a randomized controlled trial. *Journal of the American Medical Association,* **276**, 1957–63.
203. Combs, G.F. (2001) Selenium in global food systems. *British Journal of Nutrition,* **85**, 517–47.
204. Reilly, C. (1997) Dietary selenium: a call for action. *British Nutrition Foundation Nutrition Bulletin,* **22**, 85–87.
205. Klein, E.A., Lippman, S.M., Thompson, I.M. *et al.* (2003) The selenium and vitamin E prevention trial. *World Journal of Urology,* **21**, 21–7.
206. Clark, L.C. & Jacobs, E.T. (1998) Environmental selenium and cancer: risk or protection? *Cancer Epidemiology, Biomarkers and Prevention,* **7**, 847–8.
207. Vinceti, M., Rothman, K.J., Bergomi, M. *et al.* (1998) Commentary re: Vinceti *et al.*, Excess melanoma incidence in a cohort exposed to high levels of environmental selenium. *Cancer Epidemiology, Biomarkers and Prevention,* **7**, 851–2.
208. Combs, G.F. (2001) Selenium in global food systems. *British Journal of Nutrition,* **85**, 517–47.
209. Combs, G.F. (2001) Impact of selenium and cancer-prevention findings on the nutrition–health paradigm. *Nutrition and Cancer,* **40**, 6–11.

210. Ip, C. (1998) Lessons from basic research in selenium and cancer prevention. *Journal of Nutrition,* **128**, 1845–54.
211. Turner, R.J. & Finch, J.M. (1991) Selenium and the immune response. *Proceedings of the Nutrition Society,* **50**, 275–85.
212. Arthur, J.R., McKenzie, R.C. & Beckett, G.J. (2003) Selenium in the immune system. *Journal of Nutrition,* **133**, 1457S–9S.
213. Reilly, C. (1991) *Selenium in Food and Health,* pp. 180–94. Chapman & Hall/Blackie, London.
214. Pence, B.C., Delver, E. & Dunn, D.M. (1994) Effects of dietary selenium on UVB-induced skin carcinogenesis and epidermal antioxidant status. *Journal of Investigative Dermatology,* **102**, 759–61.
215. Toews, G.B., Bergstresser, P.R., & Streilein, J.W. (1980) Epidermal Langerhans cell density determines whether contact hypersensitivity or unresponsiveness follows skin painting with DNFB. *Journal of Immunology,* **124**, 445–53.
216. Rafferty, T.S., Norval, M., El-Ghorr, A. *et al.* (2003) Dietary selenium levels determine epidermal Langerhans cell numbers in mice. *Biological Trace Element Research,* **92**, 161–72.
217. Arthur, J.R., McKenzie, R.C. & Beckett, G.J. (2003) Selenium in the immune system. *Journal of Nutrition,* **133**, 1457S–9S.
218. Serfass, R.E. & Ganther, H.E. (19754) Defective microbial activity in glutathione peroxidase deficient neutrophils of Se deficient rats. *Nature (London),* **116**, 816–22.
219. Vilette, S., Kyle, J.A.M., Brown, K.M. *et al.* (2002) A novel single nucleotide polymorphism in the 3′ untranslated region of human glutathione peroxidase 4 influences lipoxygenase metabolism. *Blood Cells, Molecules, and Disease,* **29**, 174–8.
220. Arthur, J.R. (2003) Selenium supplementation: does soil supplementation help and why? *Proceedings of the Nutrition Society,* **62**, 393–7.
221. Broome, C.S., McArdle, F., Kyle, J.A.M. *et al.* (2002) Functional effects of selenium supplementation in healthy UK adults. *Free Radical Biology and Medicine,* **33**, S261.
222. Peretz, A.M., Néve, J., Desmet, J. *et al.* (1991) Lymphocyte response is enhanced by supplementation of elderly subjects with selenium-enriched yeast. *American Journal of Clinical Nutrition,* **53**, 1323–8.
223. Kiremidjian-Schumacher, L., Roy, M., Wishe, H. *et al.* (1994) Supplementation with selenium and human immune cell functions. II. Effects of cytotoxic lymphocytes and natural killer cells. *Biological Trace Elements Research,* **41**, 115–27.
224. Hawkes, W.C. & Hornbostel, L. (1996) Effects of dietary selenium on mood in healthy men living in a metabolic research unit. *Biological Psychiatry,* **39**, 121–8.
225. Benton, D. (2002) Selenium intake, mood and other aspects of psychological functioning. *Nutritional Neuroscience,* **5**, 363–74.
226. Rayman, M.P. (2000) The importance of selenium to human health. *Lancet,* **356**, 233–41.
227. Finley J. & Penland, J. (1998) Adequacy or deprivation of dietary selenium in healthy men: clinical and psychological findings. *Trace Elements in Experimental Medicine,* **11**, 11–27.
228. Kaplan, B.J., Crawford, S.G., Gardner, B. *et al.* (2002) Treatment of mood lability and explosive rage with minerals and vitamins: two case studies in children. *Journal of Child and Adolescent Psychopharmacology,* **12**, 205–19.
229. Sher, L. (2002) Role of selenium depletion in the effects of dialysis on mood and behaviour. *Medical Hypotheses,* **59**, 89–91.
230. Benton, D. (2002) Selenium intake, mood and other aspects of psychological functioning. *Nutritional Neuroscience,* **5**, 363–74.
231. Anon (1993) Oxidative stress and human disease: a broad spectrum of effects. *Antioxidant Vitamins Newsletter,* **7**, 12.
232. Burk, R.F. (1988) Selenium deficiency in search of a disease. *Hepatology,* **8**, 421–3.

233. Eye Disease Control Study Group (1993) Antioxidant status and neovascular age-related macular degeneration. *Archives of Ophthalmology,* **111**, 104–9.
234. Flatt, A., Pearce, N., Thomson, C.D. *et al.* (1989) Reduced selenium in asthmatic subjects in New Zealand. *Thorax,* **45**, 95–9.
235. Dworkin, B., Newman, L.J., Berezin, S. *et al.* (1987) Low blood selenium levels in patients with cystic fibrosis compared to controls and healthy adults. *Journal of Parenteral and Enteral Nutrition,* **11**, 38–41.
236. Money, D.F.L. (1970) Vitamin E and selenium deficiencies and their possible aetiological role in sudden death in infants syndrome. *New Zealand Journal of Science,* **71**, 32–4.
237. Rhead, W.J., Cary, E.E., Allaway, W.H. *et al.* (1972) The vitamin E and selenium status of infants and the sudden infant death syndrome. *Bioinorganic Chemistry,* **1**, 289–95.
238. Néve, J. (2000) New approaches to assess selenium status and requirement. *Nutrition Reviews,* **58**, 363–9.
239. Johnson, P.E. (1996) New approaches to establish mineral element requirements and recommendations: an introduction. *Journal of Nutrition,* **126**, 2309S–11S.
240. Food and Nutrition Board, Institute of Medicine (2000) *Dietary Reference Intakes for Vitamin C, Vitamin E, Selenium, and Carotenoids,* pp. 284–324. National Academy Press, Washington, DC.
241. National Health and Medical Research Council (1987) *Recommended Dietary Intakes for Use in Australia.* Australian Government Publishing Services, Canberra.
242. National Research Council (1989) *Recommended Dietary Allowances,* 10th ed. National Academy Press, Washington, DC.
243. World Health Organisation (1992) *Trace Elements in Human Nutrition.* World Health Organisation, Geneva.
244. Néve, J. (2000) New approaches to assess selenium status and requirement. *Nutrition Reviews,* **58**, 363–9.
245. Levander, O.A. & Whanger, P.D. (1996) Deliberations and evaluations of the approaches, endpoints and paradigms for selenium and iodine dietary recommendations. *Journal of Nutrition,* **126**, 2427S–34S.
246. Thomson, C.D. (2003) Proposed Australian and New Zealand nutrient reference values for selenium and iodine. *Journal of Nutrition, Supplement,* **133**, 278E (Abstract).
247. Thomson, C.D. (2002) personal communication.
248. Rayman, M.P. (1997) Dietary selenium: time to act. *British Medical Journal,* **314**, 387–8.
249. COMA (1998) *Statement from the Committee on Medical Aspects of Food and Nutrition Policy on Selenium. Food Safety Information Bulletin No.* **93**. Department of Health, London.
250. Arthur, J.R. (2003) Selenium supplementation: does soil supplementation help and why? *Proceedings of the Nutrition Society,* **62**, 393–7.
251. Combs, G.F. (2001) Selenium in global food systems. *British Journal of Nutrition,* **85**, 517–47.
252. Clark, L.C., Combs, G.F, Jr., Turnbill. B.W. *et al.* (1996) Effects of selenium supplementation for cancer prevention in patients with carcinoma of the skin: a randomized controlled trial. *Journal of the American Medical Association,* **276**, 1957–63.
253. Rayman, M. & Clark, L. (1999) Selenium in cancer prevention. In: *Trace Elements in Man and Animals* 10 (eds. A.M. Roussel, R.A. Anderson & A.E. Favier). Kluwer Academic/Plenum, New York.
254. World Health Organisation (1996) Selenium. In: *Trace Elements in Human Nutrition,* pp. 105–22. World Health Organisation, Geneva.
255. Department of Health (1991) *Dietary Reference Values for Food Energy and Nutrients for the United Kingdom.* Report on Health and Social Subjects 41. HMSO, London.

256. Vinceti, M., Rothman, K.J., Bergomi, M. *et al.* (1998) Commentary re: Vinceti *et al.*, Excess melanoma incidence in a cohort exposed to high levels of environmental selenium. *Cancer Epidemiology, Biomarkers and Prevention,* **7**, 851–2.
257. Poirier, K.A. (1994) Summary of the derivation of the reference dose for selenium. In: *Risk Assessment for Essential Elements* (eds. W. Mertz, C.O. Abernathy & S.S. Olin), pp. 157–66. International Life Sciences Institute, Washington, DC.
258. Schrauzer, G.N. (2000) Selenomethionine: a review of its nutritional significance, metabolism and toxicity. *Journal of Nutrition,* **130**, 1653–6.
259. Arthur, J.R. Selenium supplementation: does soil supplementation help and why? *Proceedings of the Nutrition Society*, **62**, 393–7.

Chapter 6
Chromium

6.1 Introduction

Chromium is widely distributed in the earth's crust, though usually at very low levels of concentration. It has many industrial uses, both in its metallic form and in various compounds. For many years, its complex chemistry and physical properties have been the subject of considerable research. A glance at any of the scientific literature data bases will show that interest continues today among chemists and metallurgists. In contrast, until quite recently, the biology of chromium has been, at best, an interest of small groups of specialists. Though its toxicity to industrial workers had been known for many years[1], it was not until the 1950s that chromium's potential role as an essential human nutrient began to be recognised[2]. This recognition gave rise to a flurry of activity, and an appreciable number of studies of the physiology of chromium deficiency and the effects of chromium supplementation followed, but little was published on the structure, function and mode of action of the biologically active form of the metal[3]. Moreover, interest in its metabolic role did not appear to extend to any great extent into the ranks of mainstream nutrition.

The situation changed to a marked extent during the past decade when studies on all aspects of the biology of chromium began to appear in the literature. The important role that the metal plays, especially in carbohydrate and lipid metabolism, is now recognised, as is its essentiality to many other metabolic activities, developments that have led to the metal being included in the new US RDAs. As we shall see, before such progress could be made, what at one time seemed to be the almost insurmountable problem of how to analyse chromium in biological samples at very low levels of concentration had been resolved[4].

6.2 Chemistry of chromium

Chromium has an atomic weight of 52 and is element number 24 in the periodic table. It is a heavy metal, with a density of 7.2, with a high melting point of approximately 1860°C. It is a very hard, white, lustrous metal and is extremely resistant to corrosion. Chromium is one of the transition metals, and can occur in nine different oxidation states, from −2 to +6. However, only the ground 0, and the +2, +3 and +6 states are of practical importance. The most stable state is Cr(III) in a series of chromic compounds, such as the oxide Cr_2O_3, chloride $CrCl_3$ and sulphate $Cr_2(SO_4)_3$.

In higher oxidation states, almost all chromium compounds are oxo-forms and are potent oxidising agents. The Cr(VI) compounds include the chromates CrO_4^{2-} and the dichromates $Cr_2O_7^{2-}$. Important industrial compounds of this type include lead, zinc, calcium, and barium chromates. From the biological point of view, hexavalent chromium is of particular importance due to its toxicity and its oxidising properties.

The relatively unstable Cr(II) chromous ion is rapidly oxidised under normal conditions to the Cr(III) form. Few of the other forms of chromium, such as Cr(IV) and Cr(V) occur naturally or, if they do, are not of biological significance.

6.3 Distribution, production and uses of chromium

Though chromium is widely distributed in various chemical forms in rocks and soils, its only commercial ore is chromite, $FeOCr_2O_3$, a mixed ore that can contain up to 55% chromic oxide. It occurs in commercial quantities in only a few places in the world, especially in South Africa and Russia. The ore is reduced in a furnace with carbon to produce ferrochrome, a carbon-containing alloy of chromium and iron. The ferrochrome can be further processed to produce pure chromium.

Chromium has many industrial uses. More than half is used in the metallurgical industries, mainly for the production of steel and a variety of alloys. Because of its high resistance to oxidation, chromium is used as an electroplated coating and in stainless steel. Chromium compounds are used in large quantities to make refractory materials for lining furnaces and kilns. They also find employment as tanning agents, pigments, catalysts, timber preservatives, as well as in some household detergents and in pottery glazes, paper and dyes[5].

A use of chromium compounds, which can be of some importance from the point of view of human intake of the metal, is as an additive in water to prevent corrosion in industrial and other cooling systems. It has been suggested that this use could account for a significant amount of environmental contamination from industrial emissions. As we shall see, the use of chromium salts as a 'passivation' agent on tin plate accounts for the sometimes high levels in tinned foodstuffs[6].

6.4 Chromium in food and beverages

Until relatively recently, because of unresolved difficulties in the analysis of chromium at low levels of concentration, available data on levels of the metal in foods and beverages were limited and often unreliable. Indeed, as was noted in a UK Department of Health report, values for levels published prior to 1980 should be viewed with caution[7]. Even today, though analytical procedures are now greatly improved, information on chromium levels in foods and diets is limited[8].

Chromium levels are usually very low in foods and beverages, in the absence of contamination, as can be seen in Table 6.1. This information on levels in UK foods, was gathered as part of the 1991 UK Total Diet Study. In the report, it was noted that in many of the samples analysed, chromium was found at or below the 0.1 mg/kg limit of detection (LOD) of the ICP-MS analytical method used by the MAFF scientists[9]. The highest levels were found in meat, whole grains, legumes and nuts, though seldom at levels above 0.5 mg/kg. Brewer's yeast is one of the best food sources of the element, though levels can vary

Table 6.1 Chromium in UK foods.

Food group	Mean concentration (mg/kg fresh weight)
Bread	0.1
Miscellaneous cereals	0.1
Carcass meat	0.2
Offal	0.1
Meat products	0.2
Poultry	0.2
Fish	0.2
Oils and fats	0.4
Eggs	0.2
Sugar and preserves	0.2
Green vegetables	0.2
Potatoes	0.1
Other vegetables	0.1
Canned vegetables	0.1
Fresh fruit	<0.1
Fruit products	<0.1
Beverages	<0.1
Milk	0.3
Dairy products	0.9
Nuts	0.7

Adapted from Ysart, G., Miller, P., Crews, H. *et al.* (1999) Dietary exposure estimates of 30 elements from the UK Total Diet Study. *Food Additives and Contaminants*, **16**, 391–403.

widely between different samples[10]. Chromium-enriched yeast is widely used as a nutritional supplement for humans as well as animals[11]. There have been reports of high levels of chromium in black pepper and other spices, as well as in raw sugar[12].

Though water may contain chromium, especially if it is affected by industrial emissions, it is unlikely to make a significant contribution to dietary intake of the element. The usual chemical form of chromium in drinking water is Cr(VI), which is more soluble than hydrated Cr(III) oxide. WHO drinking-water standards, which have been adopted by the EU, set a maximum permitted level of 50 μg/l for Cr(VI). Chromium levels in tap water in several European cities range from 1.0 to 5.0, with a mean of 2.0 μg/l[13].

Higher than normal levels of chromium can occur in certain food crops, as a result of the use of sewage sludge to treat agricultural soils. Because of this, some countries have introduced legislation to limit this practice. In the UK, the Department of the Environment has set a guideline limit of 400 mg/kg in sludge-amended soil. This is about 10 times greater than levels that occur naturally in most agricultural soils[14].

6.4.1 Adventitious chromium in foods

Much of the chromium in the diets of many people comes, not from natural sources, but from accidental contamination as adventitious chromium. Canned and other processed foods often contain chromium taken up from steel cooking utensils and storage vessels, including cans. Stainless steel, which is widely used in food-processing equipment and fittings, may contain chromium, as well as other metals besides iron. All of these can migrate from the steel into food, the amount transferred depending particularly on the length of contact time between the food and the metal[15]. The processing temperature and pH are also of importance in this regard. The level of chromium in red cabbage pickled in 4% acetic acid (vinegar) in a stainless steel vessel, for example, has been reported to be 72 μg/kg, compared with about 10 μg/kg in the fresh vegetable[16].

The 'passivation treatment', in which chromic acid or another chromium compound is used to increase the lacquer adherence and resistance to oxidation of tinplate, can contribute significantly to chromium levels in canned foods. It has been calculated that if all the chromium on the inner surface of a 454-g can migrated into the contents, this would result in a final concentration of about 400 μg/kg in the food[17]. Lacquering is used to protect the can contents from this pick-up from the tinplate. It has been found that the concentration of chromium in fruit and vegetables (with an average chromium content of 9 μg/kg) doubled to 18 μg/kg when the food was canned[18].

6.5 Dietary intakes of chromium

Daily dietary intakes of 30 mg or more were reported in some of the earlier reports on levels of chromium in diets published in the 1930s[19]. However, with the development of more reliable analytical procedures, reported intakes today are much lower. The daily mean adult intake in the UK was found to be 0.1 mg in the 1997 TDS, with 0.17 mg for the 97.5th percentile[20]. Similar levels of intake have been reported in recent years in other technologically advanced countries, for example, the US (0.25 mg)[21], Japan (0.89 mg)[22] and Denmark (0.5 mg)[23].

6.6 Absorption and metabolism of chromium

The mechanisms of absorption and transport of chromium are still uncertain. Absorption appears to be an active process and not simple diffusion. The process is affected by a variety of factors. Total uptake is inversely related to the amount of chromium in food ingested. Absorption is significantly reduced by the presence of phytate and enhanced by ascorbic acid[24]. There also appears to be competition for uptake between chromium and other metals, including zinc, iron, manganese and vanadium[25]. Overall, the rate at which chromium is absorbed from the gut is low, ranging from 0.5 to 3%. Different chemical compounds of Cr(III) have been shown to be absorbed from the gut at different rates. For example, chromium oxide is poorly absorbed compared with chromium chloride hexahydrate and chromium acetate hydroxide[26]. Cr(VI) compounds are absorbed more rapidly than are those of Cr(III)[27].

Once absorbed from the GI tract, chromium is believed to be transported in blood bound to transferrin, in competition with iron[28]. The mechanisms whereby this occurs are still uncertain. It has been shown *in vitro* that addition of chromium to blood results in the loading of transferrin with Cr(III). However, under these conditions, the metal also binds to albumin. Recent reports on the effects of insulin on iron transport and the relationship between haemochromatosis and diabetes suggest that transferrin is the major physiological transport agent[29].

The adult human body is estimated to contain a total of between 4 and 6 mg of chromium. This is stored to a limited extent in organs, including kidney, spleen and testes. Tissue chromium levels decrease with age. Excretion is mainly in urine, with a small amount in faeces[30].

6.6.1 Essentiality of chromium

The essentiality of chromium for humans is now widely accepted, though with reservations by some investigators[31]. In the late 1950s, Schwarz and Mertz showed that rats fed a chromium-deficient diet based on *Torula* yeast were unable to remove glucose efficiently from their blood. The condition was reversed by feeding them a diet rich in chromium(III)[32]. The chromium was believed to function in an organic complex, the 'glucose tolerance factor' (GTF), which potentiates the action of insulin[33]. The chromium is an integral part of the GTF which is a dinicotinic acid–glutathione complex. Though GTF has been extracted from brewer's yeast, and other apparently biologically active chromium complexes have been detected in other organisms, none of them has yet been fully characterised[34].

6.6.1.1 Chromium and glucose tolerance

In humans, evidence for an essential role for chromium comes from observations on patients undergoing TPN. Some who developed diabetic symptoms that were refractory to insulin responded to treatment with chromium[35]. There is evidence that chromium deficiency is associated with elevated blood glucose levels. A reduction in blood levels and an increase in chromium excretion in urine have been found to occur in adult-onset diabetes[36]. Improvements in glucose tolerance have been shown to occur in elderly persons who are given chromium supplements. However, a meta-analysis of 20 reports of randomised clinical trials on the use of chromium in the management of type II diabetes concluded that the results showed no effect of chromium on glucose or insulin in non-diabetic subjects and that the data for persons with diabetes were inconclusive[37]. In contrast, a recent study in India of persons with type II diabetes, found that chromium supplementation resulted in a significant improvement in glycaemic control[38]. There is evidence that chromium supplementation improves blood lipid levels in elderly persons[39]. Chromium appears to participate in lipoprotein metabolism, and a low chromium status may result in decreased levels of high-density cholesterol. Improved chromium status may also reduce factors associated with cardiovascular disease as well as with diabetes[40]. It has been shown that in post-menopausal women, chromium status, as well as glucose and lipid metabolism, were improved by hormone replacement therapy (HRT)[41].

6.6.2 Mechanism of action of chromium

There is evidence that the mechanism of action of chromium at the molecular level depends on a unique chromium-binding oligopeptide, a low moleular weight chromium-binding substance (LMWCr) to which the name chromodulin has been given[42]. Chromodulin has a molecular weight of approximately 1500 Da and is made up of residues of the four amino acids, cysteine, glycine, glutamic and aspartic[43]. The oligopeptide can bind four equivalents of CrIII ions. It has been isolated and purified from a wide range of mammals. Using isolated rat adipocytes, it has been shown that chromodulin has the ability to potentiate the effects of insulin on the conversion of glucose into carbon dioxide or lipid[44]. The stimulation is directly dependent on the chromium content of the chromodulin[45]. The effect on insulin has not been shown to occur with any chromium complex other than chromomodulin[46].

Evidence from studies of the effects of chromium on glucose transport and of the insulin dose-response in rat adipocytes suggests a role for chromium as chromodulin in signal transduction. Of particular interest in this regard has been the recognition that chromodulin brings about, among other effects, an insulin-sensitive stimulation of insulin receptor tyrosine kinase activity[47]. On the basis of these and other observations, a mechanism for the activation of insulin receptor kinase activity by chromodulin in response to insulin has been proposed by Vincent[48]. He believes that the action of chromodulin can best be seen as part of an autoamplification system of insulin signalling. Insulin, which is released into the blood in response to an increase in blood sugar levels, binds to an external subunit of the transmembrane protein insulin receptor of an insulin-sensitive cell and in doing so converts the receptor from an inactive to an active form[49]. At the same time, a rise in plasma insulin levels causes a movement of chromium from the blood to insulin-dependent cells, most probably mediated by ferritin. There, the chromium is bound to apochromodulin, which appears to be stored in the cytosol and nucleus of insulin-dependent cells[50]. The apochromodulin is converted into active chromodulin, which can then bind to the insulin-stimulated insulin receptor, helping to maintain its active conformation and amplifying insulin signalling. When the insulin concentration drops, chromodulin is released from the receptor and leaves the cell, and thus its stimulation of insulin action ceases.

6.6.3 Chromium and athletic performance

There is considerable interest, especially among athletes and sports nutritionists, in the possibility that chromium can increase lean body mass and decrease percentage body fat. Many studies have been conducted to investigate the relationship of chromium with exercise and fitness. However, results are equivocal[51]. While it has been claimed that the use of chromium supplements by athletes can compensate for losses caused by exercise, reduce fat and increase lean body mass, a recent study has concluded that the role of chromium in supporting performance is not well established, and there is a need for further studies before the long-term use of chromium supplements for athletic purposes can be encouraged[52]. It has also been pointed out that there is need for caution, since the most popular form of chromium in dietary supplements, chromium picolinate (chromium (III) tris-picolinate) appears to be absorbed in a different fashion from dietary chromium[53]. Moreover, the chromium picolinate complex is remarkably stable, appears to pass unchanged through the jejunum and is incorporated into cells in its original form. There, it can be reduced by ascorbate and other reducing agents. The resulting chromous complex can interact with oxygen to generate the hydroxyl radical and cause significant DNA cleavage[54].

6.7 Assessing chromium status

Reliable biomarkers of dietary chromium and chromium status are lacking, and hence there are serious problems in assessing these parameters. Apart from difficulties in estimating chromium at the low levels normally in biological materials, there is the added problem that plasma chromium levels are normally so low as to be near the limit of detection[55].

6.7.1 Blood chromium

Plasma and serum chromium levels are not considered to be useful indicators of chromium status, both because of the low levels normally present[56] and because there does not seem to be equilibrium between tissue stores and blood chromium concentrations[57]. However, serum levels may be an indicator of status when chromium intakes are relatively high, for example in industrial workers exposed to the element[58], and following prolonged intake of chromium supplements[59].

It has been suggested that what is known as 'the relative chromium response', which is the change in serum chromium levels after a glucose load, may be used to assess functional levels of chromium. Though there is some doubt whether this is a reliable index of status, supplementation with chromium at physiological levels and testing for an improvement in glucose tolerance is a widely used method for detecting chromium deficiency[60].

6.7.2 Measurements of chromium in urine and hair

Urinary excretion has been used in several studies to measure chromium status[61]. There are conflicting views on the relationship of urinary chromium to dietary intake[62]. It has been suggested that if chromium excretion is expressed in terms of creatinine, rather than volume, a more reliable indication of status may be obtained[63].

Hair chromium levels have been suggested as a measure of long-term exposure to chromium. However, the technique is subject to the uncertainties associated with hair sampling and analysis as a measure of trace metals in the human body[64].

None of the above procedures offer an absolutely reliable method for estimating chromium status or for determining chromium deficiency. The only method available at present for performing the latter operation with any degree of certainty is to carry out carefully designed intervention trials with small quantities of supplemental chromium and depletion trials coupled with careful measurements of dietary and urinary chromium levels[65].

6.8 Chromium requirements

In the absence of any reliable objective measure of chromium status, the UK's Panel on Dietary Reference Values in its 1991 Report, rather than setting an RNI for the element, proposed as a safe and adequate intake 25 μg/d for adults and between 0.1 and 1.0 μg/kg body weight/d for children and adolescents.[66] For the same reason, the US NRC, in its 10th (1989) edition of the RDAs, tentatively recommended an ESADDI of between 50 and 200 μg/d for adults[67]. A decade and more later, there is still uncertainty about chromium requirements, and there is no RDA/RNI for chromium. However, on the basis of observed intakes of different population groups, it has been possible to set an AI for chromium, as shown in Table 6.2[68]. The AI is believed to cover the needs of all individuals in the

Table 6.2 US recommendations for chromium (μg/d)

Life-stage group	Adequate Intake
Infants	
0–6 months	0.2
7–12 months	5.5
Children	
1–3 years	11
4–8 years	15
Males	
9–13 years	25
14–18 years	35
19–30 years	35
31–50 years	35
50–70 years	30
>70 years	30
Females	
9–13 years	21
14–18 years	24
19–30 years	25
31–50 years	25
50–70 years	20
>70 years	20
Pregnancy	
≤18 years	29
19–30 years	30
31–50 years	30
Lactation	
≤18 years	44
19–30 years	45
31–50 years	45

For healthy breastfed infants, the AI is the mean intake. The AI for other life-stage and gender groups is believed to cover the needs of all individuals in a group, but because of the lack of data, the percentage of individuals covered by this intake cannot be specified with confidence.

Adapted from: Food and Nutrition Board National Academy of Sciences (2002) *US Dietary Reference Intakes: Elements.* http://www4.nationalacademies.org/10M/10MHome.nst/pages/Food+and+Nutrition+Board

different life-stage groups, but, as the explanatory notes to the table make clear, 'lack of data prevent being able to specify with confidence the percentage of individuals covered by this intake'. In the circumstances, it would appear that the wisest course for those seeking guidance on dietary requirements for chromium is to follow the advice given in the 10th (1989) edition of the RDAs, that, 'until more precise recommendations can be made, the consumption of a varied diet, balanced with regard to other essential nutrients, remains the best assurance of an adequate and safe chromium intake'[69].

6.9 Chromium supplementation

It was estimated some years ago that approximately 10 million Americans bought chromium supplements at a price of $150 million each year, which made chromium the largest-selling mineral supplement, after calcium, in the US[70]. Consumption of chromium supplements has probably not decreased in the intervening years. Sales are encouraged by advertisers' claims about the benefits of the trace metal, for example in promoting weight loss and lean muscle mass development, especially in athletes[71]. The absence of an RNI and the continuing use in promotional literature, as well as by some nutritionists, of the ESADDI of 50–200 μg/d, has also led to the belief that 90% of people suffer from chromium deficiency. As a result, it is suggested, most people may be at risk of poor glucose tolerance and may develop maturity-onset diabetes and cardiovascular disease[72].

Several different types of chromium supplements are available for over-the-counter sales. These include the inorganic Cr(III) compound, chromium chloride ($CrCl_3$), as well as the probably more bioavailable organic compounds, chromium nicotinate and chromium picolinate[73]. A supplement containing GTF, the chromium–dinicotinic acid–glutathione complex, derived from yeast, is also available.

There is debate about the safety of some of these supplements. Trivalent chromium, the form of the element used in supplements, is considered to be one of the least toxic nutrients[74], in contrast to the hexavalent chromium, which is extremely toxic[75]. However, concern has been raised by reports of toxic effects of ingestion of Cr(III) in the form of chromium picolinate. This has been found, in animal experiments, to be clastogenic at a low level of intake[76]. In contrast, other investigations have found chromium picolinate to be non-toxic in humans; nor have there been any documented toxic effects of supplemental chromium[77]. It has been suggested that, in the case of chromium picolinate, it is the picolinate and not the Cr(III) that is responsible for the chromosome damage[78].

References

1. Akasuka, K. & Fairhall, L.T. (1934) The toxicology of chromium. *Journal of Industrial Toxicology and Hygiene*, **16**, 1–10.
2. Schwarz, K. & Mertz, W. (1959) Chromium (III) and the glucose tolerance factor. *Archives of Biochemistry and Biophysics*, **85**, 292–303.
3. Vincent, J.B. (2000) The biochemistry of chromium. *Journal of Nutrition*, **130**, 715–8.
4. Veillon, C. & Patterson, K.Y. (1999) Analytical issues in nutritional chromium research. *Journal of Trace Element Experimental Research*, **12**, 99–109.

5. Burrows, D. (1983) *Chromium: Metabolism and Toxicity*. CRC Press, Boca Raton, FL.
6. Rowbottom, A.L., Levy, L.S. & Shuker, L.K. (2000) Chromium in the environment: an evaluation of exposure of the UK general population and possible adverse health effects. *Journal of Toxicology and Environmental Health – Part B: Critical Reviews*, **3**, 145–78.
7. Department of Health (1991) *Dietary Reference Values for Food Energy and Nutrients in the United Kingdom*, pp. 181–2. HMSO, London.
8. Tinggi, U., Reilly, C. & Patterson, C. (1997) Determination of manganese and chromium in foods by atomic absorption spectrometry after wet digestion. *Food Chemistry*, **60**, 123–8.
9. Ysart, G., Miller, P., Crews, H. *et al.* (1999) Dietary exposure estimates of 30 elements from the UK Total Diet Study. *Food Additives and Contaminants*, **16**, 391–403.
10. Mordenti, A., Piva, A. & Piva, G. (1997) The European perspective on organic chromium in animal nutrition. In: *Biotechnology and the Feed Industry. Proceedings of Alltech's 13th Annual Symposium* (eds. T.P. Lyons & K.A. Jacques), pp. 227–40. Nottingham University Press, Nottingham, UK.
11. Hegoczki, J., Suhajda, A., Janzso, B. & Vereczkey, G. (1997) Preparation of chromium enriched yeasts. *Acta Alimentaria*, **26**, 345–58.
12. Saner, G. (1986) The metabolic significance of dietary chromium. *Nutrition International*, **2**, 213–20.
13. EEC (1980) *Council Directive Relating to the Quality of Water Intended for Human Consumption, 80/778*. European Economic Community, Brussels.
14. Ministry of Agriculture, Fisheries and Food (1998) *Cadmium, Mercury and Other Metals in Food. 53rd Report of the Steering Group on Chemical Aspects of Food Surveillance*. The Stationery Office, London.
15. Whitman, W.E. (1978) Interactions between structural materials in food plants, and foodstuffs and cleaning agents. *Food Progress*, **2**, 1–2.
16. Offenbach, E.G. & Pi-Sunyer, F.X. (1983) Temperature and pH effects on the release of chromium from stainless steel into water and fruit juices. *Journal of Advances in Food Chemistry*, **31**, 89–92.
17. Hoare, W.E., Hedges, E.S. & Barry, B. (1965) *The Technology of Tinplate*. Arnold, London.
18. Anderson, R.A. (1988) Chromium. In: *Trace Metals in Food* (ed. K.T. Smith), pp. 231–47. Dekker, New York.
19. Murthy, G.K., Rhea, U. & Peeler, J.R. (1971) Chromium in the diet of schoolchildren. *Environmental Science and Technology*, **5**, 436–42.
20. MAFF (1999) *MAFF-1997 Total Diet Study – Aluminium, Arsenic, Cadmium, Chromium, Copper, Lead, Mercury, Nickel, Selenium, Tin and Zinc. Food Surveillance Information Sheet No. 191*. Ministry of Agriculture, Fisheries and Food, London.
21. Anderson, R.A., Bryden, N.A. & Polansky, M.M. (1992) Dietary chromium intake: freely chosen diets, institutional diets, and individual foods. *Biological Trace Elements Research*, **32**, 117–21.
22. Mertz, W., Toepfer, E.W., Roginski, E.E. & Polansky, M.M. (1994) Present knowledge of the role of chromium. *Federation Proceedings*, **33**, 2275–80.
23. Petersen, A. & Mortensen, G.K. (1994) Trace elements in shellfish on the Danish market. *Food Additives and Contaminants*, **11**, 365–73.
24. Seaborn, C.D. & Stoecer, B.J. (1992) Effects of ascorbic acid depletion and chromium status on retention and urinary excretion of ^{51}chromium. *Nutrition Research*, **12**, 1229–34.
25. Hill, C.H. (1976) Mineral interrelationships. In: *Trace Elements in Human Health and Disease* (ed. A. Prasad), pp. 201–10. Academic Press, New York.
26. Juturu, V., Komorowski, J.R., Devine, J.P. & Capen, A. (2003) Absorption and excretion of chromium from orally administered chromium chloride, chromium acetate and chromium oxide in rats. *Trace Elements and Electrolytes*, **20**, 23–8.

27. Anderson, R.A. (1998) Effects of chromium on body composition and weight loss. *Nutrition Reviews*, **56**, 266–70.
28. Hopkins, L.L. & Schwarz, K. (1964) Chromium (III) binding to serum proteins, specifically siderophilin. *Biochimica et Biophysica Acta*, **90**, 484–91.
29. Vincent, J.B. (2000) The biochemistry of chromium. *Journal of Nutrition*, **130**, 715–8.
30. Mertz, W. (1969) Chromium occurrence and function in biological systems. *Physiological Reviews*, **49**, 162–239.
31. Holm, R.H., Kennepohl, P. & Solomon, E.I. (1996) Structural and functional aspects of metal sites in biology. *Chemical Reviews*, **96**, 2239–314.
32. Schwarz, K. & Mertz, W. (1959) Chromium (III) and glucose tolerance factor. *Archives of Biochemistry and Biophysics*, **85**, 292–5.
33. Mertz, W., Roginski, E.E. & Schwarz, K. (1961) Effect of trivalent chromium on glucose uptake by epididymal fat tissues of rats. *Journal of Biological Chemistry*, **236**, 318–22.
34. Vincent, J.B. (1999) Mechanisms of chromium action: low molecular-weight chromium binding substance. *Journal of the American College of Nutrition*, **18**, 6–12.
35. Anderson, R.A. (1995) Chromium and parenteral nutrition. *Nutrition*, **11**, 83–6.
36. Morris, B.W., MacNeill, S., Hardisty, S.A. *et al.* (1999) Chromium homeostasis in patients with type II (NIDDM) diabetes. *Journal of Trace Elements in Medicine and Biology*, **13**, 57–61.
37. Althuis, M.D., Jordan, N.E., Ludington, E.A. & Wittes, J.T. (2002) Glucose and insulin responses to dietary chromium supplements: a meta-analysis. *American Journal of Clinical Nutrition*, **76**, 148–55.
38. Ghosh, D., Bhattacharya, B., Mukherjee, B. *et al.* (2002) Role of chromium supplementation in Indians with type 2 diabetes mellitus. *Journal of Nutritional Biochemistry*, **13**, 690–7.
39. Offenbacher, E.G. & Pi-Sunyer, F.X. (1980) Beneficial effects of chromium-rich yeast on glucose tolerance and blood lipids in the elderly. *Diabetes*, **29**, 919–25.
40. Anderson, R.A. (1995) Chromium, glucose tolerance, diabetes and lipid metabolism. *Journal of the Advancement of Medicine*, **8**, 37–50.
41. Roussel, A.M., Bureau, I., Favier, M. *et al.* (2002) Beneficial effects of hormonal replacement therapy on chromium status and glucose and lipid metabolism in postmenopausal women. *Maturitas*, **42**, 63–9.
42. Vincent, J.B. (2000) The biochemistry of chromium. *Journal of Nutrition*, **130**, 715–8.
43. Davis, C.M. & Vincent, J.B. (1997) Chromium oligopeptide activates insulin receptor tyrosine kinase activity. *Biochemistry*, **36**, 4382–5.
44. Davis, C.M. & Vincent, J.B. (1997) Chromium in carbohydrate and lipid metabolism. *Journal of Biological Inorganic Chemistry*, **2**, 675–9.
45. Yamamoto, A., Wada, O. & Manabe, S. (1989) Evidence that chromium is an essential factor for biological activity of low-molecular-weight-chromium-binding substance. *Biochemistry and Biophysics Research Communications*, **163**, 189–93.
46. Vincent, J.B. (2000) The biochemistry of chromium. *Journal of Nutrition*, **130**, 715–8.
47. Davis, C.M., Royer, A. & Vincent, J.B. (1997) Synthetic multinuclear chromium assembly activates insulin receptor kinase activity: functional model for low-molecular-weight chromium-binding substance. *Inorganic Chemistry*, **36**, 5316–20.
48. Vincent, J.B. (2000) The biochemistry of chromium. *Journal of Nutrition*, **130**, 715–8.
49. Saltiel, A.R. (1994) The paradoxical regulation of protein phosphorylation in insulin action. *Federation of American Societies of Experimental Biology Journal*, **8**, 1034–40.
50. Morris, B.W., MacNeill, S., Stanley, K., Gray, T.A. & Fraser, R. (1993) The inter-relationship between insulin and chromium in hyperinsulinaemic euglycaemic clamps in healthy volunteers. *Journal of Endocrinology*, **139**, 339–45.
51. Kobla, H.V. & Volpe, S.L. (2000) Chromium, exercise, and body composition. *Critical Reviews in Food Science and Nutrition*, **40**, 291–308.

52. Lukaski, H.C. (2001) Magnesium, zinc, and chromium nutrition and athletic performance. *Canadian Journal of Applied Physiology*, **26**, S13–22.
53. Vincent, J.B. (2000) The biochemistry of chromium. *Journal of Nutrition*, **130**, 715–8.
54. Speetjens, J.K., Collins, R.A., Vincent, J.B. & Woski, S.A. (1999) The nutritional supplement chromium (III) tris(picolinate) cleaves DNA. *Chemical Toxicology*, **12**, 483–7.
55. Granadillo, V.A., de Machado, L.P. & Romero, R.A. (1994) Determination of total chromium in whole blood, blood components, bone, and urine by fast furnace program electrothermal atomization AAS and using neither analyte information nor background correction. *Analytical Chemistry*, **66**, 3624–31.
56. Veillon, C. (1989) Analytical chemistry of chromium. *Science of the Total Environment*, **1**, 65–8.
57. Borel, J.S. & Anderson, R.A. (1984) Chromium. In: *Biochemistry of the Essential Ultratrace Elements*, pp. 175–99. Plenum, New York.
58. Randall, J.A. & Gibson, R.S. (1987) Serum and urine chromium as indices of chromium status in tannery workers. *Proceedings of the Society of Experimental Biology and Medicine*, **185**, 16–23.
59. Anderson, R.A., Bryden, N.A. & Polansky, M.M. (1985) Serum chromium in human subjects: effects of chromium supplementation and glucose. *American Journal of Clinical Nutrition*, **41**, 571–7.
60. Gibson, R.S. (1990) *Principles of Nutritional Assessment*, pp. 137–8. Oxford University Press, Oxford.
61. Offenbacher, E.G., Spencer, H., Dowling, H.J. & Pi-sunyer, F.X. (1986) Metabolic chromium balances in men. *American Journal of Clinical Nutrition*, **44**, 77–82.
62. Anderson, R.A. & Bryden, N.A. (1985) Chromium intake, absorption and excretion of subjects consuming self-selected diets. *American Journal of Clinical Nutrition*, **41**, 1177–83.
63. Paustenbach, D.J., Panko, J.M., Fredrick, M. *et al.* (1997) Urinary chromium as a biological marker of environmental exposure: what are the limitations? *Regulations of Toxicology and Pharmacology*, **26**, S23–34.
64. Gibson, R.S. (1990) *Principles of Nutritional Assessment*. Oxford University Press, Oxford.
65. Anderson, R.A., Polansky, M.M., Bryden, N. & Canary, J.J. (1991) Supplemental-chromium effects on glucose, insulin, glucagon, and urinary chromium losses in subjects consuming low-chromium diets. *American Journal of Clinical Nutrition*, **54**, 909–916.
66. Department of Health (1991) *Dietary Reference Values for Food Energy and Nutrients in the United Kingdom*, pp. 181–2. HMSO, London.
67. National Research Council (1989) *Recommended Dietary Allowances*, 10th ed., pp. 241–3. National Academy Press, Washington, DC.
68. Food and Nutrition Board, Institute of Medicine (2002) *Dietary Reference Intakes for Vitamin A, Vitamin K, Arsenic, Boron, Chromium, Copper, Iodine, Iron, Manganese, Molybdenum, Nickel, Silicon, Vanadium, and Zinc*. National Academies Press, Washington, DC. http:/books.nap.edu/books/0309072794/html/19.html
69. National Research Council (1989) *Recommended Dietary Allowances*, 10th ed., pp. 241–3. National Academy Press, Washington, DC.
70. Nielsen, F. H. (1996) Controversial chromium: does the superstar mineral of the mountebanks receive appropriate attention from clinicians and nutritionists? *Nutrition Today*, **31**, 226–33.
71. Hellerstein, M.K. (1998) Is chromium supplementation effective in managing type II diabetes? *Nutrition Reviews*, **56**, 302–6.
72. Brewer, S. (2003) *The Essential Guide to Vitamins and Minerals*, pp. 45–6. Market Vision/ Healthspan, St Peter Port, Guernsey, UK.
73. Clarkson, P.M. (1997) Effects of exercise on chromium levels: is supplementation required? *Sports Medicine*, **23**, 341–9.

74. Mertz, W., Abernathy, C.O. & Olin, S.S. (1994) *Risk Assessment of Essential Elements*, pp. 29–38. ILSI Press, Washington, DC.
75. Kaufman, D.B., Nicola, W. & McIntosh, R. (1970) Acute potassium dichromate poisoning. *American Journal of the Diseases of Childhood*, **119**, 374–6.
76. Stearns, D.M., Wise, J.P., Sr., Patierno, S.R. & Wetterhahn, K.E. (1995) Chromium (III) picolinate produces chromosome damage in Chinese hamster ovary cells. *Federation of American Societies of Experimental Biology Journal*, **9**, 1643–8.
77. Anderson, R.A, Bryden, N.A. & Polansky, M.M. (1979) Lack of toxicity of chromium chloride and chromium picolinate. *Journal of the American College of Nutritionists*, **16**, 273–9.
78. Hatcock, J.N. (1997) Vitamin and minerals: efficacy and safety. *American Journal of Clinical Nutrition*, **66**, 427–37.

Chapter 7
Manganese

7.1 Introduction

Until relatively recently, little attention was paid to the metal manganese by biological scientists. If considered at all, it was almost exclusively as a toxin, responsible for what was known as 'manganese madness' suffered by workers exposed to the metal's fumes. Even today, though its essentiality to health is recognised, to judge by the small number of papers about it published in the nutritional literature or presented at scientific meetings, manganese attracts only limited interest among life scientists. Consequently, there are large gaps in our knowledge of its biological role. There are inadequate data on body composition and metabolism of the metal on which to base dietary recommendations. However, what is known indicates that the metal has important roles to play in mammalian metabolism and health, which no doubt will be made clear by further research.

7.2 Production and uses of manganese

Manganese is a 'modern' metal, though its principal ore, pyrolucite (manganese dioxide), was known to the ancients as a pigment. It is an almost ubiquitous constituent of the environment, making up about 0.1% of the earth's crust. It also occurs in substantial deposits in many countries. It is the twelfth most common element, and the second most common heavy metal, after iron. Manganese was first isolated in 1774 by the Swedish chemist, Johan Gahn, by heating pyrolucite with charcoal. By the late nineteenth century, manganese was being refined and used in substantial quantities in the manufacture of particularly strong and workable steel. Today, nearly 90% of all manganese produced each year is used in this way. It is also used to make other types of alloys for a wide variety of industrial applications, for example in electrical accumulators. Manganese compounds are used in pigments and glazes, as well as domestic and pharmaceutical products. A recent use has been as a replacement of alkyllead additives in petroleum and of lead in shotgun cartridges.

7.3 Chemical and physical properties of manganese

Manganese is number 25 in the periodic table of the elements It has an atomic weight of 54.94. Its chemical and physical properties are, in many respects, similar to those of iron, which it immediately precedes in the first transition series. Like iron, it is a reactive element, for example, dissolving readily in dilute, non-oxidising acids, igniting in chlorine to form $MnCl_2$, and reacting with oxygen to form Mn_3O_4. It can also combine directly with boron, carbon, sulphur, silicon and phosphorus.

Manganese has several oxidation states, +7, + 4, + 3 and +2. The most characteristic of these, especially in biological complexes, is the divalent Mn(II). This forms a series of manganous salts with all common anions, most of which are soluble in water and crystallise as hydrates. It also forms a series of chelates with EDTA and other agents. Mn(III) is of particular importance *in vivo*. Mn(IV) compounds are of little importance, except for the dioxide (MnO_2). Mn(VI) is found only in the manganate ion (MnO_4). Mn(VII) is best known in the permanganate ion (MnO_4^{2-}). Potassium permanganate is a common and widely used compound, traditionally known to many as the wine-red aqueous solution, Condy's fluid. Permanganates are powerful oxidising agents. Manganese forms several organo-compounds. One used in recent years industrially, as a substitute for alkyllead as an anti-knock additive in petroleum fuels, is methylcyclopentadienyl manganese tricarbonyl.

7.4 Manganese in food and beverages

Manganese is present in all biological tissues, usually at low concentrations. Reported levels in foods in different countries are very similar. Data for the UK, as shown in Table 7.1, are close to those from other countries such as the US[1]. Interestingly, in spite of similarities in environmental distribution and chemistry between the two metals, in contrast to iron, cereals and cereal products are among the richest food sources of manganese, with low levels in meat and offal. Green leafy vegetables are also good sources. An interesting and, in the context of a tea-drinking nation, important finding is that tea is a major dietary source of manganese for many in the UK. Dry tea leaves can contain between 350 and 900 mg/kg, and the beverage itself 7.1–38.0 mg of manganese per kilogram[2].

7.5 Dietary intake of manganese

In the UK, the mean daily dietary intake of manganese is 4.5 mg[3], about half of which is believed to be derived from tea[4]. US intakes appear to be somewhat lower, averaging 2.85 and 2.21 mg for 25–30 year-old men and women, respectively, over the years 1982–91[5]. Similar intakes have been recorded in several European countries, such as Belgium and Spain[6]. However, intakes can vary greatly, depending mainly on the presence or absence in the diet of rich sources of the metal and, in some cases, on levels of environmental pollution. Intakes of up to 200 mg/d have been recorded among residents of Groote Eylandt, an island in the Gulf of Carpentaria in the north of Australia, where one of the world's richest open cast manganese mines is worked[7].

7.6 Absorption and metabolism of manganese

Manganese absorption from food in the GI tract is low, but there is considerable variation between individuals. Normally, only a small percentage of dietary manganese is absorbed.

Table 7.1 Manganese in UK foods.

Food group	Mean concentration (mg/kg fresh weight)
Bread	8.0
Miscellaneous cereals	6.8
Carcass meat	0.14
Offal	2.8
Meat products	1.4
Poultry	0.17
Fish	1.1
Oils and fats	0.02
Eggs	0.31
Sugar and preserves	1.5
Green vegetables	2.0
Potatoes	1.9
Other vegetables	1.6
Canned vegetables	1.8
Fresh fruit	2.0
Fruit products	2.2
Beverages	2.7
Milk	0.03
Dairy products	0.27
Nuts	15

Adapted from Ysart, G., Miller, P., Crews, H. *et al.* (1999) Dietary exposure estimates of 30 elements from the UK Total Diet Study. *Food Additives and Contaminants*, **16**, 391–403.

There is some evidence that manganese absorption can be affected by the presence of phytate. Animal studies have shown that replacement of cow's milk with soy formula, which is rich in phytate, can reduce manganese absorption significantly[8].

A retention rate for manganese of 3% has been reported, with a range of 0.6–9.2% in adult men[9]. Absorption takes place along the length of the small intestine The process appears to be an active process and is related to the manganese status of the body. Once absorbed, the manganese quickly leaves the blood, and some is concentrated in liver and other organs. Excretion is rapid mainly in bile in faeces, with only a small amount in urine[10].

7.6.1 Metabolic functions of manganese

Manganese is recognised as an essential micronutrient for mammals, including humans. It is involved in the formation of bone and in the metabolism of amino acids, cholesterol and carbohydrates. It is a component of several enzymes, including arginase, glutamine synthetase, phosphoenolpyruvate decarboxylase, hexokinase, xanthine oxidase and manganese superoxide dismutase. Glycosyltransferases and xylosyltransferases, which are involved in proteoglycan synthesis and thus in bone formation, are sensitive to manganese status. Manganese is also an activator of a number of enzymes, though in most cases, these can also be activated by other metals, especially magnesium[11]. Because the Mn(II) ion is very similar in size and charge density to Mg(II) and Zn(II), it can replace magnesium in pyruvate carboxylase and zinc in zinc superoxide dismutase, with negligible effects on their activities[12].

7.6.2 Manganese deficiency

Manganese deficiency has been observed in a number of experimental animals. Signs of deficiency included impaired growth and reproduction as well as alterations in lipid and carbohydrate metabolism, including impaired glucose tolerance. Defects of skeletal development have also been observed[13]. There are few reports of manganese deficiency in humans. In one case, a volunteer who received a purified diet containing 0.1 mg of manganese per day, was reported to have developed transient dermatitis and hypercholesterolaemia. Other volunteers on a low manganese intake developed similar symptoms[14]. Decreased plasma manganese levels have been reported to be associated with the development of osteoporosis in women. An improvement in bone density followed supplementation of the diet with minerals, including manganese[15].

Apart from these few observations, little has been documented in the clinical literature about manganese deficiency. There is some evidence that certain types of stress accentuate dietary manganese insufficiency. Ethanol toxicity, for example, is known to increase superoxide production and can be counteracted by manganese superoxide dismutase, thus placing an increased demand on manganese stores.[16]

Because of the long recognised connection between manganese and toxicity, especially in the case of industrial workers who developed 'manganese madness' after exposure to metal fumes, the relation between manganese and brain function has attracted a good deal of attention. It has been shown that manganese is supplied to the brain via both the blood–brain and blood–cerebrospinal fluid barriers. Transferrin appears to be involved, along with other carriers, in the transport of manganese into the brain. Once across the brain barriers, much of the manganese is bound to proteins, especially to glutamine synthetase in astrocytes. There is evidence that some manganese probably exists in the synaptic vesicles in glutaminergic neurons and is dynamically coupled to the electrophysiological activity of the neurons. It is possible that release of this manganese into the synaptic cleft influences synaptic neurotransmission. Dietary deficiency of manganese, which may enhance susceptibility to epileptic function, appears to affect manganese homeostasis of the brain, probably followed by alteration of neural activity[17].

7.6.3 Manganese toxicity

Though manganese has long been recognised as a toxic element to industrial workers exposed to fumes of the metal, it is considered to be one of the least toxic through oral intake. This has been attributed to the fact that even when excess manganese is consumed, absorption is very low, and what is absorbed is rapidly and efficiently excreted in bile and urine[18]. There have been no reports of toxicity as a result of consuming manganese in food as part of a normal diet.

High levels of manganese, taken into the body, for example, by inhalation of metal fumes or in total parenteral nutrition fluids, are highly toxic. Excess manganese in the brain, especially in the basal ganglia, can affect motor and cognitive function; continued accumulation causes severe extrapyramidal neurological and psychiatric disease[19], with symptoms similar to those of Parkinson's disease[20]. Some of these symptoms have been observed in miners and metallurgical workers, as well as in non-mining local residents exposed to environmental pollution from manganese mining operations[21].

Recent research has produced evidence that astrocytes are a site of early brain dysfunction and damage in manganese toxicity. Astrocytes have been shown to possess a high affinity, high capacity, specific transport system for manganese that facilitates its uptake and sequestration in mitochondria. There, the manganese causes disruption of oxidative phosphorylation as well as a number of other functional changes, including impairment of glutamate transport, alterations of the glycolytic enzyme glyceraldehyde-3-phosphate dehydrogenase and production of nitric oxide. As a result of these effects, energy metabolism is compromised, there are changes in cellular morphology, reactive oxygen species are produced, and there is an increase in extracellular glutamate concentration[22].

TPN patients with chronic obstructive liver disease or being fed intravenously following gastrointestinal surgery may also be at risk of toxicity, depending on how much manganese is in the infusion fluid. Such patients lack the normal means of excreting excess manganese. Elevated blood manganese levels, with evidence of deposition in brain, have been observed in some instances where patients were given manganese-supplemented TPN[23]. A high incidence of hypermanganesaemia has been reported in children on TPN, even though they were given the standard manganese dose. The condition was associated with impaired liver function. Manganese deposition in brain was seen in a small number of cases. As a consequence of such findings, a reduction in levels of manganese in parenteral formulas for children on long-term TPN has been recommended[24]. Because of uncertainty about the correct dose in infusion fluid used in home parenteral nutrition, there is concern that some patients undergoing this treatment may accumulate undesirable levels of manganese[25].

7.7 Assessment of manganese status and estimation of dietary requirements

There is at present no accurate index or reliable biomarker for evaluating manganese status[26] and consequently dietary requirements. Methods used successfully with other trace nutrients have not proved satisfactory in the case of manganese. Balance studies are problematic because of the rapid excretion of manganese into bile and because manganese balances do not appear to be proportional to manganese intakes[27]. Though serum and plasma concentrations have been reported to respond to dietary intake, findings are not always consistent, and concentrations appear to be sensitive to large variations in manganese intake. Similarly, though levels in urine are responsive to severe manganese deficiency, there is controversy on the use of urine levels for assessment of status when typical amounts are consumed[28].

Activities of a number of manganese-dependent enzymes have been suggested as markers of status. However, so far, none have proved totally satisfactory for the task. Arginase, which has been shown to be depressed in livers of manganese-deficient experimental animals[29], is affected by a number of other dietary factors, besides manganese, as well as by liver disease[30]. Possibly of more use is manganese-superoxide dismutase (MnSOD). Activity of the enzyme is low in manganese-deficient animals[31]. In women, MnSOD activity in lymphocytes has been increased by manganese supplementation. However, other factors, including alcohol consumption, can also affect activity of the enzyme.[32]

Table 7.2 US recommendations for manganese (mg/d).

Life-stage group	Adequate Intake
Infants	
0–6 months	0.003
7–12 months	0.6
Children	
1–3 years	1.2
4–8 years	1.5
Males	
9–13 years	1.9
14–18 years	2.2
19–30 years	2.3
31–50 years	2.3
50–70 years	2.3
>70 years	2.3
Females	
9–13 years	1.6
14–18 years	1.6
19–30 years	1.8
31–50 years	1.8
50–70 years	1.8
>70 years	1.8
Pregnancy	
≤18 years	2.0
19–30 years	2.0
31–50 years	2.0
Lactation	
≤ 18 years	2.6
19–30 years	2.6
31–50 years	2.6

For healthy breastfed infants, the AI is the mean intake. The AI for other life-stage and gender groups is believed to cover the needs of all individuals in a group, but because of the lack of data, the percentage of individuals covered by this intake cannot be specified with confidence.

Adapted from: Food and Nutrition Board National Academy of Sciences (2002) *US Dietary Reference Intakes: Elements.* http://www4.nationalacademies.org/10M/10MHome.nst/pages/Food+and+Nutrition+Board

It has recently been proposed that manganese status can be assessed accurately by making use of magnetic resonance imaging (MRI) to measure manganese levels in brain[33]. While this may be of use in limited situations, such as with hospital patients, because of the need for MRI measurements, it is highly unlikely ever to be in general use for assessing manganese status.

7.7.1 Manganese dietary requirements

Though deficiency has been produced in experimental animals and in a small number of human volunteers given low manganese diets, these are contrived cases, and there is no evidence that manganese deficiency ever occurs in healthy persons consuming a diet containing reasonable amounts of cereals and other vegetable foods. There is little, if any, reason, therefore, to doubt the statement of the UK's Panel on DRVs, that current population intakes of manganese are adequate[34]. In the absence of adequate data on body composition and of detailed studies of turnover and metabolism, which would have allowed determination of an RNI for manganese, the Panel had recourse to a pragmatic approach in determining DRVs for the element. In place of an RNI, they set a Safe Intake (SI) of above 1.4 mg/d for adults and above 16 μg/d for infants and children.

Until 2001, the US did not have a DRV for manganese. A provisional daily dietary manganese intake for adults of 2.0–5.0 mg was included in the 10th edition of the *Recommended Dietary Allowances* published in 1989[35]. This ESADDI was based, in the absence of adequate data which would allow estimation of an RDI, on observed current intakes and on the apparent lack of manganese deficiency as a practical nutritional problem in adults. Though there is still a need for additional data, the 2002 revision of the US Dietary Reference Intakes has replaced the ESADDI with recommendations for Adequate Intakes (AI), as shown in Table 7.2[36].

References

1. Pennington, J.A.T. & Schoen, S.A. (1996) Total Diet Study: estimated dietary intakes of nutritional elements, 1982–91. *International Journal of Vitamin and Nutrition Research*, **66**, 350–62.
2. Wenlock, R.W., Buss, D.H. & Dixon, E.J. (1979) Trace nutrients 2: manganese in British foods. *British Journal of Nutrition*, **41**, 253–61.
3. Gregory, J., Foster, K., Tyler, H. & Wiseman, M. (1990) *The Dietary and Nutritional Survey of British Adults*. HMSO, London.
4. Nielsen, F.H. (1994) Ultratrace elements. In: *Modern Nutrition in Health and Disease* (eds. M.E. Shils, J.A. Olsen & M. Shike), pp. 275–7. Lea & Febiger, Philadelphia.
5. Pennington, J.A.T. & Schoen, S.A. (1996) Total Diet Study: estimated dietary intakes of nutritional elements, 1982–91. *International Journal of Vitamin and Nutrition Research*, **66**, 350–62.
6. Van Dokkum, W. (1995) The intake of selected minerals and trace elements in European countries. *Nutrition Research Reviews*, **8**, 271–302.
7. Cawte, J. & Florence, M. (1987) Environmental sources of manganese on Groote Eylandt, Northern Territory. *Lancet*, **i**, 62.

8. Lönnerdal, B. (2002) Phytic acid–trace element (Zn, Cu, Mn) interactions. *International Journal of Food Science and Technology*, **37**, 749–58.
9. Davidson, L., Cederblad, A. & Lonnerdal, R. (1989) Manganese retention in man: a method of estimating manganese absorption in man. *American Journal of Clinical Nutrition*, **49**, 170–9.
10. Testolini, G., Ciapellano, S., Alberto, A. *et al.* (1993) Intestinal absorption of manganese – an *in vitro* study. *Annals of Nutrition and Metabolism*, **37**, 289–94.
11. Nielsen, F.H. (1994) Ultratrace elements. In: *Modern Nutrition in Health and Disease* (eds. M.E. Shils, J.A. Olsen & M. Shike), pp. 275–7. Lea & Febiger, Philadelphia.
12. Stillman, M.J. & Presta, A. (2000) Characterizing metal ion interactions with biological molecules – the spectroscopy of metallothionein. In: *Molecular Biology and Toxicology of Metals* (eds. R.K. Zalups & J. Koropatnick), pp. 4–8. Taylor & Francis, London.
13. Keen, C.L., Ensuna, J.L., Watson, M.H. *et al.* (1999) Nutritional aspects of manganese from experimental studies. *Neurotoxicology*, **20**, 213–23.
14. Friedman, B.J., Freeland-Graves, J.H., Bales, C.W. *et al.* (1987) Manganese balance and clinical observations in young men fed a manganese-deficient diet. *Journal of Nutrition*, **117**, 133–43.
15. Freeland-Graves, J. & Turnlund, J.R. (1996) Deliberations and evaluations of the approaches, endpoints and paradigms for manganese and molybdenum dietary recommendations. *Journal of Nutrition*, **126**, 2435S-40S.
16. Nielsen, F.H. (1994) Ultratrace elements. In: *Modern Nutrition in Health and Disease* (eds. M.E. Shils, J.A. Olsen & M. Shike), pp. 275–7. Lea & Febiger, Philadelphia.
17. Takeda, A. (2000) Manganese action in brain function. *Brain Research Review*, **41**, 79–87.
18. Underwood, E.J. (1977) *Trace Elements in Human and Animal Nutrition*, 4th ed., pp. 170–81. Academic Press, New York.
19. Leach, R.M. & Harris, E.D. (1997) Manganese. In: *Handbook of Nutritionally Essential Mineral Elements* (eds. B.L. O'Dell & R.A. Sunde), pp. 335–56. Dekker, New York.
20. Takeda, A. (2000) Manganese action in brain function. *Brain Research Review*, **41**, 79–87.
21. Cawte, J., Hams, G. & Kilburn, C. (1987) Mechanisms in a neurological ethnic complex in Northern Australia. *Lancet*, **i**, 61.
22. Normandin, L. & Hazell, A.S. (2002) Manganese neurotoxicity: an update of pathophysiologic mechanisms. *Metabolic Brain Disease*, **17**, 375–87.
23. Iwase, K., Higaki, J., Mikata, S. *et al.* (2002) Manganese deposition in basal ganglia due to perioperative parenteral nutrition following gastrointestinal surgeries. *Digestive Surgery*, **19**, 174–83.
24. Fell, J.M.E., Reynolds, A.P., Meadows, N. *et al.* (1996) Manganese toxicity in children receiving long-term parenteral nutrition. *Lancet*, **347**, 1218–21.
25. Takagi, Y., Okada, A., Sando, K. *et al.* (2002) Evaluation of indexes of *in vivo* manganese status and the optimal intravenous dose for adult patients undergoing home parenteral nutrition. *American Journal of Clinical Nutrition*, **75**, 112–8.
26. Takagi, Y., Okada, A., Sando, K. *et al.* (2002) Evaluation of indexes of *in vivo* manganese status and the optimal intravenous dose for adult patients undergoing home parenteral nutrition. *American Journal of Clinical Nutrition*, **75**, 112–8.
27. Greger, J.L. (1998) Dietary standards for manganese: overlap between nutritional and toxicological studies. *Journal of Nutrition*, **128**, 368S-71S.
28. Greger, J.L., Davis, C.D., Suttie, J.W. & Lyle, B.J. (1990) Intake, serum concentrations, and urinary excretion of manganese by adult males. *American Journal of Clinical Nutrition*, **51**, 457–461.
29. Paynter, D.I. (1980) Changes in activity of the manganese superoxide dismutase enzyme in tissues of the rat, with changes in dietary manganese. *Journal of Nutrition*, **110**, 437–47.

30. Dreosti, I.E., Manuel, S.J. & Buckley, R.A. (1982) Superoxide dismutase (EC 1.15.1.1), manganese and the effect of ethanol in adult and foetal rats. *British Journal of Nutrition*, **48**, 205–10.
31. Davis, C.D., Wolf, T.L. & Greger, J.L. (1992) Varying levels of manganese and iron affect absorption and gut endogenous losses of manganese by rats. *Journal of Nutrition*, **122**, 1300–8.
32. Dreosti, I.E., Manuel, S.J. & Buckley, R.A. (1982) Superoxide dismutase (EC 1.15.1.1), manganese and the effect of ethanol in adult and foetal rats. *British Journal of Nutrition*, **48**, 205–10.
33. Takagi, Y., Okada, A., Sando, K. *et al.* (2002) Evaluation of indexes of *in vivo* manganese status and the optimal intravenous dose for adult patients undergoing home parenteral nutrition. *American Journal of Clinical Nutrition*, **75**, 112–8.
34. Department of Health (1991) *Dietary Reference Values for Food Energy and Nutrients for the United Kingdom*, p. 179. HMSO, London.
35. National Research Council (1989) *Recommended Dietary Allowances*, 10th ed., pp. 230–3. National Academy Press, Washington, DC.
36. Food and Nutrition Board National Academy of Sciences (2002) *US Dietary Reference Intakes: Elements*. http://www4.nationalacademies.org/10M/10Mhome.nst/pages/Food+and+Nutrition+Board

Chapter 8
Molybdenum

8.1 Introduction

Molybdenum is another of the 'modern' metals whose role in animal and human metabolism has been recognised relatively recently. It was first isolated in 1792 and began to be used industrially in the nineteenth century. In 1930, its first biological role was recognised, when it was found to act as a catalyst for nitrogen fixation in certain bacteria. About the same time, *teart disease* in cattle was found to be caused by ingestion of fodder with high levels of molybdenum. Then in 1943, the enzyme xanthine oxidase in rat liver was shown to be molybdenum-dependent[1]. Subsequently, other molybdoenzymes were identified, and in 1976 its essentiality for humans was accepted when the pathology of molybdenum deficiency was recognised in a patient undergoing total parenteral nutrition (TPN)[2].

8.2 Distribution and production of molybdenum

Though molybdenum is today of considerable industrial importance, especially in the production of strong, high quality steels for making heavy machines and industrial hardware, it is, in fact, one of the rarer elements. Levels in most agricultural soils are generally low, though there are some high-molybdenum areas, especially where the soil overlies certain types of molybdenum-containing shale, with consequences for grazing animals. Molybdenum occurs in several different types of ore, the most important of which is the molybdenite, MoS_2. Its only known major deposit is in Colorado in the US. To extract the metal, the ore is crushed, treated by a flotation process and roasted in air to form MoO_3.

8.3 Chemical and physical properties of molybdenum

Molybdenum belongs to Group 6 of the periodic table, along with chromium and tungsten with which it has several close chemical and physical affinities. Like them, it is a transition metal, though not in the same transition series. It is number 42 in the periodic table, a heavy metal, with a density of 9.0 and atomic weight of 95.94. It is dull, silver-white in colour, and malleable and ductile, with a high melting point of 2610°C. It is resistant to corrosion by oxygen at ordinary temperatures but when heated in air undergoes oxidation.

The chemistry of molybdenum is complex. Like other transition elements, it has a number of oxidation states, from −2 to +6. Only the higher states are of practical significance, with the lower states occurring only in organometal complexes. The most stable oxidation state is Mo(VI). The trioxide, MoO_3, is a white solid that dissolves in alkaline solutions to form molybdates, X_2-MoO_4. These tend to polymerise into polymolybdates in the form $X_6Mo(Mo_6O_{24}).4H_2O$. It seems that in blood and urine, molybdenum exists mainly as the molybdate ion. Numerous complexes of Mo(V) are known, including cyanides, thiocyanates, oxyhalides and a variety of organic chelates. Molybdenum can form alloys with other metals. The chemistry of these, like that of its organic complexes, is extensive and complicated.

8.4 Molybdenum in food and beverages

Molybdenum is found in all foods and beverages, usually at low levels of less than 1 mg/kg. Typical concentrations in a range of foodstuffs are shown in Table 8.1, which is based on data obtained in the UK Total Diet Study. Animal offal and nuts appear to be the only foodstuffs that contain relatively high levels. Mean levels of molybdenum in foods in the US are similar to those in the UK. However, there is a wide variation in levels in individual food samples. Ranges reported in a US survey were: cereals/cereal products 26–1170; meat/fish 4–1290; milk/dairy products 19–99; vegetables 5–332 μg/kg[3].

In certain conditions, such as when soil is either naturally rich in molybdenum or has been contaminated by industrial activity, certain food crops and other plants may accumulate unusually high levels of the metal. In parts of India and Armenia, residents have been reported to have abnormally high intakes of the metal as a result of eating locally produced foods grown on molybdenum-rich soil[4]. Dietary intakes of up to 15 mg/d have been reported in some of these cases[5]. High levels of molybdenum have also been detected in plants grown on soil which has been treated with sewage sludge and certain fertilisers[6].

8.5 Dietary intakes of molybdenum

Except for a few special situations, such as those described above, where foods are contaminated with molybdenum, normal intakes of the metal are low. The average intake in the UK has been reported as 0.12 mg/d, with an upper level of 0.21 mg[7]. Similar levels of daily intake are found in other countries, with 120–240 μg in the US[8], 44–260 μg in Sweden[9] and 120 μg in Finland[10]. These are generally lower than the 250–1000 μg previously reported from some other countries. These higher figures, however, appear to reflect unreliable analytical procedures rather than true intakes.

8.6 Absorption and metabolism of molybdenum

Molybdenum ingested in food is readily absorbed in the gastrointestinal tract. More than 80% is absorbed in the stomach and the remainder in the small intestine. Absorption

Table 8.1 Molybdenum in UK foods.

Food group	Mean concentration (mg/kg fresh weight)
Bread	0.20
Miscellaneous cereals	0.23
Carcass meat	0.01
Offal	1.2
Meat products	0.12
Poultry	0.04
Fish	0.03
Oils and fats	0.02
Eggs	0.08
Sugar and preserves	0.03
Green vegetables	0.15
Potatoes	0.09
Other vegetables	0.06
Canned vegetables	0.31
Fresh fruit	0.01
Fruit products	0.009
Beverages	0.003
Milk	0.03
Dairy products	0.07
Nuts	0.96

Adapted from Ysart, G., Miller, P., Crews, H. *et al.* (1999) Dietary exposure estimates of 30 elements from the UK Total Diet Study. *Food Additives and Contaminants,* **16**, 391–403.

appears to be a passive process, though there is some evidence that, at least in rat intestine, a carrier may be involved. The mechanism of molybdenum absorption and its location within the GI tract have not yet been fully worked out[11].

Retention rates within the body are low, and most of what is absorbed appears to be rapidly excreted in urine. The kidney is probably the primary site of molybdenum homeostatis regulation. The source of the small amount of molybdenum that appears in faeces is not clear but may include bilary excretion[12]. A small amount of the absorbed molybdenum is retained in liver and kidneys. Concentrations in whole blood vary widely, with an average of about 0.5 μg/l. Most of the molybdenum in erythrocytes is loosely bound to protein[13]. It is believed that plasma transport proteins for molybdenum include α-macroglobulin.

Molybdenum is an essential component of several enzymes, including xanthine oxidase and xanthine dehydrogenase, both necessary for the formation of uric acid, as well as of aldehyde oxidase involved in purine metabolism. Sulphite oxidase, which detoxifies sulphite, produced during the metabolism of S-amino acids, is also a molybdenum-dependent enzyme. Sulphite ingested in foods preserved with bisulphite or in sulphur dioxide inhaled accidentally is detoxified by the same mechanism[14].

There is evidence that in all molybdoenzymes, the metal forms part of a complex, the structure of which is not fully known. It is believed to be a small, non-protein complex containing a pterin nucleus. This ‘molybdopterin cofactor’ binds to molybdoproteins within cells[15]. The need of the body to incorporate molybdenum into a complex structure in this way gives potential for genetic abnormalities. An example is a rare lethal inborn error of metabolism that causes a combined deficiency of sulphite oxidase and xanthine oxidase activities. It is characterised by deranged cysteine metabolism and is believed to be due to a lack of the molybdopterin cofactor[16].

A close connection between the metabolism of molybdenum and of both sulphur and copper has been clearly recognised in farm animals affected by teart disease[17]. Sulphur and sulphur compounds are known to limit molybdenum absorption and retention in animals, and these are, in fact, used to treat the condition. Teart disease occurs in cattle in areas of high soil molybdenum and is brought about by ingestion of molybdenum-rich fodder. Molybdenum has been shown to prevent retention of copper in tissues and increase its excretion in urine, leading to copper deficiency[18]. While the interaction between molybdenum and copper in farm animals, especially sheep, is well established, there are still unanswered questions about a similar interaction in humans. It has been reported that a molybdenum intake of over 0.5 mg/d was associated with increased urinary copper excretion in humans[19]. However, results of another study suggest that diets very low in molybdenum do not alter copper metabolism in young men and that dietary molybdenum intake in amounts up to 1490 μg/d do not influence copper metabolism[20].

8.6.1 Molybdenum deficiency

Dietary deficiency of molybdenum has not been found to occur in humans, though it has been produced in experimental animals and is a recognised condition in farm animals under certain conditions. Iatrogenic or acquired molybdenum deficiency has been reported in a patient on prolonged TPN. The condition was characterised by defects in sulphur metabolism, accompanied by mental disturbance and coma. Administration of ammonium molybdate reversed the condition[21]. A relatively small number of cases of human molybdenum cofactor deficiency have been reported. This inborn error of metabolism is normally fatal within a short time of birth. Infants who survive have severe neurological abnormalities and other defects[22].

8.6.2 Molybdenum toxicity

Though molybdenum ingested in foods appears to be relatively non-toxic to humans, there is some evidence that high intakes of between 10 and 15 mg/d may be associated with altered metabolism of nucleotides and reduced copper absorption[23]. A possible connection between consumption of vegetables rich in molybdenum and a high incidence of gout, which may be caused by increased xanthine oxidase activity, has been reported in Armenia[24]. However, the study in which these observations were made has been criticised as inadequate[25], and other investigators have failed to find changes in uric acid levels with increased intakes of molybdenum[26]. An intake in the diet of 1490 μg/d has been shown to cause no toxic symptoms in adult men[27]. In the UK, a Safe Intake of 50–400 μg/d has been recommended[28]. In the US, the ESADDI of 75–250 μg/d was replaced in the 1990 dietary recommendations by a UL of 0.2–0.3 mg/d for children and 0.6–1.0 mg/d for males and females of nine to $>$70 years[29].

8.6.2.1 Toxicity from molybdenum in dietary supplements

Levels of molybdenum in multivitamin and mineral supplements for adults in the US have been found to include as much as 160 μg of molybdenum per tablet[30]. There is a report of acute molybdenum toxicity caused by consumption of a supplement described as 'chelated molybdenum', which contained 100 μg of molybdenum per tablet. After three weeks of consuming one tablet each day, an adult male began to show psychotic and other symptoms which were similar to those of 'manganese madness'. One year after he had ceased to take the supplement, the man still showed some signs of molybdenum toxicity[31].

8.7 Molybdenum requirements

In the absence of adequate data, there are considerable difficulties in trying to estimate dietary requirements for molybdenum[32]. Because molybdenum levels in human tissues are very low and are difficult to measure, there are few reports on plasma or serum concentrations. It is known that plasma levels increase with dietary intake, but these peak and return to basal levels within a few hours after meals. Consequently, plasma concentrations do not reflect molybdenum status[33]. Measurement of urinary levels is also unsuitable for assessing molybdenum needs. Though urinary levels rise with higher amounts in the diet, they do not reflect actual status, since, as intake increases, the percentage of the ingested molybdenum that appears in urine changes[34].

Biomarkers for molybdenum deficiency are decreased urinary levels of sulphate and uric acid, with elevated sulphite, hypoxanthine and xanthine[35]. However, while these changes are indicative of impaired activities of the molybdoenzymes, they are not fully satisfactory for measuring molybdenum status. Though, in the one reported case of human molydbenum deficiency, urinary sulphate was found to be low and sulphite was present[36], similar observations have not been made in normal, healthy people in relation to molybdenum intakes[37].

In the absence of other suitable methods, balance studies have provided the basis on which an average requirement (EAR) has been estimated by US NRC Food and Nutrition Board[38]. Balance studies are of use in establishing whether homeostasis is maintained and whether body stores are being depleted or repleted on different dietary intakes. Findings of two such controlled studies, in which specific amounts of molybdenum were provided to healthy adult males, suggested that an intake of 22 μg/d is near the minimum requirement for the element[39]. When an increment was added to allow for miscellaneous losses and for the possible presence of components that might limit the bioavailability of molybdenum in some diets, an EAR of 34 μg/d was calculated for adults. EARs for other age groups were extrapolated from the adult EARs. The EARs for all age groups except for infants are given in Table 8.2. In the case of the latter groups, AIs are given, in the absence of adequate data to allow RDAs to be estimated.

Though not a great deal is known about molybdenum toxicity in humans, it was believed that there were sufficient data to allow ULs to be estimated, as shown in the table for all age groups, with the exception of infants. These were not determinable because little is known about adverse effects of high molybdenum intakes in the

Table 8.2 US recommendations for molybdenum intake ($\mu g/d$).

Life-stage group	RDA/AI*	UL
Infants		
0–6 months	2*	ND
7–12 months	3*	ND
Children		
1–3 years	**17**	300
4–8 years	**22**	600
Males		
9–13 years	**34**	1000
14–18 years	**43**	1700
19–30 years	**45**	2000
31–50 years	**45**	2000
50–70 years	**45**	2000
>70 years	**45**	2000
Females		
9–13 years	**34**	1100
14–18 years	**43**	1700
19–30 years	**45**	2000
31–50 years	**45**	2000
50–70 years	**45**	2000
>70 years	**45**	2000
Pregnancy		
≤ 18 years	**50**	1700
19–30 years	**50**	2000
31–50 years	**50**	2000
Lactation		
≤ 18 years	**50**	1700
19–30 years	**50**	2000
31–50 years	**50**	2000

RDA: Recommended Dietary Allowances are shown in **bold.** Adequate Intakes (AIs) are shown in ordinary type followed by an asterisk. ND: not determinable due to lack of data on adverse effects in this age group and concern with regard to the lack of ability to handle excess amounts. The source of intake should be from food only to prevent high levels of intake. Adapted from: Food and Nutrition Board National Academy of Sciences (2002) *US Dietary Reference Intakes: Elements.* http://www4.nationalacademies.org/10M/10MHome.nst/pages/Food+and+Nutrition+Board

first years of life and because of concern that infants would be unable to handle such intakes[40].

The UK's Panel on Dietary Reference Values has not yet set an RNI for molybdenum in the belief that normal intakes are sufficient to meet requirements. A safe intake is believed to lie between 50 and 400 $\mu g/d$ for adults and children from one to 18 years of age, and between 0.5 and 1.5 $\mu g/kg/d$ for infants[41].

References

1. Coughlan, M.P. (1983) The role of molybdenum in human biology. *Journal of Inherited Metabolic Diseases,* **6**, S70–7.
2. Rajagopalan, K. (1987) Molybdenum – an essential trace element. *Nutrition Reviews,* **45**, 321–8.
3. Pennington, J.A.T. & Jones, J.W. (1987) Molybdenum, nickel, cobalt, vanadium and strontium in total diets. *Journal of the American Dietetics Association,* **87**, 1644–50.
4. Coughlan, M.P. (1983) The role of molybdenum in human biology. *Journal of Inherited Metabolic Diseases,* **6**, S70–7.
5. Coughlan, M.P. (1983) The role of molybdenum in human biology. *Journal of Inherited Metabolic Diseases,* **6**, S70–7.
6. Horak, O., Wilhartitz, P., Krismer, R. *et al.* (1998) Influence of fertilizer treatment on molybdenum uptake by pasture plants. In: *Trace Elements in Man and Animals – TEMA 8* (eds. M. Anke, D. Meissner & C.F. Mills), pp. 480–1. Verlag Media Touristik, Gersdorf, Germany.
7. Ysart, G., Miller, P., Crews, H. *et al.* (1999) Dietary exposure estimates of 30 elements from the UK Total Diet Study. *Food Additives and Contaminants,* **16**, 391–403.
8. Pennington, J.A.T. & Jones, J.W. (1987) Molybdenum, nickel, cobalt, vanadium and strontium in total diets. *Journal of the American Dietetics Association,* **87**, 1644–50.
9. Mills, C.E. & Davis, G.K. (1986) Molybdenum. In: *Trace Elements in Human and Animal Nutrition* (ed. W. Mertz), pp. 429–61. Academic Press, New York.
10. Varo, P. & Koivistonen, P. (1980) Mineral composition of Finnish foods XII. General discussion and nutritional evaluation. *Acta Agricultura Scandinavica,* **S22**, 165–70.
11. Nielsen, F.H. (1999) Ultratrace minerals. In: *Modern Nutrition in Health and Disease* (eds. M.E. Shils, J.A. Olsen, M. Shike & A.C. Ross), 9th ed., pp. 283–303. Williams & Wilkins, Baltimore, MD.
12. Nielsen, F.H. (1999) Ultratrace minerals. In: *Modern Nutrition in Health and Disease* (eds. M.E. Shils, J.A. Olsen, M. Shike & A.C. Ross), 9th ed., pp. 283–303. Williams & Wilkins, Baltimore, MD.
13. Versieck, J., Hoste, J., Barbier, F. *et al.* (1978) Determination of molybdenum in human serum by neutron activation analysis. *Clinica Chimica Acta,* **87**, 135–40.
14. Failla, M.L. (1999) Considerations for determining 'optimal nutrition' for copper, zinc, manganese and molybdenum. *Proceedings of the Nutrition Society,* **58**, 497–505.
15. Johnson, J.L. (1997) Molybdenum. In: *Handbook of Nutritionally Essential Mineral Elements* (eds. B.L. O'Dell & R.A. Sunde), pp. 413–38. Dekker, New York.
16. Rajagopalan, K.V. (1988) Molybdenum: an essential trace element in human nutrition. *Annual Review of Nutrition,* **8**, 401–27.
17. Williams, C.L., Wilkinson, R.G. & Mackenzie, A.M. (2003) The effect of molybdenum or iron on copper status in growing lambs. *Journal of Nutrition,* **133**, 264E.
18. Poole, D.B.R. (1982) Bovine copper deficiency in Ireland – the clinical disease. *Irish Veterinary Journal,* **36**, 169–73.
19. Deosthale, Y.G. & Gopalan, C. (1974) The effect of molybdenum levels in sorghum (*Sorghum vulgare Pers.*) on uric acid and copper excretion in man. *British Journal of Nutrition,* **31**, 351–5.
20. Turnlund, J.R. & Keyes, W.R. (2000) Dietary molybdenum: effect on copper absorption, excretion, and status in young men. In: *Trace Elements in Man and Animals 10* (eds. A.M. Roussel, R.A. Anderson & A.E. Favier), pp. 951–3. Kluwer/Plenum, New York.

21. Chiang, G., Swenseid, M.E. & Turnlund, J. (1989) Studies of biochemical markers indicating molybdenum status in humans. *Federation of American Societies of Experimental Biology,* **3**, Abstract No. 4922.
22. Johmnson, J.L., Rajagopalan, K.V. & Wadman, S.K. (1993) Human molybdenum cofactor deficiency. In: *Chemistry and Biology of Pteridines and Folates* (eds. J.E. Ayling, G.M. Nair & C.M. Baugh), pp. 373–8. Plenum, New York.
23. Department of Health (1991) *Dietary Reference Values for Food Energy and Nutrients in the United Kingdom. Report of the Panel on Dietary Reference Values of the Committee on Medical Aspects of Food Policy, Report on Health and Social Studies,* **41**, p. 178. HMSO, London.
24. Yarovaya, G.A. (1964) Molybdenum in the diet in Armenia. *Proceedings of the Sixth International Biochemical Congress, New York, Abstracts,* **6**, 440.
25. Food and Nutrition Board National Academy of Sciences (2002) *Dietary Reference Intakes: Elements.* pp. 434–5. http://www4.nationalacademies.org/10M/10Mhome.nsf/pages/Food+and+Nutrition+Board
26. Deostale, Y.G. & Gopalan, C. (1974) The effect of molybdenum levels in sorghum (*Sorgham vulgare* Pers.) on uric acid and copper excretion in man. *British Journal of Nutrition,* **31**, 351–5.
27. Failla, M.L. (1999) Considerations for determining 'optimal nutrition' for copper, zinc, manganese and molybdenum. *Proceedings of the Nutrition Society,* **58**, 497–505.
28. Department of Health (1991) *Dietary Reference Values for Food Energy and Nutrients in the United Kingdom. Report of the Panel on Dietary Reference Values of the Committee on Medical Aspects of Food Policy, Report on Health and Social Studies,* **41**, p. 178. HMSO, London.
29. Food and Nutrition Board National Academy of Sciences (2002) *Dietary Reference Intakes: Elements.* http://www4.nationalacademies.org/10M/10Mhome.nsf/pages/Food+and+Nutrition+Board
30. Failla, M.L. (1999) Considerations for determining 'optimal nutrition' for copper, zinc, manganese and molybdenum. *Proceedings of the Nutrition Society,* **58**, 497–505.
31. Momčilovič, B. (2000) Acute human molybdenum toxicity from a dietary supplement – a new member of the 'LucorMetallicum' family. In: *Trace Elements in Man and Animals 10* (eds. A.M. Roussel, R.A. Anderson & A.E. Favier), pp. 699–70. Kluwer/Plenum, New York.
32. Versieck, J., Hoste, J., Barbier, F. *et al.* (1978) Determination of molybdenum in human serum by neutron activation analysis. *Clinica Chimica Acta,* **87**, 135–40.
33. Cantone, M.C., de Bartolo, D., Gambarini, A. *et al.* (1995) Proton activation analysis of stable isotopes for a molybdenum biokinetics study in humans. *Medical Physics,* **22**, 1293–8.
34. Turnlund, J.R., Keyes, W.R., Pfeiffer, G.I. & Chiang, G. (1995) Molybdenum absorption, excretion, and retention studied with stable isotopes in young men during depletion and repletion. *American Journal of Clinical Nutrition,* **61**, 1102–9.
35. Hambidge, M. (2003) Biomarkers of trace mineral intake and status. *Journal of Nutrition,* **133**, 948S–55S.
36. Abumrad, N.N., Schneider, A.J., Steel, D. & Rogers, L.S. (1981) Amino acid intolerance during prolonged total parenteral nutrition reversed by molybdate therapy. *American Journal of Clinical Nutrition,* **34**, 2551–9.
37. Johnson, J.L., Rajagopalan, K.V. & Wadman, S.K. (1993) Human molybdenum cofactor deficiency. In: *Chemistry and Biology of Pteridines and Folates* (eds. J.E. Ayling, G.M. Nair & C.M. Baugh), pp. 373–8. Plenum, New York.
38. Olin, S.S. (1998) Between a rock and a hard place: methods for setting dietary allowances and exposure limits for essential minerals. *Journal of Nutrition,* **128**, 364S–7S.
39. Turnlund, J.R., Keyes, W.R., Pfeiffer, G.I. & Chiang, G. (1995) Molybdenum absorption, excretion, and retention studied with stable isotopes in young men during depletion and repletion. *American Journal of Clinical Nutrition,* **61**, 1102–9.

40. Food and Nutrition Board National Academy of Sciences (2002) *Dietary Reference Intakes: Elements.* http://www4.nationalacademies.org/10M/10Mhome.nst/pages/Food+and+Nutrition+Board
41. Department of Health (1991) *Dietary Reference Values for Food Energy and Nutrients in the United Kingdom. Report of the Panel on Dietary Reference Values of the Committee on Medical Aspects of Food Policy, Report on Health and Social Studies,* **41**, p. 178. HMSO, London.

Chapter 9
Nickel, boron, vanadium, cobalt and other trace metal nutrients

9.1 Introduction

Besides the seven trace metals of nutritional interest discussed in earlier chapters, and for which there is evidence of their essentiality and sufficient data to allow dietary reference values to be estimated, there are several others which are clearly of biological importance but whose essentiality is still a matter of controversy. These include three, nickel, boron and vanadium, that can be shown to have a variety of unique metabolic roles in living organisms, as well as cobalt which, unlike other metal trace nutrients, appears to be required by the human body, not as a metal in its own right, but as a component of vitamin B_{12}, cyanocobalamin.

9.2 Nickel

To the seventeenth-century miners of the Ore Mountains of Central Europe, nickel was a problem. They were looking for copper, but often found, mixed up with the copper ore, another mineral that made extraction of the metal very difficult. They called this unwanted intruder kupfer-nickel, 'Old Nick's copper', after a local bad earth spirit that plagued their workings[1]. The nickel had a refractory nature that made it difficult to extract by smelting. Modern metallurgists have long overcome the problems of extracting and using nickel industrially, but for human biologists, nickel remains a problem. Though there are numerous findings indicating that the metal is an essential nutrient for experimental animals, evidence that it is also essential for humans remains controversial. No clearly defined biochemical function has as yet been determined for the metal, nor has nickel deficiency been observed in humans. Nevertheless, there are many indications that it is only a matter of time before its essentiality for humans is established[2].

9.2.1 Chemical and physical properties of nickel

Nickel was isolated by the Swedish chemist Cronstedt in 1751, who named it after the kupernickel ore from which he obtained it. It is the 22nd most abundant element, and the seventh most abundant transition metal, number 28 in the periodic table, with an atomic weight of 58.71. It is a tough, silvery white, heavy metal. It has good thermal as well as electrical conductivity and is highly resistant to attack by air and water. Nickel forms numerous alloys with other metals. Its alloy with iron, nickel steel, is extremely tough and corrosion-resistant.

The chemistry of nickel is relatively complex. Like other transition metals, it has several oxidation states, including Ni(0), Ni(I) and Ni(II), with the divalent form being the most commonly encountered. Ni(II) forms a number of binary compounds with various non-metals, such as carbon and phosphorus. It is able to bind to many organic compounds of biological interest, including proteins and amino acids. Nickel forms an extensive series of inorganic compounds, many of which are green in colour and soluble in water.

More than two-thirds of nickel produced worldwide is used for the manufacture of 'stainless steel'[3]. This is widely used in the manufacture of food-processing equipment and containers, including 'tin cans'. Nickel compounds are important to the chemical and food industry, for example as catalysts in the hydrogenation of unsaturated fats, for use in the manufacture of margarine[4].

9.2.2 Nickel in food and beverages

Nickel is widely distributed in the environment and occurs in most soils, usually at levels between 0.5 and 3.5 mg/kg[5]. Levels in foods are low, at less than 0.2 mg/kg, as can be seen in Table 9.1. There are some exceptions, such as the tea plant, *Camillia sinensis*, which has the ability to accumulate the metal to a high level. Dried tea leaves used for beverage making, have been found to contain 3.9–8.2 mg/kg, and instant tea 14–17 mg/kg.[6] Certain culinary herbs also contain relatively high levels. The cacao bean, from which cocoa and chocolate are made, may contain up to 10 mg/kg. As a consequence, chocolate-containing confectionery can be a useful source of dietary nickel. Nuts can also contain appreciable amounts[7].

Higher than normal levels of nickel are sometimes found in processed foods. This is adventitious nickel, picked up from the stainless steel used in the manufacture of equipment and containers. Cooking in stainless steel utensils may increase the nickel content of acidic food[8]. A study carried out in The Netherlands found that appreciable amounts of nickel migrate into milk and other dairy products from stainless steel containers as a result of contact with acidic dairy products and acid cleaning agents used on dairy equipment[9].

9.2.3 Dietary intake of nickel

Normal intake of nickel in foods and beverages is very low. The mean total daily adult exposure to nickel in the UK diet has been reported to be 0.12 mg, with a maximum of 0.21 mg[10]. Results reported in other countries are similar, with 0.13 mg in Finland[11], and 0.17 mg in the US[12]. A Canadian study found that intakes had a range of 0.207–0.406 mg in adults, and 0.19–0.251 mg in infants[13]. It has been estimated that nickel intakes in Denmark could reach over 900 $\mu g/d$ because of high intakes of oatmeal, legumes, including soybeans, nuts, cocoa and chocolate[14].

9.2.3.1 Intake of nickel from dietary supplements

It has been reported that the median intake of nickel as dietary supplements by adults in the US is approximately 5 $\mu g/d$[15].

Table 9.1 Nickel in UK foods.

Food group	Mean concentration (mg/kg fresh weight)
Bread	0.10
Miscellaneous cereals	0.17
Carcass meat	0.04
Offal	0.06
Meat products	0.06
Poultry	0.04
Fish	0.08
Oils and fats	0.03
Eggs	0.03
Sugar and preserves	0.28
Green vegetables	0.11
Potatoes	0.10
Other vegetables	0.09
Canned vegetables	0.25
Fresh fruit	0.03
Fruit products	0.06
Beverages	0.03
Milk	< 0.02
Dairy products	0.02
Nuts	2.5

Adapted from Ysart, G., Miller, P., Crews, H. *et al.* (1999) Dietary exposure estimates of 30 elements from the UK Total Diet Study. *Food Additives and Contaminants,* **16**, 391–403.

9.2.4 Absorption and metabolism of nickel

There are many gaps in our knowledge of how the body handles dietary nickel. Nickel in food is poorly absorbed. Absorption can be affected by several other components of the diet, including milk, coffee, tea, orange juice and ascorbic acid[16]. Retention by the body is also low, between 3 and 6% of what is absorbed. Absorption appears to be enhanced by iron deficiency. In the blood, nickel is transported mainly bound to albumin. It seems to be fairly evenly distributed between tissues and not accumulated in any particular organ. Most organs contain less than 50 μg/kg dry weight, though the thyroid and the adrenal glands have relatively high concentrations of about 140 μg/kg dry weight[17]. Excretion is mainly in urine, with small amounts in faeces[18].

Nickel has been recognised as an essential nutrient for farm and experimental animals for some years. Its essentiality for humans is still a matter of controversy[19]. No clear biochemical function for the element has as yet been identified in humans, though there is evidence that it serves as a cofactor or structural component of several metalloenzymes similar to certain nickel-containing enzymes that have been identified in plants and micro-organisms[20]. These include urease, hydrogenase and carbon monoxide dehydrogenase. Other enzymes, including carboxylase, trypsin and coenzyme A, are activated by nickel.

Signs of nickel deficiency have not been reported in humans, though they are well recognised in other animal species. Rats deprived of nickel show depressed growth, reduced reproduction and alterations of serum lipid and glucose levels[21]. It has been suggested that because the nickel content of some human diets can be lower than the intakes that can induce such changes in animals, the metal should be considered a possibly limiting nutrient under specific human conditions[22]. It has been surmised that its essentiality may be due to the fact that nickel can interact with the vitamin B_{12}/folic acid-dependent pathway of methionine synthesis from homocysteine[23].

9.2.5 Dietary requirements for nickel

Because of the absence at the time of their deliberations (in the late 1990s) of reports of studies to determine the biological role of nickel in higher animals or humans, the US National Academy of Sciences Expert Panel on Dietary Reference Intakes decided not to establish an EAR, RDA or AI for nickel[24].

9.3 Boron

In the report on dietary reference values published by the UK Ministry of Health in 1991, the element boron received only 12 lines out of a total of more than 200 pages of text. The two final sentences of those few lines read: 'the role of B in humans is unknown and the essentiality of B remains to be demonstrated. There do not appear to be any published studies relating to the question of B toxicity'[25]. The US counterpart of the British expert panel on DRVs noted in its 2002 report that in recent years, boron has been the subject of most extensive study of its possible nutritional importance for animals and humans: 'Still, the collective body of evidence has yet to establish a clear biological function for boron in humans'[26]. These views are challenged by a number of experts who believe that there is strong evidence that boron is indeed an essential nutrient for humans, with a unique metabolic role[27].

9.3.1 Chemical and physical properties of boron

Boron-containing compounds have been known for many hundreds of years and were referred to in alchemical works as 'borax'. The element was first isolated in the early nineteenth century. It is widely distributed in low concentrations throughout the lithosphere, in a variety of combinations with oxygen. It is commercially produced from a number of ores which occur in volcanic regions and in dry lake beds.

Boron is element number 5 in the periodic table, with an atomic weight of 10.8. It is a metalloid, with predominantly non-metallic properties. It exists in two forms, as an amorphous dark brown powder, and as yellow crystals. Crystalline boron is transparent and nearly as hard as diamonds. Its electrical resistance is remarkable, in that at room temperature it is about two million times greater than at red heat. The chemical properties of boron are similar to those of silicon. It forms compounds with oxygen, hydrogen, halogens, nitrogen, phosphorus and carbon. Boron burns in oxygen to form boric oxide, B_2O_3. This dissolves in water, producing orthoboric acid, H_3BO_3. When orthoboric acid is heated in the absence of water, it is converted first into metaboric acid, HBO_2, then into tetraboric acid, $H_2B_4O_7$, and finally the oxide, B_2O_3.

9.3.2 *Uses of boron*

Among the industrially important compounds of boron are sodium tetraborate decahydrate, $Na_2B_4O_7.10H_2O$, commonly known as borax, and boron nitride, BN. This is a crystalline substance analogous to graphite, known as 'inorganic graphite'. It is extremely hard and is used as a substitute for diamonds in cutting and abrading tools. Boron also forms complexes with a variety of organic molecules of biological importance, including carbohydrates, ATP, vitamin C and steroids[28].

Boron has a number of industrial uses, in metallurgy, pigments and glazes, and, in recent decades, in the nuclear industry for manufacturing shielding and control rods for nuclear reactors[29]. Borax and boric acid have a long history of medicinal use, as antiseptics. Boron compounds were once widely used to extend the palatability as well as to preserve food[30]. In recent years, this use has been discouraged, if not totally banned, in many countries following recognition of the potentially toxic effects of boron compounds. Boron compounds continue to be widely used in various domestic products, such as washing powders and cosmetics.

9.3.3 *Boron in food and beverages*

Boron, because of its wide distribution in the environment, in part resulting from its use in many domestic products, is a normal component of the diet in significant amounts. It occurs in all food groups, as shown in Table 9.2. It occurs in highest concentrations in plant foods, especially vegetables and fruit, and lowest in animal products. Levels in foods in the UK are similar to those in the US. Particularly good sources are peanuts (17 mg/kg), peanut butter (14.5 mg/kg) and raisins (22 mg/kg)[31]. Concentrations in beverages range from 6.1 mg/kg in dry table wine to 1.8 mg/kg in apple juice and milk, 0.29 mg/kg in coffee, 0.13 mg/kg in cola drinks, 0.12 mg/kg in beer and 0.09 mg/kg in brewed tea. The median level of boron in US drinking water is 0.031 mg/l, with an upper range of 2.44 mg/l[32].

9.3.3.1 *Dietary intake of boron*

The mean adult intake of boron in the UK has been estimated to be 1.4 mg/d, with an upper range of 2.6 mg/d[33]. Intake in the US appears to be similar, averaging 1.5 mg/d[34]. Because of the volumes consumed, coffee and milk are the major contributors to boron intake in the US[35]. A recent study of boron intakes in six countries found a range of 0.43–3.45 mg/d for adult males, with the highest levels of intake in Germany and Mexico[36].

9.3.3.2 *Boron intakes by vegetarians*

Because of the relatively high levels of boron found in plant foods compared with animal products, vegetarians might be expected to have a higher than average intake. One estimate, based on a vegetarian diet, was as high as 20 mg/d[37]. However, a US study found intakes by adult vegetarians of 1.47 ± 0.70 for males and 1.29 ± 1.12 mg/d for females. Such unexpectedly low intakes may be accounted for by the fact that though vegetarians consume more boron-rich foods, their diet also includes more low-boron grain products than that of non-vegetarians[38].

Table 9.2 Boron in UK foods.

Food group	Mean concentration (μg/kg fresh weight)
Bread	0.5
Miscellaneous cereals	0.9
Carcass meat	< 0.4
Offal	< 0.4
Meat products	0.4
Poultry	< 0.4
Fish	0.5
Oils and fats	0.4
Eggs	< 0.4
Sugar and preserves	0.8
Green vegetables	2.0
Potatoes	1.4
Other vegetables	1.4
Canned vegetables	1.2
Fresh fruit	3.4
Fruit products	2.4
Beverages	0.4
Milk	< 0.4
Dairy products	0.4
Nuts	14

Adapted from Ysart, G., Miller, P., Crews, H. *et al.* (1999) Dietary exposure estimates of 30 elements from the UK Total Diet Study. *Food Additives and Contaminants,* **16**, 391–403.

9.3.3.3 Boron intakes from supplements

Boron does not appear to be widely consumed in supplemental form. The intake of boron by adults in the US has been reported to be approximately 0.14 mg/d.[39] In many of these supplements, the boron is chelated with amino acids. Inorganic boron, as sodium borate, has been used as a supplement for experimental animals[40].

9.3.4 Absorption and metabolism of boron

Studies with animals have indicated that ingested boron is rapidly taken up from the GI tract, with possibly more than 90% absorbed[41]. Most of the boron ingested appears to be hydrolysed in the gut to form $B(OH)_3$ which is easily absorbed, probably by a passive process[42]. The absorbed boron appears to be rapidly transported throughout the body. It is probably transported in blood as free boric acid, rather than as a complex. The boron is not metabolised, and most is rapidly excreted in urine. A small amount may be retained in body tissues, such as bone and spleen[43]. There is some evidence that boron is subject to some homeostatic control in the body, but this has been disputed[44]. It has been found that, in animals, blood levels are dependent on dietary intake, reflecting the very small boron pool that blood represents, as well as efficient absorption and excretion[45].

9.3.5 Boron: an essential nutrient?

Whether or not boron is an essential trace nutrient for humans remains a matter of debate. It has long been recognised that it is essential for plants, and there is growing consensus among scientists that it is of considerable nutritional significance for animals, including humans[46]. Because of its chemistry, boron can, theoretically at least, form complexes with biologically important organic molecules. Such complexes could give stability to various organic molecules of biological importance, such as carbohydrates and steroids. In plants, for example, the very complex polysaccharide rhamnogalacturonan II forms dimers through boron and is essential for plant growth. It has been suggested that the formation of similar cross-links with carbohydrates of cell surfaces may be an important function of boron in eukaryotes[47]. Boron has been shown to play a part in wound healing, possibly by promoting intracellular protease activity, particularly collagenase[48]. It also, apparently, potentiates synthesis of what is known as hsp 70 (heat shock protein 70), which protects cells against stress[49].

There is some evidence that boron may also play a regulatory role in enzymes, though no boron-containing enzyme has been identified[50]. Observations made on a variety of animals have indicated a number of activities that appear to be boron-dependent, but no sufficiently definitive pattern of effects has been shown to establish a definite biological function for the element. Defects in embryonic development of certain types of fish deprived of boron suggest that it may have a role in reproduction and development[51]. There is good experimental evidence that boron deprivation affects the composition or function of several components of the animal body, including the skeleton and brain. In boron-deficient poultry, changes in blood glucose and triglyceride concentrations have been observed. Several studies have found evidence pointing to a connection between calcium and bone metabolism[52]. However, many of these effects have only been observed in the presence of secondary nutritional stressors, such as vitamin D deficiency. Boron appears to affect calcium and magnesium positively and may be necessary for energy substrate use and membrane function[53].

A number of clinical studies have indicated that boron deficiency can occur in humans and may be of significance in relation to the development of osteoporosis in postmenopausal women. It has been shown that women who supplemented their diet with boron excreted less calcium, magnesium and phosphorus than they did before taking the supplement[54]. A connection between boron and mental function has also been suggested. Boron deprivation has been shown to adversely affect hand–eye coordination, attention, and short-term memory in humans[55]. A possible role of boron in immunity has also been suggested. Boron is believed to act by regulating the normal inflammatory process by modulating the response of key immune cells to antigens[56]. Connections between low dietary boron levels and a number of other conditions, including arthritis, prostate cancer and heart disease, have also been postulated, particularly in the popular health literature[57].

9.3.6 An acceptable daily intake for boron

There are no official recommendations or dietary reference values for boron. Nevertheless, since boron supplements are available and are consumed, especially by women who believe the element will prevent development of osteoporosis, there may be a need for some guidance on safe intakes. Since there is no evidence of boron deficiency in humans who consume a normal diet, an intake of about 1 mg/d, in line with current reported intakes in several countries, would appear to meet the needs of most healthy individuals[58]. Boron in food has, in fact, a low toxicity, most probably because almost all that is ingested is rapidly excreted. It is only when the body's controls are overwhelmed by high doses, as has been seen in a few cases of accidental poisonings, that acute toxicity occurs. Thus, a modest increase in intake is unlikely to pose any risk to health. An ADI of 0.3 mg/kg body weight/d, equivalent to about 20 mg/d for a 70-kg man, has been proposed by the US FDA on the basis of a NOAEL of 9.6 mg/kg body weight/d. The minimum lethal dose for humans is not known, though consumption of 18 g has caused the death of a male adult[59].

9.4 Vanadium

Interest in the biological effects of vanadium has grown substantially since claims were made in the 1970s that it was an essential trace element for humans[60]. In recent years, vanadium has been the subject of several books and conference proceedings, and though as yet, a functional role for it has not been identified in humans, and its essentiality remains to be proved beyond doubt, it is becoming widely accepted that the metal has important and unique roles to play in human metabolism[61].

9.4.1 Chemical and physical properties of vanadium

Vanadium is element number 23 in the periodic table, with an atomic number of 50.9. It is a relatively light metal (density 6.1), steel grey in colour, tough and corrosion-resistant. Its chemistry is complex[62]. It has a number of oxidation states, from −1 to +5, though the most common valence states are +3, + 4 and +5. The tetravalent vanadyl form (VO^{2+}) and the pentavalent vanadate ($VO_4{}^{3-}$) are the predominant forms in biological systems. Vanadium is capable of undergoing oxidation–reduction exchanges, and this suggests that at least some of its known biological activities may involve cellular redox activity[63].

9.4.2 Production and uses of vanadium

Vanadium occurs widely in the environment, though not in metallic form. In most soils, it is present at levels of about 0.1 mg/kg. It has several different ores, all of which are mixed. An important source is crude oil and fly ash from power stations. The principal use of vanadium is in alloys with other metals. The presence of even small amounts gives strength, toughness and heat resistance to steel, which is suitable for making high speed machinery and tools. Pure vanadium metal and its compounds have numerous industrial applications, as catalysts in the production of ammonia, polymers and rubber, and in ceramics, glass, paint and photography.

9.4.3 Vanadium in food and beverages

Little information is available on normal levels of vanadium in foods and diets. They are, apparently, generally low, between 1 and 30 $\mu g/kg$[64]. Levels reported in a limited number of different food groups consumed in the US are shown in Table 9.3. Among the richest food sources are skim milk, lobster, mushrooms, vegetable oils, certain types of vegetable and various cereals. Fruit, meat, fish, butter, cheese and beverages are relatively poor sources[65]. Some foods have higher levels, with, for example, up to 40 mg/kg reported in certain vegetable oils[66]. Processed foods have been reported to contain more vanadium than unprocessed foods[67].

9.4.3.1 *Dietary intakes of vanadium*

Daily intakes of vanadium from the diet of adults have been estimated in a number of countries to range from about 10 μg to 2 mg, with an intake of 13 μg in the UK[68], and 10–60 μg in the US[69]. Levels of up to 230 μg/d have been reported in adults in Japan[70]. Intakes by infants, children and adolescents in the US range from 6.5 to 11 μg/d. In the US, grains and grain products contribute between 13 and 30% of the adult intake, with beverages, at least in the case of older men, contributing between 26 and 57% of this intake[71]. Beer is a particularly good source. A German study found that daily intake by men , at 33 $\pm$ 35 μg, was about twice that of women, at 14 $\pm$ 11 μg, and was due to 28 μg provided by beer[72].

9.4.3.2 *Intake of vanadium from dietary supplements*

The median intake of vanadium as dietary supplements in the US has been estimated to be 9 μg/d[73]. Intakes by certain individuals can be much higher[74]. Various vanadium compounds are commonly used by some athletes in the belief that vanadium can increase muscle mass and enhance physical ability. Though the evidence for this is not strong, some athletes are known to consume as much as 60 mg/d of vanadyl sulphate. Vanadyl sulphate, as well as sodium metavanadate, at intakes of up to 125 mg/d, have been used as a supplement for diabetic patients[75]. Such high intakes, which can result in gastrointestinal distress, are required because of the very low absorption and tissue uptake of inorganic vanadyl and vanadate compounds. A number of oxovanadate complexes with a higher solubility have been investigated and show promise of improved uptake and tissue retention[76].

Table 9.3 Vanadium in US foods.

Food group	Mean (μg/kg fresh weight)	Range
Cereals/cereal products	23	0–150
Meat/fish	10	0–120
Vegetables	6	0–72
Milk	1	0–6

Based on data from Pennington, J.A.T. & Jones, J.W. (1987) Molybdenum, nickel, cobalt, vanadium and strontium in total diets. *Journal of the American Dietetics Association*, **87**, 1644–50.

9.4.4 Absorption and metabolism of vanadium

The absorption of ingested vanadium in the GI tract is poor, with as little as 2% believed to enter the bloodstream. Daily absorption by an adult is estimated to be between 5 and 10 μg[77]. Absorbed vanadium appears to be converted into the vanadyl cation, which can complex with ferritin and transferrin in plasma[78]. Vanadium is found at extremely low levels in biological tissues, including blood, though there does seem to be some accumulation in liver, kidney and bone[79]. Excretion of accumulated vanadium is rapid and occurs through the kidneys.

There is growing evidence that vanadium is an essential nutrient for animals, possibly including humans[80]. It has been shown in experimental animals to be able to mimic the action of insulin and diminish hyperglycaemia by increasing glucose transport activity and improving glucose metabolism.[81]. Vanadium deficiency has been found to be associated with stunted growth, impaired reproduction, altered red blood cell formation and iron metabolism, changes in blood lipid levels and hard tissue formation. It has also been found that vanadium can alter the activity of a number of enzymes, including Na–K-ATPases involved in muscle contraction, and thus may regulate the sodium pump by means of a redox mechanism[82]. It also appears to have a role in relation to serine/threonine kinases, phosphatases and receptors for insulin.[83] Whether these effects occur also in humans has not been established.

9.4.5 Vanadium toxicity

Vanadium in food has, apparently, a low level of toxicity. Entry into the body by other routes, however, can cause serious consequences. Pentavalent vanadium is the most toxic, and the toxicity of vanadium compounds usually increases with the valency. Most of the effects result from local irritation of the eyes and upper respiratory tract rather than systemic toxicity. There can also be other undesirable effects, including neurotoxic and hepatotoxic damage[84].

9.4.6 Vanadium requirements

In the absence of identification of a clear biological role in humans, an EAR, RDI and AI are yet to be established for vanadium in the US. For similar reasons, there is no vanadium RNI in the UK. An absolute requirement is believed to be 1–2 μg/d.

9.5 Cobalt

Cobalt is one of the most fascinating of the biological trace elements, with several unusual facets. Its name was derived from the German word for goblin, and was coined by the medieval miners of the Ore Mountains of Thuringia and Saxony. Just as they did with nickel, they looked on cobalt as a useless and evil metal, because its presence in mixed ores prevented the extraction of other metals; they named it after 'Kobold', the evil earth spirit[85].

Cobalt is a relatively rare element, making up about only 0.001% of the lithosphere. It occurs in animals, including man, in minute amounts. Daily intake is not much more than 0.1 μg, yet it is an essential trace element. It is an integral part of vitamin B_{12}, or cobalamin, of which the body contains not much more than 5 mg. However, if there is less than this, pernicious anaemia can develop. Its role in vitamin B_{12} appears to be cobalt's main, if not sole, function in animals. Intake to meet nutritional requirements must be as part of the preformed vitamin – the metal itself will not suffice. Indeed, in more than minute amounts, cobalt itself can be toxic.

9.5.1 Chemical and physical properties of cobalt

Cobalt was first isolated in 1739 by Georg Brandt, another of the great Swedish chemists of the eighteenth century. It is element number 27 in the periodic table, with an atomic weight of 58.9. It is a hard, brittle, bluish-white metal, with magnetic properties similar to those of iron. The metal is fairly unreactive and dissolves only slowly in dilute acids. Like other transition metals, it has several oxidation states, but only states 2 and 3 are of practical significance. Co(II) forms a series of simple and hydrated cobaltous salts with all common anions. Few cobaltic, Co(III), salts are known, since oxidation state 3 is relatively unstable. However, numerous stable complexes of both the cobaltous and the cobaltic forms are known.

9.5.2 Production and uses of cobalt

Cobalt occurs in the earth's crust in association with other elements, especially arsenic. However, its chief commercial source is the residue left after electrolytic refining of nickel, copper and lead. World demand for cobalt has been increasing rapidly in recent decades, due to its increasing use in chemical applications (primarily in portable rechargeable batteries)[86].

The principal use of cobalt is for the production of high-strength 'superalloys'. The addition of cobalt to steel results in greater hardness and alters its magnetic properties. Combined with aluminium and nickel, it produces an alloy used to make strong permanent magnets for radios and electronic devices. When alloyed with chromium and tungsten, it is used to make hard-edged metal cutting and surgical instruments. Cobalt is also used in glass and pottery. The artificially produced isotope, Cobalt-60 (^{60}Co), is used as a source of γ-rays in radiotherapy and as a medical tracer.

9.5.3 Cobalt in food and beverages

Information on levels of cobalt in foods and diets is not plentiful. Data from the UK indicate that levels in most foods are very low, at < 0.1 mg/kg, as can be seen in Table 9.4. The highest levels are found in offal meat and nuts. It has been reported that another good source of cobalt is yeast extract, sold under such brand names as Marmite (in the UK) and Vegemite (in Australia). Surprisingly, though generally dairy products are low in cobalt, an Italian study found that the concentration range in cheese was 1.6–32 μg/kg.

Table 9.4 Cobalt in UK foods.

Food group	Mean concentration (μg/kg fresh weight)
Bread	0.02
Miscellaneous cereals	0.01
Carcass meat	0.004
Offal	0.06
Meat products	0.008
Poultry	0.003
Fish	0.01
Oils and fats	0.003
Eggs	0.002
Sugar and preserves	0.03
Green vegetables	0.009
Potatoes	0.02
Other vegetables	0.006
Canned vegetables	0.01
Fresh fruit	0.004
Fruit products	0.005
Beverages	0.002
Milk	0.002
Dairy products	0.004
Nuts	0.09

Adapted from Ysart, G., Miller, P., Crews, H. *et al.* (1999) Dietary exposure estimates of 30 elements from the UK Total Diet Study. *Food Additives and Contaminants,* **16**, 391–403.

The average daily intake in the UK is about 0.3 mg. This is about the same as the estimated daily intakes in the US (150–600 μg)[87] but considerably higher than that reported in Finland (13 μg)[88] and Belgium (26 μg)[89].

The use of cobalt-containing food additives has been known to increase dietary levels considerably. Formerly, cobalt salts were sometimes added to beer to improve its foaming qualities[90]. The practice is no longer permitted because of fears that an excessive intake of cobalt was responsible for an epidemic of cardiac failure in certain groups of heavy drinkers, some of whom were ingesting the equivalent of 8 mg of cobalt sulphate each day. An investigation concluded that the cobalt alone was not responsible for the epidemic and that two other factors, a high alcohol intake and a dietary deficiency of protein and/or thiamin, played a part in the incident[91]. The use of cobaltous salts as an additive in human foods has been banned by the USFDA.

9.5.4 Absorption and metabolism of cobalt

Reports by different investigators on levels of absorption of cobalt from the diet present a confusing picture, with estimates ranging from 5 to 45%[92]. The variation may, in fact, be due to nutritional and other factors that affect levels of absorption, such as the iron status of the body[93] and the chemical form of the element in the diet[94]. The human body contains little more than 1 mg of cobalt, with about a fifth of this stored in the liver.[95] Excretion is mainly in urine.

No functions of cobalt in human nutrition, other than as an integral part of vitamin B_{12}, have been clearly established. This is a large, complicated molecule in which a single atom of cobalt sits at the centre of a porphyrin-like corrin ring. Neither animals, including humans, nor higher plants are able to synthesise cobalamin, and it has to be obtained as the preformed vitamin in food. It is made by bacteria, particularly soil bacteria, that have the ability to incorporate cobalt into the corrin ring structure. The vitamin plays an important role, especially in cells where active division is taking place, such as in blood-forming tissues of bone marrow. Deficiency is responsible for the development of pernicious anaemia when abnormal cells known as megaloblasts develop. This leads to potentially fatal macrocytic anaemia. In addition, the nervous system is also seriously affected.

There are some indications that cobalt is also necessary for the synthesis of thyroid hormone, according to a report that noted an inverse relationship between cobalt levels in food, water and soil in some areas with the level of incidence of goitre in animals and humans[96]. It has recently been claimed that cobalt, rather than chromium, is the metal in GTF, the Glucose Tolerance Factor[97].

9.5.5 Dietary intake recommendations for cobalt

There are no recommended intakes for cobalt itself, but only for the cobalt-containing vitamin B_{12}, cobalamin. The UK adult RNI for vitamin B_{12} is 1.5 μg/d, which is equivalent to about 0.06 μg of cobalt.

9.5.5.1 Safe intakes of cobalt

There is no evidence that cobalt ingestion, at least at the levels normally found in the diet, has any toxic effects. Health authorities have not felt it necessary to set statutory or guideline limits for cobalt in food. However, there is a need for caution when high levels of cobalt are ingested during some medical procedures. When cobalt salts have been used as a non-specific bone marrow stimulus in the treatment of certain refractory anaemias, doses of 29.5 mg/d produced serious toxic effects, including goitre, hypothyroidism and heart failure[98]. There can also be problems with high levels of cobalt in some dietary supplements and health foods. In the UK, a Working Party on Dietary Supplements and Health Foods of MAFF warned that cobalt could have undesirable effects above a chronic dose of 300 mg/d[99].

9.6 Other possibly essential trace metals and metalloids

It is believed by a number of experienced investigators that several other metals and metalloids will be shown to be nutritionally essential for humans. This is because, though none of these elements currently satisfy all the usually accepted criteria for defining essentiality, they do satisfy a number of them. Moreover, it has been shown in several cases that if animals are deprived of one or other of these elements, they can develop recognisable symptoms of deficiency. However, none of these potentially essential elements have yet been shown to have a clearly identified and specific metabolic function in humans. Consequently, most nutritionists, and not least expert nutrition panels, are unwilling to accept their essentiality or assign them an RDA or other dietary reference value.

9.6.1 Silicon

Silicon, element number 14 in the periodic table, with an atomic weight of 28, is second only to oxygen in abundance in the world. It makes up almost a quarter of the earth's crust, which is largely composed of silicon compounds, especially its binary compounds with oxygen, the silicates. Silicon is present in every type of food and beverage, and is a normal and significant component of all diets. Estimates of dietary intakes of silicon vary widely. While one study has reported that the UK diet provides 1.2 g/d[100], and intakes of up to 129 mg/d have been recorded in some countries[101], the median intake by US adults in 1991 was reported to be 14–21 mg/d[102]. Higher intakes of up to 46 mg/d have been recorded by those who consume high-fibre diets[103].

The major sources of silicon in human diets are plant-based foods, which are richer in the element than are animal-based products. Results of the USFDA total diet study show that beverages, including beer, coffee and water contribute 55% of the US adult silicon intake, followed by grains and grain products (14%), and vegetables (8%). While refining reduces the silicon content of some foods, especially cereals, the use of silicon-containing additives such as antifoaming and anticaking agents, can increase it. However, the bioavailability of these additives is low. Much of the silicon in foods is in the form of silica, SiO_2, which remains unabsorbed after ingestion. A small amount, however, is in the form silicic acid (orthosilicic acid, H_4SiO_4) which is water-soluble and is readily absorbed.

Silicon is present throughout the human body, with particularly high concentrations in the aorta, lungs and tendons. There is some evidence that the silicon content of the aorta declines with age and that concentrations in the arterial wall decrease with the development of atherosclerosis[104]. Findings in animal experiments indicate that silicon may be required for normal development of connective tissue and of the skeleton[105]. There are suggestions that a deficiency may be related to the development of certain conditions observed especially in the elderly, such as hypertension and Alzheimer's disease. A number of studies have found evidence of a possible protective role for silicon against aluminium neurotoxicity and accumulation of aluminium in the brain[106]. A connection between silicon and selenium in relation to the control of production of free-radical formation and lipid peroxidation in animals has been postulated[107]. However, evidence in support of these views is uncertain, and a clear functional role for silicon in humans has not yet been identified[108].

9.6.2 Arsenic

Though arsenic is better known to most people for its poisonous properties, there are indications that it may play a useful, if not essential, role in humans. Arsenic is a metalloid, sharing characteristics of both non-metals and metals. It has several allotropic forms, one of which, grey arsenic, is metallic in appearance. The chemistry of arsenic is very similar to that of phosphorus and nitrogen, with which it shares membership of group 15/V in the periodic table of the elements. It forms a series of inorganic compounds, such as the trioxide (As_2O_3). This is known as 'white arsenic' and is the very poisonous compound that has featured often in suicides and homicides. Arsenic also forms organic compounds, such as arsenobetaine ($CH_3As^+CH_2COO^-$). These are of considerable biological interest, since they make up the bulk of total arsenic found in foods, especially in marine products, and are far less toxic than inorganic forms of the element[109].

Arsenic is widely distributed in the earth's crust. It occurs in soils, waters, both fresh and marine, and almost all plants and animals. It has many industrial applications, especially in the chemical industry, as well as in pharmaceutical and agricultural products, uses that accounted for the fact that arsenic was formerly second only to lead as a poison in the farm and household[110].

Arsenic is to be found in most foods and beverages. Natural levels in foods rarely exceed 1 mg/kg, except in seafoods, including some seaweeds. Levels detected in UK foods in the 1994 total diet study ranged from 2 to 10 μg/kg for all food groups, with relatively high levels of 4.3 mg/kg in fish[111]. Indeed, as has been shown also in other studies, the total dietary intake of arsenic is usually positively related to the quantities of fish and other seafoods consumed[112]. The population exposure to total arsenic in 1997 was 63 μg/d, with a mean adult exposure of 120 μg/d, and a 97.5th percentile of 420 μg[113]. In the US, a mean adult daily arsenic intake of 38 μg has been reported[114], compared with 150 μg in New Zealand and 286 μg in the Basque region of Spain[115]. In all these cases, fish consumption accounted for most of the arsenic in the diet.

Arsenic is detectable in almost all potable waters, with concentrations usually ranging from 0 to 200 μg/l, with a mean of 0.5 μg/l[116]. Natural groundwater, such as is obtained from wells and springs, sometimes contains exceptionally high levels of arsenic and can be responsible for what is known as 'regional endemic chronic arsenicism'[117]. In parts of Bangladesh, where water is drawn from deep tube wells to avoid surface water which may be disease-contaminated, levels of up to 100 μg/l and in some cases 1 mg/l, have been recorded, with serious implications for the health of large sections of the population[118].

Arsenic in all its forms is readily absorbed from the GI tract. It is then transported rapidly to lungs and other organs, and later to skin, hair and nails, where it is bound to keratin. After about 24 hours, the organs begin to release their arsenic, which is excreted in urine. Skin, hair and nails, however, retain their arsenic, and levels may increase with further intake of arsenic[119].

After absorption, inorganic arsenic compounds are first reduced and then methylated in the liver to generate organic compounds that can be excreted through the kidneys. Organic arsenic compounds, in contrast, are not metabolised but are rapidly excreted from the body[120]. Arsenic, especially in its inorganic form, but even to a lesser extent the organic forms, is highly toxic, and its ingestion can cause both acute and chronic poisoning[121]. However, it has been argued that in spite of its evident toxicity, arsenic is an essential nutrient for humans[122]. Arsenic deprivation in animals has been shown to cause depressed growth and abnormal reproduction[123]. It also may play a metabolic role in cells, possibly as an activator of certain enzymes, and can act as a substitute for phosphate in certain reactions[124]. Other functions with which arsenic may be involved are methionine metabolism[125] and the regulation of gene expression[126]. However, whether such findings justify the inclusion of arsenic among the essential trace metal nutrients is still far from certain.

9.6.3 Other as-yet unconfirmed essential trace metals and metalloids

The three international bodies WHO, FAO and IAEA, followed by most nutritionists, as well as by expert committees worldwide, consider an element to be essential when reduction of its exposure below a certain limit results consistently in a reduction in a physiologically important function, or when the element is an integral part of an organic structure performing a vital function in the organism[127]. It has been suggested that this definition is too narrow and that, even if a clear biological function cannot be identified for an element, it can still be considered an essential nutrient if it meets other criteria. Suggested criteria include evidence of growth inhibition in animals maintained on a diet deficient in the element[128], observed beneficial, if not essential, effects in animals and humans[129], consistent changes in tissue concentrations in response to changing levels in the diet[130], and the possibility that essentiality is an adaptive and not a static property of an element[131]. On the basis of these criteria, the addition of a number of additional trace metals to the list of essential trace nutrients has been proposed. These include lithium, aluminium, titanium, zirconium, scandium and yttrium, as well as the heavy metals cadmium and lead.

Lithium is probably the most likely of these elements to be essential for human life. It is a light alkali metal, in group 1 of the periodic table, along with sodium, potassium, rubidium and caesium. Chemically, it resembles sodium and potassium, though its salts are not as soluble as those of the other two metals. It is found in all foods, at low levels, normally less than 0.1 mg/kg. The mean daily adult intake in the UK has been estimated to be 17 μg[132]. Lithium is absorbed efficiently in the GI tract and is excreted mainly in urine. Though there is some evidence that lithium may have an essential role in some animals, this has not been confirmed[133]. It has been suggested that the element's known therapeutic efficacy in the treatment of psychoses depends on its effect on the distribution of electrolytes[134]. It has been argued that lithium plays a protective role against brain deterioration with ageing and thus is essential to humans[135].

Evidence in support of the essentiality of the other metal candidates is even less convincing than for lithium. Apart from their ubiquitous distribution, normally at very low levels, in the environment and in human tissues, in most cases there is little more than speculation to justify their inclusion among the essential trace metals. However, even for the hardline sceptic, it is difficult not to have sympathy with the view of Horowitz, who queries whether a major part of the periodic table is really unessential for life[136]. Perhaps, as he says, what is needed is further interpretation of the variety of metabolism in species diversity, its changes through evolution and the movement of various forms of elements in terms of compartments. When that is done, perhaps we will see that many more trace metals besides the small number for which RDAs are currently assigned are, in fact, essential nutrients for humans.

References

1. Tylecote, R.F. (1976) *A History of Metallurgy*, pp. 148–9. The Metals Society, London.
2. Nielsen, F.H. (1990) Newer essential trace elements. In: *Present Knowledge in Nutrition*, (ed. M.L. Brown), 6th ed., pp. 294–307. Nutrition Foundation, Washington, DC.

3. Tylecote, R.F. (1976) *A History of Metallurgy*, pp. 148–9. The Metals Society, London.
4. Lancashire, R.J. (2003) *Nickel Chemistry*. http://wwwchem.uwimona.edu.jm:1104/courses/nickel.html
5. Mitchell, R.L. (1945) Trace elements in soil. *Soil Science*, **60**, 63–75.
6. Smart, G.A. & Sherlock, J.C. (1987) Nickel in foods and diets. *Food Additives and Contaminants*, **4**, 61–71.
7. Ellen, G., Van Den Bosch-Tibbesma, J. & Douma, F.F. (1987) Nickel in food. *Zeitschrift für Lebensmittel Unterforschung*, **179**, 145–56.
8. Christensen, O.B. & Moller, H. (1978) Release of nickel from cooking utensils. *Contact Dermatitis*, **4**, 343–6.
9. Koops, J., Klomp, H. & Westerbeek, D. (1982) Spectroscopic determination of nickel and furildioxime with special reference to milk and milk products and to the release of nickel from stainless steel by acidic dairy products and by acid cleaning. *Netherlands Milk and Dairy Journal*, **36**, 333–5.
10. Ysart, G., Miller, P., Crews, H. *et al.* (1999) Dietary exposure estimates of 30 elements from the UK Total Diet Study. *Food Additives and Contaminants*, **16**, 391–403.
11. Varo, P. & Koivistonen, P. (1980) Mineral composition of Finnish foods XII. General discussion and nutritional evaluation. *Acta Agricultura Scandinavica*, **S22**, 165–70.
12. Nielsen, F.H. (1984) Fluoride, vanadium, nickel, arsenic and silicon in total parenteral nutrition. *Bulletin of the New York Academy of Medicine*, **60**, 177–95.
13. Dabeka, R.W. & McKenzie, A.D. (1995) Survey of lead, cadmium, fluoride, nickel, and cobalt in food composites and estimations of dietary intakes of these elements by Canadians in 1986–88. *Journal of the Association of Official Analytical Chemists*, **78**, 897–909.
14. Nielsen, F.H. & Flyvholm, M. (1983) Risks of high nickel intake with diets. In: *Nickel in the Human Environment* (ed. F.W. Sunderman), pp. 333–8. IARC Scientific Publications No. 53. International Agency for Research on Cancer, Lyon, France.
15. National Academy of Sciences (2002). *Dietary Reference Intakes for Vitamin A, Vitamin K, Arsenic, Boron, Chromium, Copper, Iodine, Iron, Manganese, Molybdenum, Nickel, Silicon, Vanadium and Zinc*. http://www.nap.edu/openbook/0309072794/html/523.html
16. Patriarca, M., Lyon, T.D. & Fell, G.S. (1997) Nickel metabolism in humans investigated with an oral stable isotope. *American Journal of Clinical Nutrition*, **66**, 616–21.
17. Rezuke, W.N., Knight, J.A. & Sunderman, F.W. (1987) Reference values for nickel concentrations in human tissues and bile. *American Journal of Industrial Medicine*, **11**, 419–26.
18. Barceloux, D.G. (1999) Nickel. *Journal of Toxicology – Clinical Toxicology*, **37**, 239–58.
19. Ysart, G., Miller, P., Crews, H. *et al.* (1999) Dietary exposure estimates of 30 elements from the UK Total Diet Study. *Food Additives and Contaminants*, **16**, 391–403.
20. Przybyla, A.E., Robbins, J., Menton, N. & Peck, H.D. (1992) Structure–function relationships among the nickel-containing hydrogenases. *Microbiological Review*, **8**, 109–35.
21. Barceloux, D.G. (1999) Nickel. *Journal of Toxicology – Clinical Toxicology*, **37**, 239–58.
22. Hunt, C.D. & Stoecker, B. (1996) Deliberations and evaluations of the approaches, endpoints and paradigms for boron, chromium and fluoride dietary recommendations. *Journal of Nutrition*, **126**, 2241–51.
23. Uthus, E.O. & Poellot, R.A. (1996) Dietary folate affects the response of rats to nickel deprivation. *Biology of Trace Elements Research*, **52**, 23–35.
24. National Academy of Sciences (2002). *Dietary Reference Intakes for Vitamin A, Vitamin K, Arsenic, Boron, Chromium, Copper, Iodine, Iron, Manganese, Molybdenum, Nickel, Silicon, Vanadium and Zinc*. http://www.nap.edu/openbook/0309072794/html/523.html
25. Department of Health (1991) *Dietary Reference Values for Food Energy and Nutrients for the United Kingdom*, pp. 191–2. HMSO, London.

26. National Academy of Sciences (2002). *Dietary Reference Intakes for Vitamin A, Vitamin K, Arsenic, Boron, Chromium, Copper, Iodine, Iron, Manganese, Molybdenum, Nickel, Silicon, Vanadium and Zinc.* http://www.nap.edu/openbook/0309072794/html/510.html
27. Nielsen, F.H. (2000) The dogged path to acceptance of boron as a nutritionally important mineral element. In: *Trace Elements in Man and Animals 10* (eds. A.M. Roussel, R.A. Anderson & A.E. Favier), pp. 1043–7. Kluwer/Plenum, New York.
28. Nielsen, F.H. (1988) Boron – an overlooked element of potential nutritional importance. *Nutrition Today,* **2**, 4–7.
29. Woods, W.G. (1994) An introduction to boron – history, sources, uses and chemistry. *Environmental Health Perspectives,* **102**, 5–11.
30. Nielsen, F.H. (1994) Ultratrace minerals. In: *Modern Nutrition in Health and Disease* (eds. M.E. Shils, J.A. Olsen & M. Shike), 8th ed., Vol. 1, pp. 272–4. Lea & Febiger, Philadelphia, PA.
31. Rainey, C.J., Nyquist, L.A., Christensen, R.E. *et al.* (1999) Daily boron intake in the American diet. *Journal of the American Dietetics Association,* **99**, 335–40.
32. Murray, F.J. (1995) A human health risk assessment of boron (boric acid and borax) in drinking water. *Regulatory Toxicology and Pharmacology,* **22**, 221–30.
33. Ysart, G., Miller, P., Crews, H. *et al.* (1999) Dietary exposure estimates of 30 elements from the UK Total Diet Study. *Food Additives and Contaminants,* **16**, 391–403.
34. Rainey, C.J., Nyquist, L.A., Christensen, R.E. *et al.* (1999) Daily boron intake in the American diet. *Journal of the American Dietetics Association,* **99**, 335–40.
35. Murray, F.J. (1995) A human health risk assessment of boron (boric acid and borax) in drinking water. *Regulatory Toxicology and Pharmacology,* **22**, 221–30.
36. Rainey, C., Nyquist, L., Casterline, J. & Herman, D. (2000) Estimation of dietary boron intake in six countries. In: *Trace Elements in Man and Animals 10* (eds. A.M. Roussel, R.A. Anderson & A.E. Favier), pp. 1053–6. Kluwer/Plenum, New York.
37. Coughlin, J.R. (1996) Inorganic borates: chemistry, human exposure, and health and regulatory guidelines. *Journal of Trace Elements in Experimental Medicine,* **9**, 137–51.
38. Draper, A., Lewis, J., Malhortra, N. & Wheeler, E. (1993) The energy and nutrient intakes of different types of vegetarians: a case for supplements? *British Journal of Nutrition,* **69**, 3–19.
39. National Academy of Sciences (2002). *Dietary Reference Intakes for Vitamin A, Vitamin K, Arsenic, Boron, Chromium, Copper, Iodine, Iron, Manganese, Molybdenum, Nickel, Silicon, Vanadium and Zinc.* http://www.nap.edu/openbook/0309072794/html/513.html
40. Wilson, J.H. & Ruszler, P.L. (1997) Effects of boron on growing pullets. *Biology of Trace Element Research,* **56**, 287–94.
41. Murray, F.J. (1995) A human health risk of boron (boric acid and borax) in drinking water. *Regulatory Toxicology and Pharmacology,* **22**, 221–30.
42. da Silva, F.J. & Williams, R.J. (1991) *The Biological Chemistry of the Elements: The Inorganic Chemistry of Life*, pp. 58–63. Oxford University Press, Oxford.
43. Nielsen, F.H. (1987) Other elements. In: *Trace Elements in Human and Animal Nutrition* (ed. W. Mertz), pp. 415–63. Academic Press, San Diego, CA.
44. Samman, S., Naghii, M.R., Lyons-Wall, P.M. & Verus, A.P. (1998) The nutritional and metabolic effects of boron in humans and animals. *Biology of Trace Elements Research,* **66**, 227–35.
45. Price, C.J., Strong, P.L., Murray, F.J. & Goldberg, M.M. (1998) Developmental effects of boric acid in rats related to maternal blood boron concentrations. *Biology of Trace Elements Research,* **66**, 359–72.
46. Schauss, A. (1995) *Minerals and Human Health: The Rationale for Optimal and Balanced Trace Element Levels*, pp. 18–19. Life Sciences Press, New York.
47. Young, V. (2003) Trace element biology: the knowledge base and its application for the nutrition of individuals and populations. *Journal of Nutrition,* **133**, 1581S–7S.

48. Benderdour, M., Hess, K., Dzondo-Gadet, M. *et al.* (1997) Effects of boric acid solution on cartilage metabolism. *Biochemistry and Biophysics Research Communications*, **234**, 263–8.
49. Oberringeer, M., Baum, H.P., Jung, V. *et al.* (1995) Differential expression of heat shock protein 70 in healing and chronic human wound tissue. *Biochemistry and Biophysics Research Communications*, **214**, 1009–14.
50. Hunt, C.D. (1998) Regulation of enzymatic activity: one possible role of dietary boron in higher animals and humans. *Biology of Trace Elements Research*, **66**, 205–25.
51. Rowe, R.I. & Eckhert, C.D. (1999) Boron is required for zebrafish embryogenesis. *Journal of Experimental Biology*, **202**, 1649–54.
52. Newnham, R. (1994) Essentiality of boron for healthy bones and joints. *Environmental Health*, **102**, 59–63.
53. Hunt, D. (1996) Biochemical effects of physiological amounts of dietary boron. *Journal of Trace Elements in Experimental Biology*, **9**, 391–403.
54. Beattie, J.H. & Peace, H.S. (1993) The influence of a low-boron diet and boron supplementation on bone, major mineral and sex hormone metabolism in postmenopausal women. *British Journal of Nutrition*, **69**, 871–84.
55. Penland, J. (1998) The importance of boron nutrition for brain and psychological function. *Biology of Trace Element Research*, **66**, 299–317.
56. Hunt, C.D. (2000) Dietary boron is a physiological regulator of the normal inflammatory response. In: *Trace Elements in Man and Animals 10* (eds. A.M. Roussel, R.A. Anderson & A.E. Favier), pp. 1071–6. Kluwer/Plenum, New York.
57. Raloff, J. (2003) Boosting boron could be beneficial. http://www.sciencenews.org/20010414/fob1.asp
58. Schauss, A. (1995) *Minerals and Human Health: The Rationale for Optimal and Balanced Trace Element Levels*, pp. 18–19. Life Sciences Press, New York.
59. Murray, F.J. (1995) A human health risk assessment of boron (boric acid and borax) in drinking water. *Regulatory Toxicology and Pharmacology*, **22**, 221–30.
60. Nriagu, G.U. (1998) *Vanadium in the Environment. Part 2: Health Effects.* Wiley, New York.
61. McNeill, J.H. (2000) Insulin enhancing effects of vanadium. In: *Trace Elements in Man and Animals 10* (eds. A.M. Roussel, R.A. Anderson & A.E. Favier), pp. 491–6. Kluwer/Plenum, New York.
62. Barceloux, D.G. (1999) Vanadium. *Journal of Toxicology – Clinical Toxicology,* **37**, 265–78.
63. Tracey, A.D. & Crans, D.E. (1998) *Vanadium Compounds: Chemistry, Biochemistry and Therapeutic Applications.* American Chemical Society, New York.
64. Myron, D.R., Givand, S.H. & Nielsen, F.H. (1977) Vanadium content of selected foods as determined by flameless atomic absorption spectroscopy. *Journal of Agriculture and Food Chemistry*, **25**, 297–300.
65. Badmev, V., Prakash, S. & Majeed, M. (1999) Vanadium: a review of its potential role in the fight against diabetes. *Journal of Alternative and Complementary Medicine* **5**, 273–91.
66. Schroeder, H.A. & Nason, A.P.(1971) Trace element analysis in clinical chemistry. *Clinical Chemistry* **17**, 461–74.
67. Myron, D.R., Givand, S.H. & Nielsen, F.H. (1977) Vanadium content of selected foods as determined by flameless atomic absorption spectroscopy. *Journal of Agriculture and Food Chemistry,* **25**, 297–300.
68. Evans, W.H., Read, J.I. & Caughlin, D. (1985) Quantification of results for estimating elemental dietary intakes of lithium, rubidium, strontium, molybdenum, vanadium and silver. *Analyst,* **110,** 873–86.
69. Clarkson, P.M. & Rawson, E.S. (1999) Nutritional supplements to increase muscle mass. *Critical Reviews in Food Science and Nutrition,* **39,** 317–328.

70. Tsalev, D.L. (1984) *Atomic Absorption Spectrometry in Occupational and Environmental Health Practice*, p. 273. CRC Press, Boca Raton, FL.
71. Pennington, J.A.T. & Jones, J.W. (1987) Molybdenum, nickel, cobalt, vanadium, and strontium in total diets. *Journal of the American Dietetics Association,* **87**, 1644–50.
72. Anke, M., Illing-Güunther, H., Gürtler, H. *et al.* (2000) Vanadium – an essential element for animals and humans? In: *Trace Elements in Man and Animals 10* (eds. A.M. Roussel, R.A. Anderson & A.E. Favier), pp. 221–5. Kluwer/Plenum, New York.
73. Pennington, J.A.T. & Jones, J.W. (1987) Molybdenum, nickel, cobalt, vanadium, and strontium in total diets. *Journal of the American Dietetics Association,* **87**, 1644–50.
74. Hight, S.C., Anderson, D.L., Cunningham, W.C. *et al.* (1993) Analysis of dietary supplements for nutritional, toxic, and other elements. *Journal of Food Composition and Analysis,* **6,** 121–39.
75. Boden, G., Chen, X., Ruiz, J., van Rossum, G.D. & Turco, S. (1996) Effects of vanadyl sulfate on carbohydrate and lipid metabolism in patients with non-insulin-dependent diabetes mellitus. *Metabolism,* **45**, 1130–5.
76. Thompson, K.H., McNeill, J.H. & Orvig, C. (2000) Design of new oxovanadium (IV) complexes for treatment of diabetes, bioavailability, speciation, and tissue targeting considerations. In: *Trace Elements in Man and Animals 10* (eds. A.M. Roussel, R.A. Anderson & A.E. Favier), p. 539. Kluwer/Plenum, New York.
77. Myron, D.R., Zimmerman, T.J. & Shuler, T.R. (1978) Intake of nickel and vanadium by humans: a survey of selected diets. *American Journal of Clinical Nutrition,* **31,** 527–31.
78. Sabbioni, E., Marafante, E., Amantini, I., Bertalli, I. & Birattari, C. (1978) Similarity in metabolic patterns of different chemical species of vanadium in the rat. *Bioinorganic Chemistry,* **8**, 503–15.
79. Patterson, B.W., Hansard, S.I., Ammerman, C.B. *et al.* (1986) Kinetic model of whole-body vanadium metabolism: studies in sheep. *American Journal of Physiology,* **251**, R325–32.
80. Nielsen, F.H. & Uthuis, E.O.(1990) The essentiality and metabolism of vanadium. In: *Vanadium in Biological Systems* (ed. N.D. Chasteen), pp. 51–62. Kluwer, New York.
81. Cam, M.C., Rodrigues, B. & McNeill, J.H. (1999) Distinct glucose lowering and beta cell protective effects of vanadium and food restriction in streptozocin-diabetes. *European Journal of Endocrinology,* **141,** 546–554.
82. Golden, M.H.N. & Golden, B.E. (1981) Trace elements. Potential importance in human nutrition with particular reference to zinc and vanadium. *British Medical Bulletin,* **37**, 31–6.
83. Berner, Y.N., Shuler, T.R. & Nielsen, F.H. (1989) Selected ultratrace elements in total parenteral nutrition solutions. *American Journal of Clinical Nutrition,* **50,** 1079–83.
84. Thompson, K.H., Battell, M. & McNeill, J.H. (1998) Toxicology of vanadium in mammals. In: *Vanadium in the Environment* (ed. K.H. Thomson), pp. 21–38. Wiley, New York.
85. Schmutzer, R.E. (1993) Welcome remarks. *Trace Elements in Man and Animals – TEMA 8* (eds. M. Anke, C.F. Meissner & C.F. Mills), pp. 1–2. Verlag Media Touristik, Gersdorf, Germany.
86. Manousoff, M.M. (1998) Cobalt's calm before the storm. *American Metal Market,* 27 January, 1–3. http://www.amm.com/ref/hot/COBALT98.HTM
87. Schroeder, H.A., Nason, A.P. & Tipton, I.H. (1967) Essential trace elements in man: cobalt. *Journal of Chronic Disease,* **20,** 869–90.
88. Varo, P. & Koivistonen, P. (1980) Mineral composition of Finnish foods XII. General discussion and nutritional evaluation. *Acta Agricultura Scandinavica,* **S22,** 165–70.
89. Robberecht, H.J., Hendrix, P., Cauwenbergh, R. & Deelstra, H.A. (1994) Daily dietary manganese intake in Belgium, using duplicate portion sampling. *Zeitschrift für Lebensmittel Untersuchung und Forschung,* **199,** 446–8.
90. Anon. (1968) Epidemic cardiac failure in beer drinkers. *Nutrition Reviews,* **26,** 173–5.
91. Grinvalsky, H.T. & Fitch, D.M. (1969) A distinctive myocardiopathy occurring in Omaha, Nebraska: pathological aspects. *Annals of the New York Academy of Science,* **156,** 544–65.

92. Toskes, P.P., Smith, G.W. & Conrads, M.E. (1973) Cobalt absorption in sex-linked anaemic mice. *American Journal of Clinical Nutrition,* **26,** 435–7.
93. Wahner-Roedler, D.L., Fairbanks, V.F. & Linman, J.W. (1975) Cobalt excretion tests as an index of iron absorption and diagnostic test for iron deficiency. *Journal of Laboratory and Clinical Medicine,* **85,** 253–8.
94. Werner, E. & Hansen, C.H. (1991) Measurement of intestinal absorption of inorganic and organic cobalt. In: *Trace Elements in Man and Animals 7* (ed. B. Momčilovič), pp. 11/16–11/17. IMI, University of Zagreb, Zagreb, Croatia.
95. Yamagata, N., Muratan, S. & Moriit, T.(1962) The cobalt content of the human body. *Journal of Radiation Research,* **3,** 4–8.
96. Blokhima, R.I. (1970) Cobalt and goitre. In: *Trace Element Metabolism in Animal* (ed. C.F. Mills), pp. 426–32. Livingstone, Edinburgh.
97. Silió, F., Santos, A. & Ribas, B.(1999) The metallic component of the glucose tolerance factor, GTF. Cobalt against chromium. In: *Trace Elements in Man and Animals 10* (eds. A.M. Roussel, R.A. Anderson & A.E. Favier), pp. 540–1. Kluwer, New York.
98. Smith, R.M. (1987) Cobalt. In: *Trace Elements in Human and Animal Nutrition* (ed. W. Mertz), Vol. 1, pp. 143–83. Academic Press, London.
99. Ministry of Agriculture, Fisheries and Food (1998) *Cadmium, Mercury and Other Metals in Food, 53rd Report of Steering Group on Chemical Aspects of Food Surveillance.* The Stationery Office, London.
100. Hamilton, E.I. & Minski, M.J. (1972) Abundance of the chemical elements in man's diet and possible relations with environmental factors. *Science of the Total Environment,* **1**, 375–94.
101. Shimbo, S., Hayase, A., Murakami, M. *et al.* (1996) Use of a food composition database to estimate daily dietary intake of nutrient or trace elements in Japan, with reference to its limitations. *Food Additives and Contaminants,* **13**, 775–86.
102. Pennington, J.A. (1991) Silicon in foods and diets. *Food Additives and Contaminants,* **8**, 97–118.
103. Kelsay, J.L., Behall, K.M. & Prather, E.S. (1979) Effect of fiber from fruits and vegetables on metabolic responses of human subjects II. Calcium, magnesium, iron and silicon balances. *American Journal of Clinical Nutrition,* **32**, 1876–80.
104. Carlisle, E.M. (1986) Silicon. In: *Trace Elements in Human and Animal Nutrition* (ed. W. Mertz), 5th ed., Vol. 2, pp. 375–94. Academic Press, New York.
105. Perry, C.C. & Keeling-Tucker, T. (2000) Biosilification: the role of the organic matrix in structure control. *Journal of Biological Inorganic Chemistry,* **5**, 537–50.
106. Carlisle, E.M. & Curran, M.J. (1987) Effects of dietary silicon and aluminium levels in rat brain. *International Journal of Alzheimer's Disease and Related Disorders,* **1**, 83–7.
107. Atroshi, F., Sankari, S., Westerholm, H. *et al.* (1991) Silicon, selenium and glutathione peroxidase in bovine mastitis. In: *Trace Elements in Man and Animals 7* (ed. B. Momčilovič), pp. 31/6–31/7. IMI, University of Zagreb, Zagreb, Croatia.
108. Van Dyck, K., Robberecht, H., Van Cauwenbergh, R., Vlaslaer, V. & Deelstra, H. (2000) Indications of silicon essentiality in humans: serum concentrations in Belgian children and adults, including pregnant women. *Biological Trace Elements Research,* **77**, 25–32
109. Edmunds, J.S. & Francesconi, K.A. (1993) Arsenic in seafoods: human health aspects and regulations. *Marine Pollution,* **26**, 665–74.
110. Buck, W.B. (1978) Toxicity of inorganic and aliphatic organic mercurials. In: *Toxicity of Heavy Metals in the Environment* (ed. F.W. Oehme), pp. 357–69. Dekker, New York.
111. Ysart, G., Miller, P., Crews, H. *et al.* (1999) Dietary exposure estimates of 30 elements from the UK Total Diet Study. *Food Additives and Contaminants,* **16**, 391–403.
112. Department of Health (1991) *Dietary Reference Values for Food Energy and Nutrients for the United Kingdom,* pp. 191–2. HMSO, London.

113. Ministry of Agriculture, Fisheries and Food (1999) *Food Surveillance Information Sheet, Number 191*. Food Standards Authority, London.
114. Gunderson, E.L. (1995) FDA Total Diet Study, July 1986–April 1991. Dietary intakes of pesticides, selected elements and other chemicals. *Journal of the Association of Official Analytical Chemists International,* **78**, 1353–63.
115. Vannort, R.W., Hannah, M.L. & Pickston, L. (1995) *1990/1991 New Zealand Total Diet Study. Part 2. Contaminant Elements*. New Zealand Health, Wellington.
116. Bowen, H.J.M. (1966) *Trace Elements in Biochemistry*, pp. 103–7. Academic Press, London.
117. Borgono, J.M. & Greiber, R. (1972) *Trace Substances in Environmental Health* (ed. D. Hemphill), Vol. 5, pp. 13–24. University of Missouri Press, Columbia, MO.
118. Battacharya, R., Chaterjee, D., Nath, B. *et al.* (2003) High arsenic ground water: mobilization, metabolism and mitigation – an overview in the Bengal Delta Plain. *Molecular and Cellular Biochemistry,* **253**, 347–55.
119. Stoeppler, M. & Vahter, M. (1994) Arsenic. In: *Trace Element Analysis in Biological Specimens* (eds. R.F.M. Herber & M. Stoeppler), pp. 291–320. Elsevier, Amsterdam.
120. Clarkson, T.W. (1983) Molecular targets of metal toxicity. In: *Chemical Toxicology and Clinical Chemistry of Metals* (eds. S.S. Brown & J. Savory), pp. 211–26. Academic Press, London.
121. Ratnike, R.N. (2003) Acute and chronic arsenic toxicity. *Postgraduate Medical Journal,* **79**, 391–6.
122. Nielsen, F.H. (1990) Other trace elements. In: *Present Knowledge in Nutrition* (ed. M.L. Brown), pp. 294–307. International Life Sciences Institute, Washington, DC.
123. Anke, M., Groppel, B. & Krause, U. (1991) The essentiality of the toxic elements cadmium, arsenic and nickel. In: *Trace Elements in Man and Animals – 7* (ed. B. Momčilovič), pp. 11/6–11/8. IM I, University of Zagreb, Zagreb, Croatia.
124. Uthus, E.O., Poellot, R., Brossart, B. & Nielsen, F.H. (1989) Effects of arsenic deprivation on polyamine content in rat liver. *Federation of American Societies of Experimental Biology Journal,* **3**, A1072.
125. Uthus, E.O. & Poellot, R. (1992) Effect of dietary pyridoxine on arsenic deprivation in rats. *Trace Elements,* **10**, 339–47.
126. Meng, Z. & Meng, N. (1994) Effects of inorganic arsenicals on DNA synthesis in unsensitized human blood lymphocytes *in vitro*. *Biological Trace Elements Research,* **42**, 201–8.
127. Mertz, W. (1998) Review of the scientific basis for establishing the essentiality of trace elements. *Biological Trace Elements Research,* **66**, 185–91.
128. Anke, M., Angelow, L., Müller, M. & Glei, M. (1993) *Trace Elements in Man and Animals – TEMA 8* (eds. M. Anke, D. Meissner & C.F. Mills), pp. 180–8. Verlag Media Touristik, Gersdorf, Germany.
129. Nielsen, F.H. (1998) The justification for providing dietary guidance for the nutritional intake of boron. *Biological Trace Elements Research,* **66**, 319–30.
130. Van Dyck, K., Robberecht, H., Van Cauwenbergh, R., Vlaslaer, V. & Deelstra, H. (2000) Indications of silicon essentiality in humans: serum concentrations in Belgian children and adults, including pregnant women. *Biological Trace Elements Research,* **77**, 25–32
131. Horovitz, C.T. (1988) Is the major part of the periodic table really unessential for life? *Journal of Trace Elements and Electrolytes in Health and Disease,* **2**, 135–44.
132. Ysart, G., Miller, P., Crews, H. *et al.* (1999) Dietary exposure estimates of 30 elements from the UK Total Diet Study. *Food Additives and Contaminants,* **16**, 391–403.
133. Mertz, W. (1993) The history of the discovery of the essential trace elements. In: *Trace Elements in Man and Animals – TEMA 8* (eds. M. Anke, D. Meissner & C.F. Mills), pp. 22–8. Verlag Media Touristik, Gersdorf, Germany.

134. Mertz, W. (1986) Lithium. In: *Trace Elements in Human and Animal Nutrition,* Vol. 2, pp. 391–7. Academic Press, London.
135. Perez-Granados, A.M. & Vaquero, M.P. (2002) Silicon, aluminium, arsenic and lithium: essentiality and human health implications. *Journal of Nutrition, Health and Aging,* **6**, 154–62.
136. Horovitz, C.T. (1988) Is the major part of the periodic table really unessential for life? *Journal of Trace Elements and Electrolytes in Health and Disease,* **2**, 135–44.

Index